Early Intervention in Natural Environments

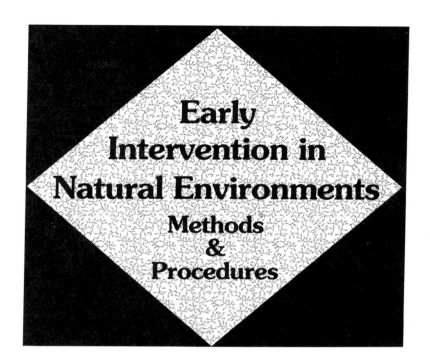

Early Intervention in Natural Environments
Methods & Procedures

Mary Jo Noonan
University of Hawaii, Manoa

Linda McCormick
University of Hawaii, Manoa

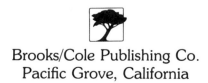

Brooks/Cole Publishing Co.
Pacific Grove, California

Brooks/Cole Publishing Company
A Division of Wadsworth, Inc.

Printed in the United States of America

10   9   8   7   6   5   4   3   2   1

Library of Congress Cataloging-in-Publication Data

Noonan, Mary Jo.
    Early intervention in natural environments : methods and
procedures / Mary Jo Noonan, Linda McCormick.
        p.   cm.
    Includes bibliographical references and index.
    ISBN 0-534-14442-X
    1. Handicapped children—Education (Preschool)   2. Handicapped
children—Rehabilitation. 3. Handicapped children—Services for.
I. McCormick, Linda.   II. Title.
LC4019.2.N66 1993
371.91—dc20   92-33628
                                                                          CIP

Sponsoring Editor: *Vicki Knight*
Editorial Assistant: *Heather L. Graeve*
Production Editor: *Marjorie Z. Sanders*
Manuscript Editor: *Judy Johnstone*
Permissions Editor: *May Clark*
Interior Design: *Terri Wright*
Cover Design: *Sharon L. Kinghan*
Cover Photo: *Georgia Lynn Yamashita*
Art Coordinator: *Susan Haberkorn*
Interior Illustration: *Matrix Communications*
Interior Photographs: *Joanne Yuen*
Typesetting: *Graphic World*
Cover Printing: *Phoenix Color Corporation*
Printing and Binding: *Malloy Lithographing, Inc.*

To our personal cheerleaders,
Lon and Hank;

and our special keikis,
Beau,
Casey,
Corey,
Jordan,
Susannah,
and Taylor

Preface

As more and more infants and young children with special needs are served in natural environments, we have come to realize that intervention strategies based on methods used in restrictive clinical settings are neither effective nor practical. Part H and Section 619 of Part B of the Individuals with Disabilities Education Act (IDEA) have heightened this awareness and stimulated a nationwide movement to serve infants and young children with disabilities in the natural environments that the family chooses (childcare settings, homes, and preschools), using play and other developmentally appropriate activities as learning opportunities. In addition to significantly increasing early intervention services, this landmark legislation is responsible for unprecedented personnel shortages. There is a critical national shortage of personnel with skills and competencies to meet the unique needs of infants and young children with disabilities (and those at risk for developmental delays) and their families.

Early intervention in Natural Environments draws from 30 years of research and technology in best practices to promote learning in infants and young children with disabilities. It provides precise, detailed descriptions of empirically validated best practices. This is a practical and comprehensive, easy-to-read introductory methods text that addresses the fundamental issues associated with implementing the legislative mandates.

Rather than following the traditional organization by developmental domains, we have organized this text according to key concepts, functions, and arrangements in the early intervention process. Each chapter covers critical recent developments in early intervention methods and procedures for infants, toddlers, and preschoolers and their families.

Chapter 1 provides an introduction to the history of early intervention perspectives and policies with emphasis on the provisions of recent legislation.

Chapter 2 describes teaming skills and strategies and presents basic premises and procedures for service coordination.

Chapters 3 and 4 deal with assessment and program planning: Chapter 3 describes infant assessment processes and development of the IFSP, and Chapter 4 describes preschool assessment processes and development of the IEP.

Chapter 5 provides guidelines for implementation of a naturalistic curriculum model.

Chapter 6 considers generic instructional procedures.

Chapter 7 describes more specialized methods in the basic skill domains of communication, social, physical development, and self-care.

Chapter 8 describes naturalistic teaching approaches and procedures, including data collection strategies.

Chapter 9 deals with planning and implementation of group instruction.

Chapters 10 and 11 provide guidelines for arranging the physical and social environment: Chapter 10 describes environmental arrangements to promote interaction, while Chapter 11 describes environmental arrangements to promote independence.

Chapter 12 reviews the major service delivery models and program management (including special provisions to address safety and health issues).

Chapter 13, the final chapter, discusses the important transitions in early childhood and outlines procedures to facilitate smooth transitions.

 # Acknowledgments

To thank the many children, family members, mentors, colleagues, and friends who have been our teachers throughout the years would require a separate book. We would like to give formal recognition to these individuals for direct assistance: Pattie Nishimoto, Josie Woll, Joanne Yuen, Jean Johnson, Nancy Ratokalou, Pam Musick, Wendy Tada, Jennifer Kilgo, Sandra E. Wood, Patti D. S. Yamamoto, and Suzanne Delaney.

In addition, we appreciate the assistance of the manuscript reviewers: David W. Anderson, Bethel College; Susan M. Benner, University of Tennessee at Knoxville; Martha J. Cook, University of Alabama; Vivian I. Correa, University of Florida; Jennifer Kilgo, Virginia Commonwealth University; Andrea P. McDonnell, University of Utah; Issaura Barrera Metz, University of New Mexico; Diane M. Sainato, Ohio State University; and Mary Kay Zabel, Kansas State University.

Mary Jo Noonan
Linda McCormick

About the Authors

MARY JO NOONAN is an Associate Professor of Special Education at the University of Hawaii and Coordinator of the Graduate Teacher Preparation Program for Students with Severe Disabilities. She is the director of an early childhood demonstration and outreach project focused on transitions from infant to preschool programs. She has worked extensively throughout the Pacific Basin in special education teacher training and public school program development. She is the author of many articles and textbook chapters concerning early childhood special education and the education of students with severe/multiple disabilities.

LINDA MCCORMICK is a Professor of Special Education at the University of Hawaii and Coordinator of the Early Childhood Special Education Teacher Training Program. She is also director of an infant specialist training project and chairperson of the Hawaii Interagency Coordinating Council. She is a consultant to numerous public and private agencies in Hawaii and elsewhere in the Pacific Basin. She has authored and co-authored many articles and chapters and several textbooks in special education.

Brief Contents

Contents

3 The IFSP Process 43

4 IEP Development 91

5 Naturalistic Curriculum Model

129

6 Basic Instructional Principles

163

7 Specialized Instructional Techniques   199

8 **Intervention in Natural Environments**   **237**

 9 **Group Instruction**   **267**

12 **Program Organization and Management** **331**

 13 **Transitions** **349**

Early Intervention Perspectives, Policies, and Practices

1. Discuss the history of concern for early intervention, and important legislation affecting services for infants and young children with disabilities.

1. Describe the major provisions of Part H and Part B–Section 619, of the Individuals with Disabilities Education Act (IDEA).

3. Describe service delivery models for early intervention.

4. Identify current best practices in early intervention.

*T*here is broad consensus that early identification and appropriate intervention are essential to maximize skill development and reduce or alleviate the need for special services when a child enters school (Guralnick, 1989). Recent legislation encouraging early intervention described in this chapter has increased demands for curricula and teaching techniques and made staff training for early intervention personnel a high priority.

Validated practices and procedures are available. The challenge lies in increasing their application and dissemination. Early interventionists need to know (a) how to select a theoretical model, (b) which procedures are most effective and with whom they are effective, and (c) how to achieve broad and lasting effects. The major purpose of this text is to present basic information and instructions for achieving these competencies.

This first chapter provides a brief introduction to the history of early intervention perspectives and policies, with special emphasis on recent legislation. The final section provides an outline for the remainder of the text.

History of Concern for Early Intervention

Early childhood special education (ECSE) is a relatively young field with a distinguished "family history." In addition to its roots in regular early childhood education, compensatory education, and special education for school-age children, ECSE draws heavily from the accumulated theory and methods in psychology, human development, nursing, and sociology (Peterson, 1987). Space limitations preclude extensive review of the many forces that have shaped and directed the field; we highlight only a few of the major historical events.

Changing Perspectives

Descriptions of persons concerned with the special needs of young children can be traced back many centuries. Among the more notable progenitors of ECSE were Piaget, Itard, and Montessori, researchers and practitioners who committed their lives to understanding and affecting the course of early development.

Jean-Marc Itard is credited with having developed the first intervention procedures and practices for a child with disabilities. Itard was a physician and an authority on diseases of the ear and the education of the deaf. He advocated an "interactionist" perspective—holding that learning potential is affected by both the environment and physiological stimulation. This was a radical position 200 years ago.

Itard tested his theory with Victor, the "wild boy of Aveyron." In 1798, Victor (estimated to be about 12 years old) was found living with wolves in the woods near Aveyron, France. He used no language and behaved more like an animal than a human. Itard developed and implemented an intensive intervention program for Victor. It included (a) an instructional sequence derived from normal development,

(b) individualized instruction, (c) sensory stimulation, (d) systematic instruction gradually moving from simple to more complex tasks, and (e) activities to build independence and functional skills. Even by today's standards Itard's procedures would come under the heading of "best practices."

In Italy, about a hundred years later, another physician, Maria Montessori, drew upon the work of Itard and others. Her earliest work was with children who were mentally retarded and living in an institution in Rome. Later she opened a school for young children who lived in Rome's tenements.

Montessori subsequently contributed many volumes describing her philosophy and practices. She believed that children pass through a series of sensitive periods when they are especially atuned to particular aspects of learning. She designed learning activities and materials (which she called a *prepared environment*) to match these sensitive periods. Maria Montessori died in 1952. To this day, programs incorporating Montessori's ideas proliferate in the United States and elsewhere around the world.

A progenitor closer in time to the present was Jean Piaget. Until his death in 1980 (at the age of 84), Piaget dedicated his life to elucidating the course of cognitive development. Among his most important contributions was the notion that the thinking and reasoning processes of children are not quantitatively different from those of adults: They are *qualitatively* different. The thinking of children changes dramatically as they develop from infancy to adulthood.

Piaget argued that the task of childhood is construction of cognitive skills and processes that are applied over and over in different situations. Piaget's first research subjects were his own three infants. He observed and carefully recorded every aspect of their cognitive development with brilliantly insightful inferences as to the processes involved. Later he observed the problem solving and reasoning of older children. It was Piaget's contention that learning entails active discovery rather than listening or watching. All early childhood programs in this country owe some debt to the Piagetian tradition.

Europeans were not the only contributors to the history of ECSE. A classic research study in Iowa in the thirties stimulated a closer look at the role of the environment in development (and intelligence) (Skeels & Dye, 1939). The Iowa research began when Dr. Harold Skeels, a psychologist, was asked by the superintendent of an orphanage to find a placement for two little girls, 18 months and 2 years old. Born out of wedlock to mothers who had mental retardation, these infants had IQs of 35 and 46 respectively.

Skeels pursuaded the state mental retardation institution to find temporary space for the girls until they could be accommodated in an orphanage. They were placed on wards with women labeled as mentally deficient.

It is not surprising that the infants were the focus of much loving attention on their respective wards. What was surprising was that, when they were tested two years later, they demonstrated dramatic IQ gains, placing them near normal intelligence. They were subsequently placed in foster homes.

Skeels was intrigued. To explore the findings further, he arranged to move 13 more children from the orphanage to the state institution. The children were all under age 3 and all but two were classified as mentally retarded (average IQ 64).

(Classification criteria were less stringent then.) They were placed on a ward with adolescent mentally retarded women, and each child was assigned a surrogate mother. The teenage surrogate mothers were given some training in how to hold, feed, talk to, and play with the children, and some toys and other educational materials were made available. Otherwise they were on their own.

A comparison group of 12 children remained in the orphanage where they received adequate medical and health services but little individual attention. All but two of these children functioned in the normal range. The average IQ of the two children who were classified as mentally retarded was 86.

Again there were impressive IQ gains. Data collected 18 to 36 months later showed that the children who had been assigned to the adolescent ward had made a mean gain of 27.5 IQ points. All were adopted. Children who remained in the orphanage showed a mean loss of 26.2 IQ points.

Follow-up data collected by Skeels in 1966, 25 years after the original study, were equally remarkable. He was able to locate and determine the adult status of all 25 children. Eleven of the 13 children in the experimental group had married and only one of the marriages had ended in divorce. The ten marriages had produced nine children, all of normal intelligence. The median educational level for this group was 12th grade, and members of this group had some college. All were either employed or worked as homemakers. Jobs ranged from professional and business work to domestic service.

The findings for the children who remained in the orphanage were discouraging. One had died, and four others were still institutionalized. The median level of education for children in this group was third grade. All but one of the seven noninstitutionalized adults were working as unskilled laborers.

Skeels' results were not met with immediate acceptance by the professional community. Several prominent psychologists maintained that Skeels' data reflected a statistical rather than an educational phenomenon (Goodenough & Maurer, 1961). They insisted that it was inconceivable that children suffering from an irreversible condition such as mental retardation could demonstrate positive change.

Skeels' findings held up and were replicated many times. Indeed, countless studies since the 1930s have confirmed the importance of a stimulating environment for development.

Dr. Samual Kirk's research in the late fifties strengthened arguments for early stimulation. Kirk measured the effects of two years of preschool experience on the social and cognitive development of 43 children (IQs ranging from 40 to 85). Fifteen of these children lived in an institution and attended a nursery school; the other 28 lived at home and attended a preschool program. The control group made up of 38 children (26 lived at home and 12 in an institution) did not have the benefits of either nursery school or preschool. Results showed gains of between 10 and 30 points on the IQ tests for the children who received early intervention and substantial losses for children who had neither nursery school nor preschool (the control group). The differences between the groups were maintained over a period of years.

Other notable research during this era attested to the damaging effects of sensory deprivation. Spitz (1945, 1946, 1947) studied children reared in depriving environments. He compared infants from two institutional environments— a foundling home and a nursery attached to a reformatory for delinquent girls. The infants in the foundling home received very little stimulation or social attention. Their mothers were socially well-adjusted but unable to support themselves and their children. The infants in the nursery were cared for by their mothers, who were described by various labels, including socially maladjusted, mentally retarded, physically handicapped, psychopathic, or criminal.

Infants in the foundling home, where stimulation was minimal, showed progressive declines in developmental ability. At 2 to 3 months of age their mean developmental quotient (DQ) was 131. By the time they were 10 to 12 months, their mean DQ had fallen to 72. Additionally, there was weight loss and they were characterized as withdrawn, weepy, and overly susceptible to infection. The mean DQ of babies in the reformatory nursery remained at approximately the same level (despite what Spitz described as undesirable genetic backgrounds). Spitz attributed the developmental losses of the babies in the foundling home to lack of mothering.

Goldfarb (1945, 1949, 1955) also compared groups of infants in two different environments. One group of babies spent the first years of life in an institution before being placed in foster homes. Children in the other group were institutionalized for only a very short time (less than a year) before being placed in foster homes. Conditions in the institution were described as sterile, nonstimulating, and lacking in adult-child interaction. Goldfarb tested all of the children when they were between the ages of 10 and 14. Those children who had spent their first three years institutionalized were deficient in cognitive development as well as speech and language. They were socially immature and unpopular with peers. Additionally, they demonstrated hyperactivity, short attention span, and poor academic performance. Children who had spent only the early months in the institution appeared to be developing normally.

In addition to this important research, there were two books by well-respected writers that strengthened arguments for the benefits of early intervention. J. McVicker Hunt (1961) published *Intelligence and Experience,* an extensive review of research on intellectual development and environmental influences. Hunt promoted Piaget's theoretical perspectives on cognitive development as an alternative to the traditional psychometric approach that was popular in the early 1960s. Hunt's two major recommendations are as viable today as they were then. He recommended (a) focusing on the early years because they are the most critical for later development, and (b) optimizing young children's interactions with the environment to accelerate intellectual development.

Benjamin Bloom's (1964) classic work, *Stability and Change in Human Characteristics,* was equally persuasive. Presenting the results of an extensive review of longitudinal studies on human development, Bloom argued that the data supported several conclusions regarding the role of early experience. First, human characteristics are shaped by early experiences. Second, environment and early experience are critical because human development is cumulative. And finally, initial learning is easier than attempting to replace inappropriate behaviors, once learned, with new ones.

These pioneering efforts of the forties, fifties, and sixties were catalysts for attitudinal change and substantial later research and writing. They provided the roots for the compensatory education movement (for example, Head Start) that began in the 1960s, and for important legislation that will be discussed in the next section.

The compensatory education movement contributed significantly, both philosophically and practically, to services for young children with disabilities. Most important, the compensatory education movement established the notion of early intervention as a cost-effective means of benefiting children and families (Peterson, 1987). Possibly the most important research effort associated with the compensatory education movement was the consortium evaluation directed by Dr. Irving Lazar.

Lazar and Darlington (1978) analyzed follow-up data from children and families served by eight preschool programs. (These were programs very similar to Head Start.) Their findings demonstrated that environmental manipulations can have remarkable and lasting effects on children's abilities. Children who had attended these programs were less likely than control-group children to be placed in special education classes in elementary school. They were also less likely to be held back a grade in elementary school. Moreover, the children who had attended these early-intervention programs scored higher than control children on achievement tests in the fourth grade. (There was a favorable difference in all areas, but the difference was statistically significant only for math scores.) The early intervention children were more achievement oriented than the control children, and their mothers reported higher vocational aspirations for them. While the children Lazar and Darlington followed were not disabled, they could be considered at risk for school failure. These findings gave a tremendous boost to recognition of the field of early childhood education as a worthy endeavor.

The merger of special education, regular early childhood education, and compensatory education that began in the sixties culminated in a new discipline, early childhood special education (ECSE), in the seventies. In 1973 a new division for early childhood personnel was established with the Council for Exceptional Children (CEC), the largest professional organization for special educators in the United States. Soon thereafter the new Division for Early Childhood (DEC) began publishing the *Journal of the Division for Early Childhood* and a newsletter. The name of the DEC journal has now been changed to *Journal of Early Intervention*.

The seventies and eighties produced significant findings concerning the "malleability of development through systematic, experientially-based interventions" (Guralnick, 1988, p. 84). In addition to documenting positive early intervention effects for a range of problems and disability groups, researchers have identified specific program variables likely to significantly and positively influence intervention outcomes (Guralnick, 1988).

TABLE 1-1

Major Federal Policies in Early Childhood Special Education

1968	PL 90-538, the Handicapped Children's Early Education Assistance Act (HCEEAA), established the Handicapped Children's Early Education Program (HCEEP).
1972	PL 92-424 amended the Economic Opportunity Act to extend Head Start services to children with disabilities.
1975	PL 94-142, the Education of the Handicapped Act (EHA), established the Preschool Incentive Grants and state grant awards based on child count (3-through 5-year-olds could be included in the count).
1986	PL 99-457 amended PL 94-142 by extending the full-service mandate to preschoolers and establishing a new program for infants, toddlers, and their families (Part H).
1990	PL 101-476 changed the title of EHA to the Individuals with Disabilities Education Act (IDEA).
1991	PL 102-119, the Individuals with Disabilities Education Act Amendments, amended IDEA.

Changing Policies

Public policy is government action that reflects the current values and concerns of the people. It is interpreted and enforced by legislative actions and the judicial system. Public policy ultimately guides service priorities and activities. The increased and improved policy commitments to early intervention are a reflection of a considerable body of research, an improved level of public awareness, and advocacy efforts by many professionals and parents.

A recent article traces the impressive history of federal policy in ECSE from 1965 to the present (Hebbeler, Smith & Black, 1991). Table 1-1 presents the legislation that has most affected services for young children with disabilities.

This section will provide a brief overview of this significant legislation: (1) the Handicapped Children's Early Education Assistance Act (HCEEAA), (2) the Head Start legislation, (3) the Education of the Handicapped Act (now referred to as the Individuals with Disabilities Education Act [IDEA]), and (4) the Amendments to the IDEA.

Handicapped Children's Early Education Assistance Act (HCEEAA). In 1968 the efforts of many parents and professionals were rewarded with passage of

Public Law 90-538 (the *Handicapped Children's Early Education Assistance Act*). This law did not provide funds for services as the Head Start legislation had. Rather, its purpose was to identify effective procedures and models for serving infants and preschoolers who had disabilities, and their families as well. The initial projects funded under this legislation—the First Chance or HCEEP (Handicapped Children's Early Education Program) projects (now the Early Education Programs for Children with Disabilities [EEPCD])—continue to provide the important data base for services for infants and young children with special needs and their families.

In addition to meeting the early intervention needs of their immediate geographic areas, the First Chance projects continue to engender many replications and adaptations in other parts of the country. One of the best known of the home-based models is The Portage Project in Wisconsin (Shearer & Shearer, 1972). The Portage Project model is a cross-categorical model for rural areas. It is designed to serve children with special needs from birth to age 6. The Precise Early Education of Children with Handicaps (PEECH) at the University of Illinois, Urbana–Champaign (Karnes, 1977) is an example of a combined home- and center-based model. The Model Preschool Program at the University of Washington (Hayden & Haring, 1976) is an example of a center-based program.

Head Start Legislation.   Head Start was conceived in the 1960s as a means of helping children break out of the cycle of poverty. Head Start programs were funded under the Elementary and Secondary Education Act (ESEA) passed in 1965. This legislation was a response to research reports citing the benefits of early intervention for the cognitive and language development of disadvantaged children. The major significance of the original Head Start legislation was not the substance of the law but what it represented. It was the first indication of legislative concern for early education for children with special needs and the beginning of a national expansion and consolidation of early intervention efforts.

The original legislation made no mention of young children with disabilities but seven years later, in 1972, the doors of Head Start programs were opened to children with disabilities. PL 92-424 (Economic Opportunity Amendments) required Head Start programs to reserve at least 10% of their enrollments for preschoolers with disablities.

Education of the Handicapped Act (EHA) (PL 94-142).   In 1975, passage of PL 94-142 marked the beginning of an advocacy alliance of professionals and parents. This law mandates a free and appropriate education (FAPE), including special education and related services for all children (ages 3 to 21) with disabilities (with the exceptions described below). Educational services are to be provided in the least restrictive environment (LRE), and an individualized education plan (IEP) is to be in effect for the eligible child before special education and related services are provided.

Unfortunately, this legislation had some gaping loopholes, which resulted in less-than-desired state commitments to services for preschoolers. Congress allowed an exception to the FAPE requirements for 3- through 5-year-olds with disabilities.

States were not required to provide services to eligible children between the ages of 3 and 6 *if* their state law did not require such services (and many states did not).

PL 94-142 required public schools to identify and evaluate from birth students with suspected disabilities, but there were to be no services beginning at age 3 if that ran counter to the individual state's law or judicial ruling. Thus determination of whether children younger than age 6 were served was dependent on state policy.

There were two sources of funds to encourage provision of services for preschoolers. Those states which provided services for eligible preschoolers received some federal monies (a specific amount per child). The government also made limited incentive funds available to encourage states to provide services. Because there was not the same level of funding available for preschoolers as for school-age children, states were slow to provide services to this population and there was great variation among states with respect to the type and comprehensiveness of services.

While the gaping loopholes in PL 94-142 resulted in less-than-desired state commitments to services for preschoolers, this legislation was significant in that it represented a formal endorsement of early intervention efforts. It remains the most important milestone in the history of education for children with special needs **anyplace in the world.**

Amendments to the EHA (PL 99-457).   PL 99-457 represents the culmination of nearly 25 years of federal activity in early childhood special education. It is evidence of a deep concern at the national level for what happens to infants and young children with special needs and their families. Signed into law in 1986, PL 99-457 contains significant policy changes related to the federal government's role in supporting services for young children with disabilities. It amended and extended Part B, rectifying the shortcomings of PL 94-142 where preschoolers are concerned. It altered the funding mechanisms to encourage states to serve all eligible preschoolers, and it mandated that all eligible preschoolers be provided a free and appropriate public education (FAPE). Additionally, it established a new Part H program that provides for comprehensive services for infants and toddlers with special needs, and their families.

In 1990, the title of EHA was changed (by PL 101-476) to the Individuals with Disabilities Education Act (IDEA). The Infant and Toddlers with Disabilities program, officially referred to as Part H, became Subchapter VIII. However, in this text we will continue to use the more easily recognized term *Part H*. The IDEA was amended again in 1991; thus, the most recent legislation is PL 102-119, The Individuals with Disabilities Education Act *Amendments.*

In summary, there are three portions of the amended IDEA that are critical to the expansion and improvement of services to infants, toddlers, and preschoolers with disabilities and their families. These are Part H, Part B–Section 619, and the Early Education Program for Children with Disabilities (EEPCD). Recall that Part H was the new portion (in 1986) dealing specifically with infants and toddlers with disabilities and their families. It created a discretionary program to assist states to plan, develop, and implement a statewide system of comprehensive coordinated, multidisciplinary, interagency services for all young children with disabilities, birth to 3 years of age. Part B–Section 619 amends a previous portion of the EHA. It created enhanced incentives so that all states now provide a free and appropriate public education (FAPE) to eligible 3- through 5-year-old children with disabilities. It encourages family services and transition planning, and it states that all requirements of the state's Part B plan for special education and related services be extended to preschool-age children. Finally, the EEPCD amended previous portions of the EHA by expanding the former HCEEP projects.

Part H, the infant component of the law, is voluntary. States have the option of applying for incentive grants to help support the development of a comprehensive statewide system of services for infants and toddlers with special needs and their families. All fifty states, the District of Columbia, Puerto Rico, and the territories chose to apply for these funds. These are the Part H requirements that differ from requirements for Part B–Section 619, the preschool component of the law.

1. **Interagency coordinating council**

   Each state has a governor-appointed public agency (called a "lead agency") that is responsible for Part H planning. Each state (and territory) also has an interagency coordinating council (ICC) to advise and assist the designated lead agency in the establishment of the statewide system. The ICC is composed of service providers and agencies concerned with services to infants and toddlers with special needs, parents, and representative(s) from higher education. This council helps states achieve interagency collaboration in the planning process (and subsequently eliminate costly duplication and overlapping services).

2. **Eligibility determination**

   The law mandates that two groups of infants and toddlers are to be served—those who are developmentally delayed, and those with established conditions that typically result in developmental delays. It is left to the discretion of individual states to decide whether services will be provided for infants and toddlers who are at risk for significant future developmental problems. Definition of "developmental delay" is left up to the state or territory. States must define developmental delay and describe the procedures that will be used to determine the existence of a developmental delay in each developmental area. (*Developmentally delayed* is typically defined by the extent to which an infant or toddler falls below the normal range of development in one or more areas.) Included in the category of established conditions are infants and toddlers who have diagnosed physical or mental conditions with a high probability of resulting in developmental delay.

3. **Assignment of a service coordinator**

   The 1991 reauthorization of Part H (PL 102-119, IDEA) made a number of changes in terminology. One change was to replace the term "case management" with *service coordination* and the term "case manager" with *service coordinator*. From here on we will use this new terminology.

   Part H requires states to develop and implement service coordination as one of the services available to families. Each infant or toddler and family are assigned a service coordinator. The original legislation stated that this person should represent the discipline most relevant to the infant's, toddler's, or family's needs. The 1991 amendments broaden the category of eligible service coordinators to include any person who is qualified to carry out all of the responsibilities of service coordinator.

Service coordination is a mechanism for helping the family (a) identify the child's needs and their own resources, priorities, and concerns; (b) locate and make use of needed services; and (c) coordinate different aspects of the service delivery system. The phrasing in the legislation suggests that service coordination is conceived as an active, ongoing process, with families playing an active role in both planning and provision of services. The emphasis is on empowerment. Service coordination is intended to promote family independence and self-sufficiency, helping families mobilize their resources to better meet their own and their child's needs. Service coordination is described at length in Chapter 2.

4. Individual Family Service Plan (IFSP)

The law requires an IFSP for each family of an eligible child. The written IFSP is developed by a multidisciplinary team in coordination with the parents. The service coordinator is responsible for implementation of the IFSP and coordination with other agencies and persons identified in the IFSP. The IFSP must include:

a. a statement of the child's present level of functioning in cognitive development, communication development, social or emotional development, physical development, and adaptive development.

b. a statement of the family's resources, priorities, and concerns.

c. a statement of expected intervention outcomes, including criteria, procedures, and timelines.

d. a description of the services that the child and family need, including method, frequency, and intensity.

e. a statement of the natural environments in which early-intervention services shall be provided.

f. projected dates for initiation of services and expected duration.

g. the name of the service coordinator who will be responsible for implementation of the plan and coordination with other agencies and persons.

h. the procedures to ensure successful transition from infant services to preschool programs.

Procedures must be in place for reviewing the IFSP every 6 months and evaluating its appropriateness once a year. Additionally, there is a requirement that the contents of the IFSP be fully explained to the parents for their informed written consent. If parents do not provide consent for a particular early intervention service, then that service is not provided. Only services for which consent has been obtained can be provided.

The conceptual development and implementation of the IFSP concept is a challenge for interventionists. While the IFSP should serve as a base for the IEP (if the child is eligible for special services at age 3), it is very different

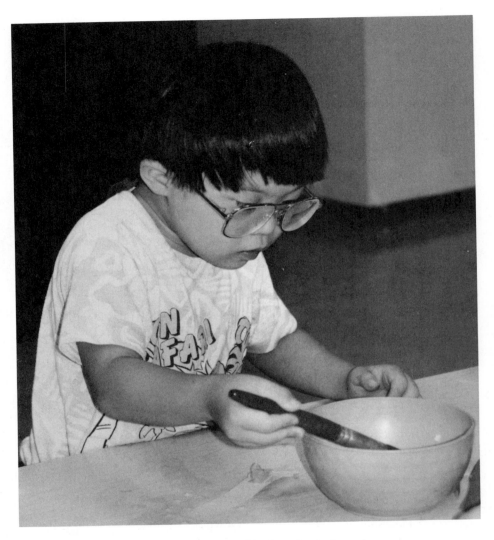

Successful transitions can be supported by fostering independence.

from the Individualized Educational Plan (IEP) that is developed for preschoolers and older children. (It is important to note here that some states and school systems also develop an IFSP for families with an eligible 3- to 5-year-old.) Development of the IFSP is discussed in Chapter 3; Chapter 4 discusses development of the IEP.

5. Transition planning

There has long been concern about easing the family stresses associated with changing programs and systems and dealing with different personnel as we ensure continuity of services for young children and their families. Part H addresses these transition concerns. As noted earlier, each IFSP must include a transition plan.

Transition planning has two goals: (a) to minimize the disruption caused by necessary changes in services, and (b) to ease subsequent adjustments to new experiences for a child and the child's family. Transitions are complicated by differences in eligibility criteria among states, as well as differences between programs for infants and toddlers and programs for preschoolers within a state (or territory). The reason that eligibility definitions differ among states is that states have flexibility in developing their eligibility definitions. Particularly where different state agencies are responsible for Part H programs and programs for preschoolers, there are likely to be different eligibility criteria within a state for the two populations. This places considerable strain on families, because children may no longer be eligible for certain services at age 3. Chapter 13 presents procedures and processes for transition planning and implementation.

6. Other services

In addition to required services (for example, a multidisciplinary assessment, a written IFSP, and transition planning), the law permits provision of certain services that will enable the infant or toddler to benefit from the other early-intervention services. These additional services *may* be provided: vision services; assistive technology devices and services; audiology services; social work services; early identification, screening, and assessment services; family support services; health services; medical services (for diagnostic and evaluation purposes); occupational therapy; physical therapy; psychological services; special education; speech pathology; and transportation.

Part B–Section 619 states that any preschool child who is eligible for special education and related services under this part is entitled to all the rights and protections guaranteed by IDEA (as well as the implementing regulations of the law). These rights and protections include free appropriate public education (FAPE), placement in the least restrictive environment, multidisciplinary evaluation, procedural safeguards, due process, and confidentiality of information.

Part B–Section 619 provides some notable refinements for preschoolers. One is the possibility of a new eligibility category: developmentally delayed. During the mid-eighties, when PL 99-457 was being developed, early interventionists and parents convinced Congress that the categories used for older school-age children were not appropriate for preschoolers (*DEC Communicator*, May–June, 1991). (Table 1-2 shows the disability categories used for older children.) Subsequently, the Senate version of the bill created a new Part B disability category, developmentally delayed, but the final version of the bill did not reflect this addition.

The 1991 amendments to IDEA (PL 102-119) corrected this oversight. States are permitted to use the category "children with disabilities" for 3- to 5-year-olds. This category may include children experiencing developmental delays in physical

---

TABLE 1-2

IDEA Eligibility Categories

Eligible children are those who need special education services *and* meet eligibility criteria associated with the specific characteristics of one of the following handicapping conditions:

1. mental retardation

2. hearing impaired (including deafness)

3. speech and language impaired

4. visually handicapped (including blindness)

5. seriously emotionally disturbed

6. orthopedically impaired

7. autistic

8. traumatic brain injury

9. health impaired

10. specific learning disability

---

development, cognitive development, communication development, social or emotional development, or adaptive development, as defined by the state and measured by appropriate diagnostic instruments.

Part B–Section 619 supports increased efforts to assist parents and strengthen their role in the development and implementation of their child's educational program. The regulations state that the IEP for an eligible preschooler may include planning for assistance to parents if it is deemed necessary to help the child benefit from special education. Also, the regulations permit inclusion of "parental training activities" as support services.

The principle of the LRE states that "children with disabilities must be educated to the maximum extent appropriate with other nonhandicapped children" (OSEP Report to Congress, 1988). This continues to pose a challenge at the preschool level in most states because there are few states that provide educational services for nonhandicapped preschoolers.

The length of the school day and the school year may be extended if local education agencies (LEAs) find this necessary in order to make use of a variety of service delivery options. Also, while preschool education programs are administered by the state education agency (SEA), LEAs may contract services from other programs (Head Start) or other agencies (Department of Health) in order to meet the requirements for provision of a full range of services.

Public Law 99-457 created new challenges in the field of early intervention. It provided clear federal initiatives on a number of issues. It represents a strong vote of public confidence for the potential benefits of early intervention services for infants and young children and their families.

Service Delivery Models

Service delivery models for early intervention range from programs designed to serve only infants or young children with disabilities, to programs that serve children in natural settings, such as homes and childcare centers. This section describes service delivery models for (a) infants and toddlers, (b) 3- to 5-year-olds, and (c) 5-year-olds.

For Infants and Toddlers

Early intervention programs for infants and toddlers may be either center-based or home-based, or some combination of the two. In *center-based* programs, families bring their infant or toddler to a program at an agency setting, where appropriate services are provided by professionals and paraprofessionals. Regular intervention sessions are scheduled either on an individual basis (for young infants) or in small groups (for toddlers). Intervention sessions may be scheduled weekly, bi-weekly, or more often, depending on family preferences and child needs. A professional in a discipline related to the infant or toddler's most significant needs is the primary interventionist. Other program staff are available for the transdisciplinary team. In some center-based programs, paraprofessionals are primary interventionists, with consultation and support provided by professionals. Parents or caregivers and family members participate in all intervention sessions; they are encouraged to imitate techniques modeled by the staff and demonstrate strategies they have found to be successful at home.

Center-based programs are typically specialized, serving only children with disabilities and their families. They are located in clinics, hospitals, health centers, churches, schools, and other easily accessible community facilities. Because many are furnished with therapeutic equipment, they often look more like a hospital therapy room than an early childhood program. Curricula varies among center-based programs but tends to follow developmental and therapeutic models.

As the name implies, the *home-based* early intervention model is implemented in the homes of infants and toddlers with disabilities. Visits are scheduled weekly or bi-weekly by a professional or a paraprofessional (or, in some cases, both). Other program staff join the primary interventionist as needed.

Home-based programs are "normalized" options, because the natural environment for most disabled infants and toddlers is the home—either their own, a relative's, or that of a childcare provider. Home-based programs are individualized to address the child's needs with whatever resources are available in the home. Instructional recommendations are practical and realistic because the interventionist has an opportunity to observe the family's lifestyle and available resources. As in the center-based model, curriculum varies from program to program but generally follows a developmental and therapeutic framework.

Regular childcare settings are viable and important service delivery options for infants and toddlers with disabilities (Bagnato, Kontos & Neisworth, 1987; Rule et al., 1987). Regular childcare settings are natural environments that provide opportunities for integration. The Americans with Disabilities Act (ADA) of 1990 (PL 101-336) requires that any private or community childcare programs serving the public must accept infants and toddlers with disabilities. Programs with physical barriers must be made accessible when such changes are not too costly, and new childcare facilities must be built to be accessible.

Childcare services may be provided by programs serving large numbers of children (ranging from 20 to a few hundred children), or in-home for a smaller number (usually 3 to 5 children). Childcare services tend to have flexible schedules, allowing families to establish a schedule based on their own needs. Some families may schedule childcare one morning per week; others schedule it from 7:30 A.M. to 5:30 P.M., Mondays through Fridays; and others may need half-day care daily.

Childcare programs are typically staffed by paraprofessionals, with a director who is an early childhood professional. Child:staff ratios in childcare centers are high, frequently 10:1 or more. Ratios are considerably lower for infants under 12 months, and for in-home childcare. Maximum child:staff ratios for childcare are usually set by local or state licensing agencies (for example, the Department of Social Services and Housing [DSSH]).

Some childcare programs focus on care rather than early education, but others are virtually indistinguishable from preschool settings. Consultation and support are provided by ECSE teachers and therapists as necessary to assist staff in meeting specialized instruction or care needs of infants and toddlers with disabilities.

For 3- to 5-Year-Olds

During the early childhood years of 3 to 5, family- or home-based childcare and center-based childcare continue to be among the service delivery models for children with and without disabilities. At age 3, however, service delivery possibilities expand to include preschool—there are segregated and integrated preschool options for children with disabilities.

Segregated Preschool Settings. Segregated preschool classes for children with disabilities are provided in most states through the public school system. Generally, the special education service delivery model for preschoolers with disabilities is a self-contained special education classroom, because the schools do not serve preschoolers who are not disabled. In some school districts, children are grouped heterogeneously; classes include children with a variety of disabilities and a range of severity levels. In others, children are grouped by severity or type of disability. Special education preschool classes follow the regular school schedule (a daily 6- to 7-hour school day), and preschoolers are expected to attend full-time (although 3-year-olds may be given an adjustment period of a few weeks while they gradually shift from a part-time schedule to a full-day schedule).

Special education preschool classrooms are staffed by certified special education teachers (in some states, there is separate ECSE certification) and a teacher's aide. Staff:child ratios are much smaller than childcare staffing ratios. In classes serving children with mild disabilities, ratios of 4:1 to 7:1 are common (one teacher, one aide, and 8 to 14 children); in classes with a heterogeneous group of children (children with a wide range of disabilities), ratios may be slightly smaller, perhaps 3:1 to 4:1; and if the classroom serves primarily children with severe or multiple disabilities, staff:child ratios may be as small as 3:1 or 2:1.

When children have a related service need they are assigned to one or more therapists. Ideally, the therapists work together as a transdisciplinary team, consulting with teachers and providing services to children in their classrooms—the "integrated therapy model" (Sternat, Messina, Nietupski, Lyon & Brown, 1977). Frequently, however, therapy services are delivered in an individual situation, either in a separate area of the special education classroom or in a therapy room.

Unfortunately, there is sometimes less family involvement and support for families in the segregated preschool service delivery model than in programs for infants and toddlers. Involvement and support may be limited to IEP development and perhaps daily written communications (that is, a communication notebook that goes back and forth between school and home).

The schedule in special education preschool classrooms is typically organized according to developmental domains with specific activities designed to address children's individual needs. As a consequence of the substantial commitment to individualized instruction, scheduling according to developmental domains, small staff:child ratios, and other disability-related accommodations, the special education preschool classroom often looks very different from a preschool classroom serving nondisabled children. Fortunately, as there is greater recognition of the benefits of providing all children with normalized experiences, special education preschool classes are beginning to adopt schedules and practices similar to those of preschool. programs that serve primarily nondisabled children (Bailey & McWilliam, 1990; Berkeley & Ludlow, 1989; Bricker, 1989; Bricker & Cripe, 1992).

Integrated Preschool Settings. Integrated preschool settings have been effective service delivery options since the early 1970s (Apolloni & Cooke, 1978; Bricker & Bricker, 1973; Guralnick, 1990a; Northcott, 1978). Integrated preschool models are staffed by early childhood professionals and paraprofessionals. There may be special education consultants or a special education teacher on the staff. The program director is typically an early childhood professional. (In some states, preschool teachers are required to be licensed or to have earned at least an Associate Degree in Child Development [CDA].) As in childcare, staff:child ratios are high, typically 1:10 or larger. The IEP for a child with disabilities enrolled in an integrated program specifies the amount and type of special assistance and related services necessary to support implementation of the child's program. Support to the preschool staff is provided through a variety of sources, including consultation, inservice training, demonstrations of specialized techniques by related services personnel and parents, and more.

Curriculum in an integrated preschool is concept-focused (for example, the Montessori curriculum) or theme and activity focused. Currently the emphasis is on "developmentally appropriate practices" (Bredekamp, 1987; Bredekamp & Shepard, 1989). What is provided in programs that emphasize developmentally appropriate practices differs from the developmental and behavioral curricula of segregated preschool service delivery models. Developmentally appropriate practices emphasize child-driven and child-guided learning and exploratory play, with children expected to select and participate in activities independently or in small groups under minimal adult supervision. This is in marked contrast to curricula in special education classes, which typically focus on discrete skill development and follow a fairly rigid progression of objectives implemented under the close supervision of adults.

Head Start.   Head Start is a unique, integrated preschool service delivery model that is required by policy to include children with disabilities (10% of the children enrolled must have disabilities). As discussed earlier in the section on legislation, Head Start is a federally sponsored program for economically disadvantaged children that was initiated in 1965. Its purpose is to provide "enrichment" experiences to prepare children for success in elementary school. The staffing, schedule, and curriculum are similar to other integrated preschool models. Head Start differs from other integrated preschool models in the level of community involvement (staffing, administrative boards, field trips, special activities), family involvement (home visits, parent volunteers), and availability of professionals from a variety of disciplines (nursing, special education, speech/language pathology). Community and family involvement make Head Start particularly sensitive to cultural differences.

Because Head Start has served children with disabilities since 1972, there is a long history of staff training and support to meet the special needs of children with disabilities (Doughty, 1985; Wolfe, Griffin, Zeger & Herwig, 1982). Most communities have a Head Start special-needs coordinator to assist in the transition of children with disabilities into the Head Start program.

For 5-Year-Olds

Segregated Kindergarten.   At age 5, most children attend kindergarten. For children with disabilities, service delivery options include a segregated special education class, an integrated kindergarten class, a resource room with partial mainstreaming in kindergarten, and Head Start. At the kindergarten level, segregated classes for children with disabilities may include children across the early elementary age span (kindergarten through second or third grade), with children assigned to classes based on the severity or category of their disabilities (learning disabled, hearing impaired, severely or multiply disabled). Heterogeneous classes with children from many disability categories (for example, mild mental retardation, learning disabilities) and severity levels are less common than at the preschool level.

Segregated special education classes serving 5-year-olds are similar to segregated special education preschool classes in staff:child ratios and scheduling. However, the curriculum may shift away from a developmental model toward pre-academics and simple academics for children with mild disabilities, and age-appropriate functional skills for children with moderate and severe disabilities. The scope of the curriculum tends to be confined to the scope of content covered on the IEPs of the children in the class. Because there are nondisabled age peers for 5-year-olds on public school campuses, there are more integration opportunities. Unfortunately, too few schools take full advantage of this. They limit integration to lunch and recess, with some joint activities such as field trips and assemblies with the kindergarten class. Parental involvement is generally the same as in the segregated preschool class, with parents participating in IEP development and (sometimes) through periodic written communications.

Integrated Kindergarten.   The integrated kindergarten service delivery model follows the mainstreaming model of elementary-level special education. The child with disabilities participates on a full-time basis in the regular kindergarten class. The staff:child ratio is larger than in most preschools, typically ranging from 1:20 to 1:30. Special education and related services personnel provide specialized intervention, consultation, or other types of support as indicated on the IEPs. Kindergarten curricula may include pre-academics and simple academics. There tends to be less family support and involvement in the integrated kindergarten class than in the segregated class.

Resource Room with Partial Kindergarten.   Because nondisabled 5-year-olds are served by the public schools in most states, the model of a resource room with partial kindergarten mainstreaming is common. A resource room is a special education classroom that serves children on a part-time basis (when they are not being mainstreamed). Children typically attend the resource room for (a) tutoring in skills and concepts with which they need special assistance, and (b) instruction addressing IEP objectives that are not covered in the regular kindergarten classroom. When children spend more than half of the school day in the regular classroom, their special education arrangement is referred to as a resource room. If children spend less than half of the day in the regular classroom, their special education arrangement is referred to as partial mainstreaming.

In the mainstreamed kindergarten class, the staff:child ratio tends to range from 1:20 to 1:30. Resource rooms are usually staffed by a special education teacher and a teacher's aide. The staff:child ratio is significantly lower and may vary throughout the day as children's mainstreaming schedules take them in and out of the resource room. Typical staff:child ratios in the resource room range from 1:3 to 1:7.

Head Start.   The Head Start service delivery model for preschool children is also an option for 5-year-olds. The program for 5-year-olds is the same as that for preschoolers, but there is more emphasis on academics (consistent with the public school kindergarten curriculum). When Head Start programs are located on or near a public school campus, part-time enrollment in Head Start and part-time enrollment in special education (either segregated special education classroom or resource room) is a viable service delivery option.

 # Current Best Practices

The history of federal initiatives in ECSE, outlined at the beginning of this chapter, provides insights into the importance of federal policy in promoting a national goal. As Hebbeler, Smith, and Black (1991) point out, our knowledge about how to provide services has grown exponentially, due in part to federally funded research and demonstration efforts.

Many of the "best practices" highlighted in this text were generated by federally funded research and demonstration activities. They include family-centered intervention, naturalistic curriculum, integration, general case instruction, group instruction, naturalistic teaching, the transdisciplinary team approach, and transition planning.

Family-Centered Intervention

The focus of services has shifted from child-centered to family-centered and family-directed intervention. Families are acknowledged as unique and able to identify their own concerns, priorities, and resources. The term *family-centered* in this context refers to particular ways of working with families as described by Dunst, Johanson, Trivette, and Hamby (1991). The beliefs and practices of family-centered services are consumer-driven and competency-enhancing. Families participate as decision-makers and partners in planning and implementing the service delivery process. Intervention goals focus on strengthening and supporting the family system as it adjusts to the needs of a member with special needs.

The family-centered focus has had a significant impact on early intervention methods. Parents or caregivers and other family members now enter into partnership with professionals in all aspects of early intervention—conducting assessment, prioritizing intervention goals, designing intervention plans, and implementing intervention.

Naturalistic/Functional Curriculum

Characteristics of a child's environments, such as the home, neighborhood, daycare center, preschool, or kindergarten, are analyzed to determine skills the child needs in order to participate in these settings. These environments are also considered when intervention strategies and contexts are selected. The trend is away from disjointed and isolated task demands toward environmental arrangements that address goals in the context of natural routines, such as dressing to go outside, preparing snacks, and clean-up activities.

Integration

Part H states that early-intervention services are to be provided in ". . . natural environments, including the home, and community settings in which children without disabilities participate" (IDEA, 1991, Sec. 672). The least restrictive environment (LRE) requirements for preschoolers are now the same as those for school-age children. The LRE requirements for school-age children state that state and local education agencies (SEAs and LEAs) must develop procedures to ensure that children with disabilities are educated to the maximum extent appropriate with children who are not disabled.

In attempting to interpret the constitutional boundaries of policy related to the LRE, the courts have ruled that children may be removed from regular educational environments "only when the nature or severity of the child's disability is such that education in regular classes with the use of supplementary aids and services cannot be achieved satisfactorily" (Turnbull & Turnbull, 1990, p. 20). Thus, the burden of proof rests with the educational agency in justifying any placement other than a regular classroom for a child with a disability. Young children with special needs should be educated in a regular preschool or kindergarten unless there is substantial evidence that instruction in the regular environment cannot be effective.

A comment added to the regulations for PL 94-142 in 1989 states that public agencies may use a variety of placement alternatives, such as full- or part-time placement in public or private preschool programs, to satisfy the LRE requirements for 3- to 5-year-olds with disabilities. It was stressed that whatever arrangements were made, the public agency must ensure that the child's placement is in the least restrictive setting in which the unique needs of the child can be met, based on the child's IEP. Integrated settings provide more competent role models, a richer curriculum, and higher expectations than segregated settings.

General Case Instruction

Traditionally, early intervention and special education have focused their initial instructional efforts on skill *acquisition,* and then later on skill *generalization.* Recently, researchers have demonstrated that generalization can be achieved concurrently with skill acquisition. Teaching generalized skills during skill acquisition is called *general case instruction.* The outcome of general case instruction is more effective and efficient intervention. If a child generalizes a new skill, the skill can be applied to a wide variety of situations across natural settings.

Group Instruction

In our efforts to provide intensive early intervention, we have tended to equate intensive instruction with individualized instruction. This practice fails to recognize (a) that most instruction in "normalized" settings occurs in group situations, and (b) that group instruction has benefits for children, families, and interventionists (more efficient use of time, opportunities for imitation). In programs guided by developmentally appropriate practice, teachers spend much of their classroom time working with children in small informal groups or individually (Kostelnik, 1992). Group instruction provides opportunities for teaching social and communication skills, as well as possibilities for incidental learning.

Naturalistic Teaching Approaches

When instruction is rigid and controlled, children with disabilities often fail to generalize newly acquired skills. Thus, there has been a shift over the past decade away from rigid and controlled procedures toward more naturalistic teaching methods such as *developmentally appropriate practice.* Many programs that service preschoolers with disabilities (both segregated and integrated programs) are following the nationally recommended methods referred to as developmentally appropriate practices (Bredekamp, 1987). These practices stress development of the "whole" child. They are child-centered, child-directed, and teacher-guided. Central to the tenets of developmentally appropriate practices is the notion that all young children should have equal opportunities to experience their surroundings, to make choices, to develop independence, and to move beyond their current skills, concepts, and strategies.

There is no intent to suggest that naturalistic teaching models (classrooms that use developmentally appropriate practices) do not have structure. Using the definition of structure put forth by Spodek, Saracho, and Davis (1991), naturalistic teaching approaches do have structure. Spodek and colleagues define structure as the extent to which teachers develop an instructional plan and subsequently organize the physical setting and social environment to support the achievement of educational goals.

Naturalistic teaching approaches are structured approaches that use natural routines and activities in natural environments as the teaching context. Naturalistic teaching methods are discussed in Chapters 5 through 11.

Transdisciplinary Team Approach

The transdisciplinary team approach is a model of team organization for assessment and intervention. Dorothy Hutchinson introduced the term *transdisciplinary* in 1974 in a description of services for atypical infants and their families. The idea evolved from a concern for limiting the handling of medically fragile infants during the assessment process (McCormick, 1990b). Possibly the greatest advantage of this approach (over the multidisciplinary or interdisciplinary approaches) is that it promotes a more integrated approach to assessment and to delivery of services (Foley, 1990). Key elements of the transdisciplinary approach are arena assessment, integrated therapy, and collaboration (discussed in Chapters 2, 3, and 4).

Transition Planning

Initially popularized as a response to the need to facilitate movement of secondary students from special education programs to postschool environments (jobs, community living arrangements), transition planning is now an accepted component of early intervention. Transition planning facilitates a positive and comfortable change process when a family and child move from one service program to another. As discussed in Chapter 13, the early childhood period is a time of many transitions for infants and young children with disabilities and their families. Major transitions include (a) from the hospital to home and infant services, (b) from infant services to preschool, and (c) from preschool to kindergarten.

Summary

This chapter has provided an introduction to the history of concern for early intervention services. Policymaking for infants and young children with disabilities and their families was shown to parallel awareness of the impact of early experiences and the environment on development. This chapter also described the various service delivery models that have evolved over the years. Finally, the chapter highlighted major trends that reflect the expanded knowledge base in early intervention. The eight trends—best practices—set the philosophical tone and at the same time introduce the remainder of the book. The perspective of this text is a naturalistic approach that integrates developmental and learning theories at the level of effective practice.

Activities

1. Find out what agency in your state is the designated "lead agency" for Part H. Contact the program in that agency responsible for planning and implementing this legislation and request a copy of the most recent state plan. Find out if your state has determined "at-risk" children to be eligible for early intervention and learn your state's eligibility definitions.

2. If you are not a member of the Council for Exceptional Children (CEC), ask someone who is a member to tell you about the organization or provide you with membership information. Consider joining the Division for Early Childhood (DEC), which is the division of CEC for persons interested in early childhood special education (ECSE).

Review Questions

1. Describe the contributions of each of these persons to the field of early intervention: Itard, Piaget, Montessori, Skeels, Kirk, Spitz, Goldfarb, Hunt, Bloom, and Lazar.
2. List the four pieces of legislation that have most affected services for infants and young children with disabilities and briefly note the major contribution of each.
3. Describe the changes to EHA provided by PL 99-457.
4. List the required components of the IFSP.
5. Explain who is eligible for services under Part H and Part B—Section 619 of IDEA.
6. Compare service delivery models for (a) infants and toddlers, (b) 3- to 5-year-olds, and (c) 5-year-olds.
7. Provide a brief explanation of what is entailed with each of these "best practices": (a) family-centered intervention, (b) naturalistic/functional curriculum, (c) integration, (d) general case instruction, (e) group instruction, (f) naturalistic teaching approaches, (g) transdisciplinary team approaches, and (h) transition planning.

Teaming, Interagency Collaboration, and Service Coordination

Objectives

1. Describe the composition of the IFSP team, the IEP team, and the three most common service delivery team approaches.

2. Discuss barriers to effective team functioning and suggest possible remedies to encourage effective teaming.

3. Discuss barriers to effective interagency collaboration and suggest ways to break down these barriers.

4. Describe the history of the concept of service coordination, models for service coordination, and functions of the service coordinator.

As discussed in Chapter 1, many of the provisions of Part H, the infant component of IDEA, are different from those for the preschool component (Part B–Section 619). Some provisions are the same. One that is the same is the requirement that professionals, parents, and caregivers and other family members work as a team in the assessment and planning processes.

Two requirements of Part H that are different are (a) the development of an Individualized Family Service Plan (IFSP) for each family of an eligible child, and (b) the requirement that a service coordinator be appointed. Recall that the original legislation used the term "case manager" for this function, and that one of the changes in terminology in the reauthorization of the act was substitution of the term *service coordinator* (IDEA Amendments, 1991). While the name changed, the functions and responsibilities assigned to the position did not.

In addition to changing the terminology, the 1991 reauthorization amends the provision in the original legislation stating that the service coordinator should be from the profession considered most relevant to the needs of the infant, toddler, or family. The 1991 amendment states that the service coordinator may be anyone who is qualified to carry out the service coordination responsibilities. This includes parents who want to assume responsibility for some or all of their own service coordination or provide service coordination for another family.

One of the major requirements of Part H is for states to develop a comprehensive system of services for infants and young children with disabilities and their families. There is enormous variability across state systems and within each system. Services range from urban child/family centers where many different types of services (childcare, therapies, health care, counseling services) are coordinated under one umbrella organization, to single-service programs with multidisciplinary staff, to rural programs where the various discipline representatives on the multidisciplinary team may be employed by different agencies (possibly located in different counties).

The considerable differences in programs within each state's comprehensive early intervention system suggest differences in the way teaming and service coordination are interpreted and, ultimately, the way these processes are implemented. However, this chapter takes the position that there is a core of basic premises and procedures that is common among most programs where teaming, interagency collaboration, and service coordination are concerned.

 ## Teaming

The rules and regulations of the legislation are specific about the membership of the IEP and IFSP teams. In addition to the caregivers and other family members, the *IFSP team* includes the service coordinator and those professionals whose disciplines best meet the child's and family's needs. More specifically, Part H regulations state that the following persons will participate in developing the IFSP: (1) the parent or parents; (2) other family members (as requested by the parent); (3) an advocate or person outside the family (as requested by the parent); (4) the interim service coordinator (someone who has been working with family since referral); (5) persons directly involved in conducting the evaluations and assessments; and (6) persons who will be providing services to the infant or toddler and the family (as appropriate).

In regard to the role of caregivers or parents and other family members on the IFSP team, McGonigel and Garland (1988) note that professionals should be less concerned with making a place for parents and other family members on the IFSP team than with developing strategies that will enable professionals to become members of the family team. The regulations concerning the IFSP process are very clear that the ultimate decision concerning services rests with the family. At least to the extent that the family desires, the IFSP process and subsequent services should constitute a "family driven" system (Nash, 1990). Professionals on the IFSP team should coordinate to provide information and professional opinion (in a manner that is not value-laden) to caregivers/family.

Most important is to provide accurate and unbiased information so that caregivers and other family members can make informed choices and decisions about what they want for their child and their family. Once the caregivers have decided what they want and need, then the professional role is one of facilitating and supporting the services.

The *IEP team* includes the caregivers/family and the child (if appropriate), a representative of the public agency who is in a supervisory capacity, the child's teacher, and a member of the evaluation team (or another individual knowledgeable about the evaluation procedures). The IEP process is different from the IFSP process in that the focus is more on deciding how and where to provide the "specially designed instruction" that the child requires.

For professionals, realizing active parent/family involvement is one of the major challenges associated with developing and implementing both the IEP and the IFSP processes. The next section will consider team approaches and teaming constructs and skills. Then we will discuss barriers to effective team functioning.

Team Models

Despite the considerable attention to teaming since the initial implementation of PL 94-142, teaming in the human services arena is still in its infancy. There is a great deal to be learned about the processes and procedures inherent in effective teaming, particularly about involving families (Nash, 1990). Data from a number of studies in the early and mid-eighties suggested that family participation on IEP teams was limited —that professionals did not seem to value parents' input to the process (Gilliam & Coleman, 1981; Winton, Turnbull & Blacher, 1985).

The three most common approaches to service delivery team organization are the multidisciplinary team approach, the interdisciplinary team approach, and the transdisciplinary team approach.

Multidisciplinary Team Model.   The multidisciplinary team approach is most commonly found in medical settings. Professionals maintain their respective discipline boundaries with only minimal, if any, coordination, collaboration, or communication across disciplines (McCormick & Goldman, 1978). Each professional assesses and attempts to remediate those aspects of the child's needs that fall within their discipline's unique province (occupational therapy, physical therapy, speech/language pathology, and so on).

Interdisciplinary Team Model.   The interdisciplinary team approach establishes formal communication channels among team members, and there is considerably more coordination and collaboration across disciplines than with a multidisciplinary team model. Typically, one team member is assigned to coordinate services. Team members generally advocate joint decision making and development of a unified intervention plan, but in practice there are often problems related to information sharing. Information often flows only one way—from team members involved in assessment to a direct service provider. There is no provision for feedback from the service provider to those responsible for assessment and intervention recommendations. This suggests lack of concern for whether the intervention recommendations are practical and functional.

Transdisciplinary Team Model.   The transdisciplinary team approach is an outgrowth of work by Dorothy Hutchinson in 1974 as part of the United Cerebral Palsy Collaborative Infant Program. It evolved from a concern for limiting the number of people who handle infants with disabilities (many of whom are medically fragile) during assessment and intervention. In practice, and philosophically, there are some very real differences between the transdisciplinary team model and the other two approaches. The most notable difference is the commitment to sharing information and skills among team members (with caregivers and parents, teachers, and related service disciplines).

Like the other models, all professionals are primarily responsible for initial assessment in their discipline. However, this is where the similarities end. With the transdisciplinary model, discipline representatives and caregivers and parents provide continued support, consultation, and direct assistance to one another and to the team member who is the direct service provider. Where infants and toddlers are concerned, the direct service provider is typically the primary caregiver or parent. With preschoolers, in most cases the direct service provider is the teacher.

Lyon and Lyon (1980) defined the relevant characteristics of the transdisciplinary team model as (a) joint functioning, (b) continuous staff development, and (c) role release. *Joint functioning* means that team members perform required services together whenever possible. Arena or conjoint assessment, which will be described in Chapters 3 and 4, is an example of joint junctioning.

Continuous staff development means that team members train one another on an ongoing basis so that the skills of all team members are always being expanded. This emphasis on continual opportunities for skill development is one of the greatest strengths of the transdisciplinary team model. *Role release* occurs when one team member assists the direct service provider in the performance of a function that is typically part of the assisting team member's role. At different times during intervention, team members role release to the direct service provider, who implements specific intervention recommendations. All team members at some point release their direct service roles to function as consultants and facilitators for the direct service provider.

Team leadership depends on the child's and the family's strengths and preferences. If the program is part of an educational system, the teacher is likely to be the team leader, coordinating the activities of all members in ways that best address individual child needs (Campbell, 1989). If the child is under age 3, the service coordinator may be the team leader or the primary service provider (depending on the family's choice). In either case, the caregivers/parents are key team members.

Barriers to Effective Teaming

Each team member has a role. Each role has a set of skills and certain expectations associated with it. Problems occur when team members do not have a clear idea what is expected of them as a team member or what to expect of others. For example, the teacher on a team may assume that the occupational therapist will take primary responsibility for assessing a child's feeding needs, while the occupational therapist may expect to be a consultant for the feeding assessment and assume that the physical therapist will conduct the assessment.

Professionals may not be clear as to the role of family members on the team, and family members may not have a clear idea what is expected of them as team members or what to expect of others. Nash (1990) suggests that teams assign one professional member to take responsibility for orienting family members to the purpose and functioning of the team as a way to help them define their roles on the team.

Ideally, each team member's role is relatively equal in power and influence (Bailey, 1984). Problems occur when one or another of the members is perceived as inferior. In response to the lack of influence and respect, the team member who is perceived to be inferior withdraws from active participation in the decision-making process.

Another barrier to effective teaming is lack of negotiation skills. Too often team members approach situations in which there is disagreement with a win-or-lose attitude. This view guarantees that at least one person will lose. When one person loses, everyone involved loses. It is critical for all team members to learn and to practice managing conflict creatively. Nash (1990) emphasizes that caregivers/ parents are more likely to let others know when they disagree with something if the team treats conflict as a normal part of team process that can lead to more satisfactory outcomes.

Additional barriers to effective team functioning include lack of leadership, professional insecurity, lack of communication skills, concerns over territoriality, lack of tolerance for philosophical differences across disciplines, use of professional jargon, and lack of time for meetings. Without a uniform philosophical approach it may be difficult for team members to reach agreement on a common goal.

Teaming Skills

Based on a review of research on teaming, Shea and Guzzo (1987) identified three requirements for effective teaming: task interdependence, outcome interdependence, and potency. *Task interdependence* is the degree to which team members interact as they pursue a goal. Early intervention team members must schedule time and take advantage of *every* opportunity to get to know one another. Initially they should concentrate on establishing areas of agreement concerning both teaming and intervention goals. Teaming will be successful to the extent that team members know and practice effective communication skills and collaborative goal setting (Bailey, 1987).

Outcome interdependence refers to the extent to which team members share in the consequences of their team efforts. Because tangible rewards are scarce, team members will generally have to rely on internal rewards. The challenge is to identify and agree upon intrinsic rewards. Persons who have different values and beliefs (common when members are from different disciplines) tend to have different intrinsic reward systems. If all team members can agree on, and place high value on, family involvement and collaborative goal setting, then demonstrations of these values will tend to be experienced as rewarding.

Potency, the third requirement for team effectiveness, is the team's belief that they have the skills and environmental supports to be effective. The value placed on family involvement and teaming by the organization or system in which the team functions will influence the extent to which these values can be successfully achieved. Organizational support gives team members the confidence to pursue their goals and accomplish the tasks at hand.

The importance of skills in communication and group process cannot be overemphasized. These skills are implicated in all activities associated with effective team functioning. Within the domains of communication and group process there are two types of skills: (1) task-oriented behaviors (problem-solving and decision-making skills), and (2) relationship-oriented skills (cooperation and collaboration skills). Task-oriented skills include the ability to:

1. Clearly identify and define the problems at hand
2. Determine potential strengths in the situation
3. Keep an open mind concerning alternative solutions
4. Develop appropriate goals and objectives
5. Search out and analyze relevant information from different sources
6. Interpret and clarify planning and implementation issues
7. Combine and summarize related constructs and ideas
8. Elicit input and consensus from others

Relationship-oriented skills include the ability to:

1. Stimulate the participation of others
2. Reconcile opposing positions in a positive manner
3. Compromise for the sake of productive discussion

4. View differences as negotiable
5. Solicit and make use of feedback
6. Clarify perceptions and feelings
7. Communicate understanding and acceptance of the opinions of others
8. Translate technical concepts into understandable terms
9. Communicate accessibility, responsiveness, and honest concern
10. Establish an atmosphere of trust, respect, and acceptance

Interagency Collaboration

Facilitating interagency collaboration is one of the most important functions of the service coordinator (Dunst & Trivette, 1989). The major reason for collaboration (at the level of individual service providers and at the agency level) is that the needs of infants and young children with disabilities and their families can be exceedingly complex and multifaceted.

The barriers to effective interagency collaboration parallel the barriers to effective teaming. Some of the most common problems are (a) competitiveness, (b) parochial interests, (c) lack of communication skills, (d) resistance to change, (e) concerns about client confidentiality, (f) inadequate knowledge about other agencies and programs, (g) negative attitudes, and (h) political naiveté.

There are no easy ways to break down these barriers, but programs such as Project IINTACT at San Diego State University provide some good ideas. Project IINTACT, a model demonstration project funded by the Handicapped Children's Early Education Program (USOE), identifies five methods for promoting successful interagency collaboration: (1) try new solutions, (2) network, (3) be responsive, (4) acknowledge and work through turf and territorial issues, and (5) communicate (Lynch & Harrison, 1986).

Doing things "the way we have always done them" is much easier than trying new solutions, but the price an agency pays for this attitude may be high in terms of the loss of opportunities for collaboration. Agencies must be prepared to explore new options, many of which will come from people in direct services positions. These persons are often the first to notice new and changing needs in the community. For example, childcare workers may realize that there are families who are homeless, with toddlers and young children who need childcare and preschool programs. Systematic documentation of these needs may generate new solutions which, in turn, can lead to mobilization of other agencies.

Networking is a way to help professionals deal with the increasing demands of their jobs while at the same time increasing interagency collaboration. Some informal networking goes on in every agency and among agencies in every community. These interactions need to be formalized so that they include all individuals who would like to participate. One idea is to start an interagency group to share information, recent research findings, and workable solutions to problems. Another possibility is to convene a group of individuals, such as an advisory group, to provide a structured forum for generating solutions to community problems.

Parents should also be included in these groups, as they bring different perspectives on the service system.

Responsiveness is a critical requisite for effective interpersonal and interagency collaboration. Some behaviors that come under the heading of responsiveness are (a) returning phone calls promptly, (b) following through on commitments, and (c) initiating prompt thank-you calls and letters.

Acknowledging turf and territorial issues is a major step in the direction of minimizing their impact. The key is for individuals and agencies to abandon their individual ego needs and allow the *group* to "own" new ideas as well as positive results. When forming interagency groups, it is important not to overlook any agency that could conceivably be interested. It is also a good idea to rotate meeting sites or find space that is on neutral ground, so that no one agency is seen as having a proprietary interest.

Finally, communication is absolutely essential for successful interpersonal collaboration and interagency collaboration. In most circumstances there is a need to create some structure for sharing information. This may entail having a facilitator help the group get organized during its early development.

In conclusion, whether the issue is collaboration among team members or interagency collaboration, someone has to start the ball rolling. Professionals and parents associated with early intervention can begin by (a) modeling the collaboration process among themselves, (b) developing a positive atmosphere for communication, and (c) arranging for collaboration to occur on a regular basis.

 ## Service Coordination

Most of the relevant literature so far uses the term "case management" for the functions subsumed under the heading of service coordination. We will substitute the term *service coordination* because, as noted earlier in the chapter, the 1991 amendments to the IDEA officially replace "case management" with *service coordination* and "case manager" with *service coordinator*. The new language is acknowledgement of widespread dissatisfaction with the term "case management." Families and professionals alike objected to the term because it suggests that children and families need to be "managed." It reflected a deficit model, implying that families of children with special needs are dependent and lacking essential childrearing knowledge and skills. The new terms have a more positive and supportive tone.

The rules and regulations for Part H define *service coordination* as "services provided to families of infants and toddlers with disabilities to assist them in gaining access to early intervention services identified in the individualized family service plan" (Federal Register, Nov. 18, 1987, p. 44355). In practice, service coordination begins even before there is an IFSP; it begins as soon as a family contacts an agency and requests early intervention services and support.

The legislation identifies the following as service coordination functions:

1. Coordinating the performance of evaluations and participating in the development of the individualized family service plan;
2. Assisting families in identifying available service providers;
3. Coordinating and monitoring the delivery of services, including the provision of early intervention services with other services that the child or family needs or is receiving, but that are not required under this part (e.g., medical services for other than diagnostic or evaluation purposes, respite care, and the purchase of personal prosthetic devices such as braces, hearing aids, and glasses); and
4. Facilitating the development of a transition plan to preschool services where appropriate. (Federal Register, Nov. 18, 1987, p. 44355)

The law provides three instructions related to service coordination. It states that (a) the IFSP must include the name of the service coordinator; (b) the service coordinator may be from the profession most immediately relevant to the infant's, toddler's, or family's needs, or it may be any person qualified to carry out service coordination responsibilities; and (c) the service coordinator is to be responsible for implementation of the plan and coordination with other agencies and persons. Service coordination is not required during the preschool years (not included in Part B–Section 619). However, recognizing the value of service coordination, many special education teachers elect to assume the functions associated with the service coordinator role.

This section begins with a brief historical perspective followed by a discussion of various models for providing service coordination and the functions associated with these models. In all cases, the emphasis is on how the functions can be performed in a manner that maximizes respect for the family and family participation.

Brief History of Service Coordination

At the broadest level, service coordination has two parts: (a) advocacy, and (b) support and assistance in organizing services and resources. While the term *service coordination* is new, the concept and practices associated with this role have been around for some time (Lowenthal, 1991). They have their roots in three separate spheres of social change in the sixties (Semon & Brashears, 1989): (1) deinstitutionalization, (2) the War on Poverty, and (3) family-centered or community-based care.

Deinstitutionalization.   Until the early seventies, the prevailing practice was to place most children and adults who had disabilities in state institutions. Many stayed in these settings for their entire lives. In 1972, Wolfensberger put forth the concept called the *normalization principle* that had a significant effect on the practice of institutionalization.

Wolfensberger (1972) defined normalization as "utilization of means which are as culturally normative as possible, in order to establish and/or maintain personal behaviors and characteristics which are as culturally normative as possible" (p. 28). The normalization principle dictates that persons with disabilities should be served in facilities and locales similar to, if not identical to, those used by persons who do not have disabilities.

The major consequence of deinstitutionalization was the return of hundreds of thousands of persons with mental and physical disabilities to their home communities for care and support. Because most had been dependent on institutional resources for many decades (sometimes from birth), they were not capable of advocating for themselves and securing appropriate services when relocated in their home communities. Coordination of services for these individuals placed enormous demands on their families and on community agencies. The logical response was to recruit or identify persons in the agencies who were to be responsible specifically for ensuring that the normalization goals of deinstitutionalization were achieved. These persons were called "case managers."

The War on Poverty.   President Kennedy's urging in the 1960s—and, subsequently, the urging of President Johnson—led to legislative action that had far-reaching effects on human services for persons living in lower socioeconomic conditions. This legislative action was called the War on Poverty. It initiated a substantial increase in the number of programs addressing the medical, financial, social, and educational needs of persons living in poverty. (Probably the best known of these programs was Head Start.) Not surprisingly, as the number of available programs increased, so did difficulties related to locating and using the available services. Again, the response was to assign specific professionals (case managers) to be responsible for organizing services and facilitating access to appropriate programs.

Family-Centered Care.   Significant advances in research and technology since the end of World War II have increased the effectiveness of medical treatment. Many children have been saved who would not have survived had they been born a decade earlier. In addition to saving lives, the new technology and appropriate support services make it possible for many youngsters with significant health care needs to live in the community with their families.

Family-centered care recognizes the family setting as the best context for nurturance. Begun in the seventies, this trend evolved to a high level of visibility in the 1980s. The success of family-centered care is dependent on case management (now called service coordination) to integrate and organize a complex system of medical and human services to support the child in living at home.

In summary, the roots of service coordination can be traced to three sources: (a) the deinstitutionalization movement of the 1960s and 1970s, (b) expansion of services associated with the War on Poverty, and (c) family-centered care made possible by technological advances, particularly in medicine. Regardless of the target population, the primary focus of service coordination is the same: (a) to support and strengthen the independence of the individual or the family, (b) to minimize the fragmentation and duplication of services, and (c) to assist in mobilizing needed resources and services.

Models of Service Coordination

Part H does not specify how service coordination functions are to be achieved, nor does it specify the service coordinator's realm of authority. For example, what activities are included in "coordinating" evaluations? Does the service coordinator

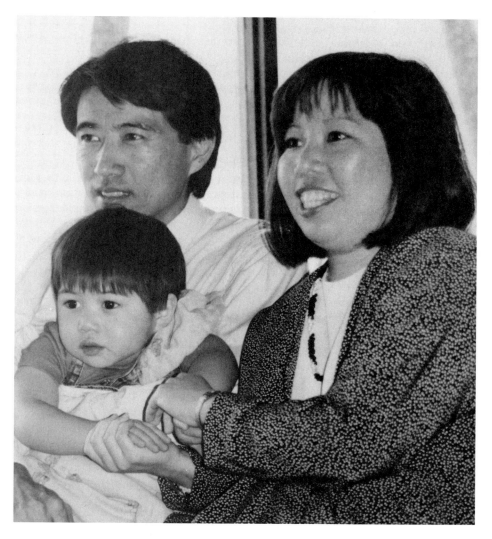

The goal is for early interventionists to become a part of the family's team.

decide which disciplines participate in the evaluation process? What does "participating in the development of the IFSP" mean? Is the service coordinator responsible for writing the IFSP document? Does the service coordinator participate in the IFSP meeting as an advocate for the family, or as facilitator of the meeting, or are both roles intended?

Implementing service coordination requires some definition and clarification of the roles of the service coordinator, family, and other team members. How these roles are defined will depend on the service coordination model that is adopted. Dunst and Trivette (1989) identify three case management/service coordination models: (a) role-focused, (b) resource procurement, and (c) client empowerment. Each model has different implications for early intervention services and outcomes.

Role-Focused Models. Role-focused approaches place major emphasis on service coordinators as organizers and integrators of needed services. Because service coordinators in these approaches assume full responsibility for managing services, they tend to usurp the family's decision-making authority. The disadvantage of these models is that families do not learn to be independent when it comes to defining goals and deciding what they need to do to achieve their goals.

Resource Procurement Models. Resource procurement models place major emphasis on identifying family needs and mobilizing resources to meet these needs. Resource procurement approaches differ from role-focused approaches in that the family is more involved in identifying needed services. The service coordinator acts as a "systems broker" rather than as a decision-maker in organizing and accessing services. However, again the assumption is that the families are not able to take primary responsibility for self-advocacy. Role-focused and resource procurement models of service coordination meet the immediate needs of families, but they do not help families learn to be optimally self-sufficient and independent.

Client Empowerment Models. Client empowerment models place major emphasis on enhancing and promoting the family's capacity for self-advocacy. Similar to the other approaches, client empowerment models emphasize coordination and integration of services. Where they differ from the other approaches is in encouraging the caregiver, parent, or family to function as independently as possible, and to assume an active role in the service coordination process. Service coordinators function as enablers, providing information, creating opportunities, and supporting and reinforcing demonstrations of family independence. With empowerment approaches, service coordination is effective only to the extent that families become more capable, competent, and self-directed as a result of the service coordinator's support.

In conclusion, there seems little question that the intent of Congress in Part H was for service coordination to be provided to families in ways designed to make them more capable of meeting their own needs and those of their children. The premises underlying empowerment models are compatible with early intervention philosophies that emphasize the importance of empowering parents as expert decision-makers for their children and their family.

An Enabling Model

The enabling model of service coordination described by Dunst and Trivette (1987, 1988, 1989) is a client (or in this case, family) empowerment model. It evolved from efforts to identify the best ways to support and strengthen family functioning. *Family empowerment* is operationally defined as family identification and recognition of needs, family deployment of competencies to obtain needed resources, and self-attributions about the role family members play in accessing resources and meeting needs. Note that family empowerment is defined by what the *family* does, not by what the service coordinator does.

Service Coordinator Functions. As noted earlier, the 1991 amendments stating that the parents may be their own service coordinators and families may provide service coordination for one another do not change the characteristics and the basic functions of the role. Dunst and Trivette (1987, 1988, 1989) suggest the following beliefs and behaviors as essential to maximizing the effectiveness of service coordinators as family enablers:

1. A positive and proactive stance toward families
2. Belief in the families' responsibility for solving problems and meeting their own needs
3. Belief that all families have the capacity to understand, learn, and manage events in their lives
4. Ability to build on family strengths, not try to "fix" deficits
5. Ability to work with families in a proactive, anticipatory fashion (rather than waiting for things to go wrong before intervening)
6. Ability to teach families the competencies they need to better negotiate their family developmental course
7. Ability to help families identify and prioritize their needs as *they* see them
8. Ability to get active family participation as part of mobilizing resources
9. Ability to use partnerships and parent-professional collaboration as the foundation for enhancing family strengths
10. Ability to provide families with the information essential to informed decision making
11. Ability to accept and support decisions made by families

Success in implementing the family enabling model is heavily influenced by the extent to which service coordinators demonstrate these attitudes and skills. In practice, all members of the service delivery team, regardless of their discipline, should demonstrate these service coordinator competencies. In addition to skills specific to their discipline, service coordinators must demonstrate empowerment and collaboration skills in order to work effectively with other team members.

Traditional functions for the case manager role included outreach, individual and family assessment, case planning, service coordination, referral, advocacy, direct casework, developing natural support systems, mobilizing resources, monitoring quality of services, public education, and crisis intervention (Wray & Wieck,

1985). These traditional functions are an integral part of the role of the service coordinator (and family enablement models), but the ways in which these functions are performed are different (Dunst & Trivette, 1989). In the family enablement model, service coordinators do not integrate or coordinate services on behalf of families; rather, they arrange for public and private service providers to become more responsive to the needs of families. Similarly, service coordinators in the enablement model do not decide what families need; instead, they help families clarify their concerns and identify their own needs. They do not mobilize resources on behalf of families; rather, they assist families in developing effective ways to access needed resources on their own. The family is not always the "doer" in all service spheres, but the family certainly is always the "decider" of what needs to be done.

These distinctions are neither trivial nor superficial. They determine whether the outcome will be families who are passive and dependent or families who are active, autonomous, and self-reliant. The functions subsumed under the heading of service coordination depend on variables related to family needs, available community services, training and personal biases of the case coordinator—and, most important, the model of service coordination that the supporting agency espouses.

The Role of the Family.   Possibly the best way to summarize the currently strong family-involvement stance is to say that the desired outcome (from the early intervention perspective) should be for the team to enable the family to take charge of the team process (to the extent that the family desires) (Lowenthal, 1991). Typically, the service coordinator determines with the parents the extent to which the parents will participate in service coordination (Garland, Woodruff & Buck, 1988). The "ideal" amount and type of family participation is an individual family matter. Participation will depend on variables such as interest, skills, comfort, and time restrictions. The family and the service coordinator work to integrate the information and skills of the entire team, ensure coordination and communication among providers, and monitor services.

Whether parents are their own service coordinators is their choice. When Able-Boone, Sandall, Loughry, and Frederick (1990) asked parents what they thought of being their own service coordinator, 23% of the parents interviewed liked the idea. Some were in fact currently serving in this role, in that they were accessing resources on their own for their child and the family. Other parents preferred to have a professional as service coordinator. They indicated that they thought the service coordinator should be a professional who could be objective in coordinating services and ensuring their quality. The greatest concern of these parents was that the service coordinator have some preparation for and experience in the role.

The family's trust in and comfort with the service coordinator is an important factor in determining the productivity of the service coordinator process. Families must have an active role in selecting a service coordinator and they must be able to change service coordinators if their needs change or if they feel that the relationship is not comfortable and productive.

Sensitivity to cultural and linguistic differences is key to effective interactions with families and successful service coordination. In one way or another, culture affects all aspects of everyone's life: It affects values, expectations, and needs. Failure to acknowledge and address the effects of cultural diversity can have damaging consequences, in that it leads to incorrect assumptions about what supports families want and need for their children with disabilities and for themselves.

Beckman and Bristol (1991) provide these suggestions for professionals concerned with infusing sensitivity to cultural diversity into early intervention programming: (a) identify your own cultural values and be aware of their influence on your professional opinions, (b) take the time to learn as much as you can about the values that are operating within the families in your program, (c) encourage and support recruitment and hiring of culturally diverse staff, and (d) develop and implement goals and objectives in a way that demonstrates respect for differing values.

How to Be a Service Coordinator

Dunst and Trivette (1989) caution against literal translation of the legislation in regard to service coordination responsibilities. Their contention is that literal translation of the statement that the service coordinator is to be responsible for implementing the plan will lead to a role-focused approach to coordination. (There is a strong likelihood that families will become passive recipients rather than active masters of the services system with a role-focused approach that is defined in terms of service coordinator functions.)

How we conceptualize and implement service coordinator practices should be guided by one overriding consideration: the importance of family empowerment as the ultimate meaningful outcome. Service coordination is effective only to the extent that it helps families become stronger, more capable, and competent.

Recall that Part H lists these specific services to be provided by the service coordinator: (1) coordinating assessments, (2) participating in the development of the IFSP, (3) assisting families in identifying available service providers, (4) coordinating and monitoring services, and (5) facilitating development of a transition plan. This section considers what these services entail.

Coordinating Assessments. Services for a family begin with the first contact with a family member. If the family does not need (or want) services at the time of initial referral, they may agree to be contacted at a later time (in a few weeks or months). Most important is for them to know that program staff are there for them and that the family will be welcomed when they decide they want services and support.

If the family is ready to begin services, the first official task after referral is pre-assessment planning. Very often this is when a service coordinator is selected.

The first responsibility of the service coordinator will be to coordinate child assessment and identification of family concerns, priorities, and resources. By law, the assessment process must be completed within 45 days after referral or initial contact.

When PL 99-457 was passed, many intervention programs began to use family assessment procedures, including instruments measuring family needs, roles, knowledge, skills, stress, environment, social support, attitudes, and coping strategies. More recently, this practice of early interventionists conducting assessments of families has been challenged. Slentz and Bricker (1992) argue that the use of clinical and research tools to assess families for early intervention services is inappropriate and may even be detrimental to the goals of the IFSP. The implicit pathological orientation of these instruments is not appropriate for early intervention programs, where the primary concern is strengthening the family to enhance and support the child's development. Moreover, it is not respectful of families. "There is little to empower families in a relationship in which professionals collect, analyze, and interpret information about family members. . . . It is not normalizing for families to share sensitive and personal information with relative strangers" (Slentz & Bricker, 1992, p. 15).

The alternative to family assessment is what Slentz and Bricker refer to as "family-guided assessment"—collection of family information that relates only to enhancing the child's development. Assessments that identify the family's interests, priorities, and concerns can be used by the families themselves and by early interventionists to meet the family's expressed needs. Families who feel they have more pressing and specific needs can request additional assessments if situations arise in the course of the working relationship that evolves between the early intervention personnel and the family.

The service coordinator assumes responsibility for ensuring that child assessments are done in a variety of settings and over as many sessions as needed to get an accurate picture of the child's skills. The service coordinator also makes sure that assessments are done in a relaxed and comfortable manner, using a variety of approaches such as interviews, questionnaires, and observations, in addition to more formal assessment instruments.

Developing the IFSP. A part of the next chapter is devoted to IFSP development, so this service coordinator function will not be discussed here. The major points to keep in mind are (a) that the IFSP is an ongoing process (not a product), and (b) that the parent-professional partnership is the key to an effective IFSP process.

Identifying Services.   It is not possible for a single agency or a single individual to meet all of the child's and family's medical, social, emotional, and educational needs. This is the reason for transdisciplinary teams and interagency agreements. As the position title implies, a major responsibility of the service coordinator is to help the family coordinate services; specifically, to (a) identify sources of support and resources, and (b) develop effective ways to access the needed resources. Used in this context, *support* means emotional, physical, informational, and instrumental resources. It could mean just being a good listener when a parent or caregiver needs someone to talk to about the difficulties of rearing a young child, or it could mean identifying medical resources or providing information about a particular disability (Dunst, Trivette & Deal, 1988). It does *not* mean making decisions. The family is always the decision-maker in these activities; the family may or may not be the doer.

There are two ways to identify existing and potential needs and sources of support. One strategy—and probably the most effective—is to use an interview format. This approach is effective if the interviewer is a good listener, knows what questions to ask, and has the knowledge and resources to make suggestions for linking families with needed support. The other methods are to use self-report or to administer a social support scale such as provided by Dunst and Trivette (1985) or Fewell (1986).

Monitoring Services.   Another component of the IFSP process (and typically a responsibility of the service coordinator) is determining criteria and timelines for evaluating whether family concerns have been addressed. Dunst and Trivette (1989) suggest evaluations of two variables: (1) the degree to which actions to obtain needed resources result in actually obtaining the resources and attaining goals, and (2) whether the family is satisfied with the process and the outcomes. They recommend using each and every contact with the family as an opportunity to evaluate progress toward resource mobilization and goal attainment. Ask the family whether they have had the opportunity to do a particular step, and how they feel about their progress toward goal attainment. This information is recorded as progress data, which are used as a basis for making changes in the plan.

Transition Planning.   Transitions can be very stressful for infants and young children with special needs and their families. Part H addresses this issue with the requirement that the IFSP must include steps to support the transition process. The service coordinator is responsible for these. Transition is discussed at length in Chapter 13.

Summary

This chapter has focused on three related topics: teaming, interagency collaboration, and service coordination. It has described the three team models—multidisciplinary, interdisciplinary, and transdisciplinary—and highlighted the relevant characteristics of the transdisciplinary team approach. Barriers to effective teaming and collaboration were discussed. Finally, the chapter presented a brief history and models of service coordination. An enabling model is recommended as most compatible with current best practices.

Activities

1. Talk with three special education teachers or therapists about the type of team organization where they work. (These may be people in your class.) Ask them what they see as barriers to effective team functioning and what they would suggest to remedy these barriers.

2. Talk with several parents (or other caregivers) about service coordination. Ask them how they feel (or would feel) about being their own service coordinator and what functions they see as most important for a service coordinator.

3. List your cultural values related to family life and childrearing. (If you have trouble articulating your own values, think about the values of your mother or father.) Consider each value separately and describe how it could affect your professional performance and the way you come across with families who have different cultural values.

Review Questions

1. List the three team models and describe how each operates.
2. List and describe at least ten barriers to effective team functioning and suggest ways to circumvent these barriers.
3. Explain the three requirements for effective teaming.
4. Compare task-oriented skills and relationship-oriented skills.
5. Discuss barriers to effective interagency collaboration and suggest ways to break down these barriers.
6. List and describe service coordinator functions as described in the rules and regulations of PL 99-457.
7. Briefly trace the history of service coordination from the sixties to the present.
8. Contrast the enabling (client empowerment) model of service coordination with traditional models and describe the beliefs and behaviors critical to the success of an enabling model.

3

The IFSP Process

Objectives

1. Present Part H requirements related to assessment and the IFSP process.

2. Discuss assessment procedures for infants and toddlers with disabilities and their families.

3. Describe the IFSP process.

*P*art H of IDEA (Individuals with Disabilities Education Act [IDEA], 1991) states that every eligible infant and toddler and their families shall receive

1. a multidisciplinary assessment of the unique strengths and needs of the infant or toddler and the identification of services appropriate to meet such needs;
2. a family directed assessment of the resources, priorities, and concerns of the family and the identification of the supports and services necessary to enhance the family's capacity to meet the developmental needs of their infant or toddler with a disability; and
3. a written individualized family service plan developed by a multidisciplinary team, including the parent or guardian. (p. 51, Sec. 677.1)

The Individual Family Service Plan (IFSP) is to include a statement of eligibility based on results of assessment of the infant's or toddler's present levels of physical development, cognitive development, communication development, social and emotional development, and adaptive development, and a statement of the family's resources, priorities, and concerns related to enhancing their child's development.

The requirements of best practices in assessment are even more stringent than the legislative mandates. Bailey (1987) argues that best practice requires the assessment process to generate these data:

1. A statement of the child's strengths and needs;
2. Information concerning the child's functional abilities (*not* test scores);
3. Description of specific abilities in all relevant developmental domains;
4. Information about the child's learning and behavioral characteristics (that is, behavioral state organization, behavioral cues, behavioral characteristics, temperament); and
5. Precise description of impairments or other limitations (for example, sensory impairment, motor impairment, chronic health problems) that are relevant to intervention planning.

As discussed later in the chapter, the selection of assessment procedures and how assessment results are interpreted and used will depend on whether information is being collected for diagnosis or eligibility determination or for development of an intervention plan.

The first part of this chapter provides an overview of the infant/toddler assessment process. Then we review the Part H mandates related to development of the IFSP and the steps in the IFSP process.

 ## Assessment Procedures

This section begins with an overview of basic assessment concepts and general assessment procedures. Then it provides an introduction to child assessment with a focus on behaviors that need to be considered in the child assessment process and approaches for collecting the necessary information.

We avoid using the term *family assessment* because it has the connotation of making a judgment. While early interventionists are comfortable with making judgments about the intervention needs of children, most are not comfortable with the idea of assessing families. Moreover, Slentz and Bricker (1992) point out that early interventionists have neither the skills nor adequate tools to assess families. Part H requires consideration of family concerns, priorities and resources: It does not require the use of formal assessment instruments such as surveys, indices, scales, and questionnaires.

Assessment directed *by* the family, not assessment *of* the family, is a more accurate description of the family's role in the assessment associated with the IFSP process. Assessment continues throughout intervention, guided and shaped by family priorities, information needs, and child characteristics, so there is no reason why family outcomes cannot be included on the IFSP as needs and concerns arise.

Collecting Information

There are three basic methods for collecting assessment information: (a) tests, (b) observations, and (c) interviews. They are differentiated by the type of information that is collected as well as by **how** data are collected.

imp!

A. **Tests.** Tests are controlled and structured procedures that attempt to elicit particular responses the child might not demonstrate spontaneously. The objective is to see how well the child performs on a particular set of standardized tasks (Bailey & Brochin, 1989).

There are three major categories of tests: norm-referenced, criterion-referenced, and curriculum-referenced. Norm-referenced tests may be standardized or nonstandardized. The instructions that accompany standardized tests specify most aspects of the assessment context, including the materials, the stimuli to be used to elicit child behaviors, and recording and score interpretation procedures. The Bayley Scales of Infant Development (Bayley, 1969) and the Battelle Developmental Inventory (Newborg, Stock, Wnek, Guidubaldi & Svinicki, 1984) are examples of standardized, norm-referenced tests.

The greatest advantages of standardized tests is the potential for comparing the child's performance with that of other children (the norm group). The greatest disadvantage of standardized tests is the possibility of results that do not accurately reflect the abilities of children with disabilities. For example, a child's responses to test items assessing cognitive ability may be seriously hampered by motor or sensory impairment.

Standardized norm-referenced tests are most often used to identify infants and young children with development delay. This is an appropriate use of these tests. However, the use of results from these tests to design interventions has serious problems. In the past decade there has been growing concern about this practice because standardized developmental tests are not designed to provide the type of information required to plan intervention goals and procedures. Certainly, standardized test results can contribute some information for formulating desired developmental outcomes, but total reliance on these tests as the only source of program planning data is not appropriate. Moreover, these tests do not provide a true picture of the skills and needs of children with sensory or motor impairments.

With any norm-referenced test (standardized or nonstandardized), the concern is how the child performs in comparison to a same-age reference group; the concern with criterion-referenced tests and curriculum-referenced tests is how the child performs relative to a predefined set of tasks or abilities. Criterion-referenced tests and curriculum-referenced tests are the most useful for planning intervention strategies.

Criterion-referenced tests provide information about the child's performance with respect to a set of skills judged important for functioning in different developmental domains or activities. The Uzgiris-Hunt Ordinal Scales of Psychological Development (Uzgiris & Hunt, 1975), an assessment of infant performance on Piaget's sensorimotor constructs, is an example of a criterion-referenced instrument. Rather than comparing the child's skills and weaknesses to those of other children, the child's performance on the test items is judged relative to the requirements of the particular items.

Curriculum-referenced tests are similar to criterion-referenced tests in that the child's skills and abilities are not compared to those of other children. Assessment with a curriculum-referenced test provides information about the child's status relative to a prespecified curriculum sequence. Examples of multidimensional criterion-referenced and curriculum-referenced procedures include:

- ◆ Early Learning Accomplishment Profile (Glover, Preminger & Sanford, 1978);
- ◆ Portage Guide to Early Education (Bluma, Shearer, Frohman & Hilliard, 1976);
- ◆ Carolina Curriculum for Handicapped Infants and Infants at Risk (Johnson-Martin, Jens & Attermeier, 1986);
- ◆ Hawaii Early Learning Profile and Activities (Furuno et al., 1979);
- ◆ Minnesota Infant Development Inventory (Ireton & Thwing, 1980).

In summary, the major difference among the three types of tests—norm-referenced, criterion-referenced, and curriculum-referenced—is the reference against which the results are judged. Norm-referenced tests compare a child's performance with that of children in a norm group; criterion-referenced tests compare a child's performance against a predetermined list of desired skills; curriculum-referenced tests assess a child's achievements relative to a given curriculum.

Observations. Observations provide a different type of information than tests do. They provide information about the way a child uses (or fails to use) relevant skills in natural contexts. Systematic observation is most valuable when there is a need for sensitive documentation of spontaneous behavior. In contrast to tests, which treat early skills as if they can be divided neatly into developmental domains such as social skills, motor skills, communication skills, and cognitive skills, observation looks at the whole child and how well the child uses his or her skills to meet expectations of the environment.

Observations may be recorded in natural environments or structured settings. In the most naturalistic observation setting a child might be observed playing with neighbor children and siblings in his own yard. The observation system might be as simple as a narrative description of who is playing, what games are played, and whether play is age appropriate. Or a child might be observed playing with a peer in a playroom especially designed for observations of play behavior. The observation system used in the more structured playroom setting could be more sophisticated, with codes for scoring a wide range of language and communication skills and social and object play behaviors. Videotaping would be a possibility for either setting to allow observations to be scored at a later time. Figure 3-1 shows an example of a checklist that could be used when observing dressing skills.

Interviews.   Interviews are the third important source of assessment information. Interviews can generate data concerning family perceptions of children's abilities, significant events in children's lives (such as transitions and medical procedures), and priorities and preferences for services. Whether the child's significant others are interviewed directly or asked to complete a checklist or rating scale, this procedure provides valuable data concerning the child's behavior in natural settings and caregiver expectations. Figure 3-2 shows an example of such a checklist.

Interviews have an advantage beyond generating information: They provide an opportunity for professionals and caregivers to get to know one another. A positive and sensitive interview sets the tone for a positive and sensitive parent-professional working relationship. Truly skillful interviewing goes beyond asking a predetermined set of questions to obtain child data and developmental information. The skilled interviewer is more than a good listener; he or she is able to communicate to caregivers that what they have to say and what they want for their child is of utmost value and importance. The skilled interviewer fosters development of the type of relationship that will ultimately lead to a productive parent-professional partnership.

There are a number of ways to go about assembling information from the family. The most popular approach is an informal meeting in which caregivers and other family members are asked to describe (a) what a typical day is like with the child, (b) what the child does well and likes to do, (c) what the child needs help with or tends to avoid, (d) recent progress or changes in the child's behavior at home, and (e) the child's interests. Table 3-1 suggests topics for a parent interview.

In summary, interviews may be structured by a list of questions or topics that are set forth on an interview form or they may be open-ended and informal. Responses may be oral or written, depending on which is more comfortable for the family. In either case, data from interviews and checklists are best used in conjunction with other assessment procedures.

	Needs physical assistance	Needs verbal prompts	Performs independently	Does child have the necessary prerequisites?	Comments
Child's name: _____ DOB: _____ Observer: _____ Date: _____					
Garments					
Cooperates with undressing (pulls arms and legs out of garment):					
Anticipates next step in dressing routine:					
Cooperates with dressing (holds out arms or puts feet into pants leg):					
Anticipates next step in dressing routine:					
Removes coat or other loose-fitting front-opening garments:					
Removes loose-fitting pants:					
Removes pull-down garments (if unfastened):					
Removes pull-over garments (if no fasteners):					
Puts on coat or other loose-fitting, front-opening garments:					
Puts on fitted coat or other front-opening garments:					
Puts on pull-up garments:					
Pulls on pull-over garments:					
Shoes and Socks					
Cooperates with putting socks/shoes on (lifts foot):					
Removes socks (when shoes have been removed):					
Removes shoes (if no laces or laces have been undone):					
Removes shoes (if no laces or laces have been undone):					
Puts socks on:					
Puts shoes on:					
Fasteners					
Unzips large zipper:					
Zips large zipper:					
Unfastens buttons and/or snaps:					
Fastens buttons and/or snaps:					
Unties bow-knots in shoes:					

Figure 3-1　Dressing observation checklist

Child's name: _____ Age: _____ Today's date: _____

Na Lei Kamili'i
(The Special Young Children)

Note: This information sheet is worded from the child's perspective to help us think in terms of information that the children might want to share.

My favorite activities are:

My least favorite activities are:

My favorite toys are:

My least favorite toys are:

My favorite foods are:

My least favorite foods are:

Figure 3-2 Example of a parent/caregiver's checklist providing information about the child's behavior in natural settings (and other family information)

(continued)

I am allergic to:

My favorite playmates are:

My family know what I like or dislike because I:

I am most cooperative when:

I help in my dressing by:

I help in my toileting by:

I help in bathing myself by:

I help in feeding myself by:

I am frightened by:

Figure 3-2—(continued)

I can be helped by:

My family would like me to join in the following activities:

My family wants me to learn to:

These are the opportunities and support my family needs:

My family makes these arrangements for my care (respite):

When they go out they leave me with: _____

_____

When they go to work they leave me with: _____

_____

My family is satisfied with these care arrangements: Yes ☐   No ☐

Explain: _____

_____

Figure 3-2—(continued)

(continued)

When I make 3, I think I would like to:

Stay home with my family ☐   Go to a babysitter ☐

Go to preschool ☐   Go to daycare ☐

These are the medications I need:

My special diet is:

I'm a really special Keiki. Here are some neat things about me that you might like to know:

University of Hawaii at Manoa
Interdisciplinary Infant Specialization: Personnel Preparation
University Affiliated Program • Special Education
1776 University Avenue • Wist 211 • Honolulu, Hawaii 96822

Developed by IIS Program Participants: Summer 1991

Figure 3-2—(continued)

TABLE 3-1
Possible Topics for Initial Interview(s)

Topics	Specifics
1. Get parents' perceptions regarding the assessment process	Ask parents: What do you see as the purpose of the assessment process? Do you feel that assessment information (collected to this time) is accurate?
2. Summarize the available information	Summarize whatever reports have been received, including date, place, evaluator/author, and results. Ask parents: What are your views on this information? What do you see as the implications of the information?
3. Review concerns	Ask parents for history of concern: When did you first suspect there might be a problem? Why? Have these problems changed? What have you tried to do to help alleviate the problem(s)?
4. Ask for pertinent family information or health history	Ask parents: Is there any family information you think might be relevant to the child's problems (e.g., moves, death in the family)? Is there any information about the physical health of siblings or other medical information you think would be relevant? (This discussion may need to be deferred until a later time, depending on the comfort level of the parents.)
5. Talk about the health of the child	Ask about growth, illnesses and treatment, operations, accidents, immunizations, etc.
6. Ask about feeding and oral behavior	In some cases all that is necessary is information about the child's appetite and food preferences and whether the child is within the norms for weight and height. In other cases, details as to possible feeding problems may be explored. Oral behavior not related to feeding that may be discussed includes thumbsucking, use of a pacifier, mouthing toys or other objects, biting, and ingestion of inedible substances.
7. Ask about independent toileting	Ask parents about the child's status and their expectations concerning this skill.
8. Ask about sleep	Ask about sleep-wake patterns, naps, and how much sleep the child gets in a 24-hour period.
9. Ask about social adaptation	Ask about the child's self-care skills, compliance with family routines and expectations, ability to follow simple directions, and participation in family outings and with visitors.

(continued)

TABLE 3-1—*(continued)*

Topics	Specifics
10. Ask about coping skills	Ask what the child does when uncomfortable, frustrated, or otherwise distressed.
11. Ask about language and communication behaviors	Ask how the child succeeds in securing desired objects and activities and what behaviors are used to indicate rejection of objects and activities. Ask what sounds or words the child is producing and what the child seems to understand.
12. Ask about preferred toys and play	Ask what kinds of toys and play materials the child likes and how the child plays with favorite toys/materials.
13. Ask about experiences outside the home	If the child is presently in a nursery setting or a day-care program, ask about experiences and friends there and how well the child meets the expectations of the setting. Ask the parents if they would like the child to be observed in that setting.
14. Ask about feelings, fears, and moods	Ask the parents to describe the variety and range of feelings the child expresses and how each is expressed (e.g., comfort, discomfort, pleasure, joy, anger, affection, hostility, sadness).
15. Wrap-up	Ask if there is other information that would help to formulate an accurate picture of the child. Provide parents with current positive impressions based on the information available at this time. Invite parents/caregivers to let you know if they have further thoughts on any of the topics discussed today or anything that should be discussed.

SOURCE: Based on Meisels, S.J. & Provence, S. (1989). *Screening and assessment: Guidelines for identifying young disabled and developmentally vulnerable children and their families.* National Center for Clinical Infant Programs, Washington, D.C.

Assessment Contexts

Beginning in the eighties, the trend has been away from professionals administering tests individually in clinical settings (a testing room or a private office) to assessment in more naturalistic assessment contexts such as the home or playroom. The defining characteristics of this more relaxed and informal approach to assessment, often referred to as *arena assessment,* are (a) communication among multidisciplinary team members as they collect data in their particular specialty domains, and (b) inclusion of both the child, the parents or caregivers, and other family members as active participants in the process (Wolery & Dyk, 1984).

A critical difference between traditional assessment and arena assessment is that in arena assessment all team members assess the child simultaneously. Team members sit in a circle on the floor or on low stools. One team member is designated as facilitator to interact with the child and elicit the child behaviors that will provide the other team members with the information they need to complete their respective assessment protocol and generate valid information about the child's skills and needs. The number of team members involved depends on the child's needs and resource constraints. There may be as few as two professionals and one or two caregivers or as many as six professionals and several generations of family members.

Arena assessment is a response to dissatisfaction with individual assessment procedures, which often yield fragmented and redundant information from different team members. The practice of assessing each developmental domain (sensorimotor, language/communication, physical, and so on) separately, as if it were truly a differentiated entity, does not provide a picture of the whole child. Another advantage of arena assessment is that it eliminates unnecessary handling where an infant is involved.

The team member with the most expertise in the infant's area of need (often the service coordinator) may act as the facilitator and primary assessor (or a family member may take this role). Other team members (including family members) sit in a circle, sharing and recording their observations. There is active exchange of information among all those present throughout the process. In the course of the assessment process, team members may ask the facilitator to attempt to elicit specific behaviors that will help them formulate an opinion about the child's skills and abilities. On occasion, team members (including family members) other than the facilitator may move to the center of the circle and administer particular items. Caregivers play a key role, providing information and refuting or confirming the representativeness of the child's responses.

Not only are arena assessment procedures different, but the products of the process are also notably different (Foley, 1990). Because professionals implement their discipline-specific assessment with minimal interaction and exchange of information, traditional multidisciplinary assessment typically yields an assortment of separate reports that are ultimately summarized in a final evaluation report. In contrast, arena assessment by a transdisciplinary team yields (a) a comprehensive report describing the functioning of the whole child in natural environments (in addition to discipline-specific information); and (b) an integrated intervention plan.

Transdisciplinary Play-Based Assessment (TPBA) by Linder (1991) is an example of an arena assessment approach. The TPBA is designed for children between the ages of 6 months and 6 years. It provides guidelines for planning and implementing observations in four domains (social/adaptive, cognitive, communication/language, sensorimotor). The guidelines are stated in the form of questions to encourage observation of the qualitative aspects of "how" the child performs—not just "if" the child performs—the task.

One professional, designated as the "play facilitator," guides the assessment process through six phases (described next). Another team member is designated as a "parent facilitator" to explain and discuss the ongoing play session with the caregivers. Before, during, and after the assessment, the caregiver(s) are encouraged to share information about the child's performance of skills in natural environments.

> **Phase 1: Unstructured play:** the play facilitator imitates, models, and expands the child's play;
>
> **Phase 2: Structured play:** the play facilitator helps the child incorporate aspects of play not initiated spontaneously in Phase 1;
>
> **Phase 3: Peer interaction:** a peer is introduced to permit observation of child-child interactions;
>
> **Phase 4: Caregiver-child interactions:** observation of caregivers-child play, separation, and reunion with the caregivers;
>
> **Phase 5: Motor play:** observation of structured and unstructured motor play;
>
> **Phase 6: Snack:** observation of oral motor performance and other developmental skills.

Linder (1991) strongly recommends videotaping the play session. In addition to providing confirmation data for postsession analysis, a videotape provides a record that can later be used by staff and caregivers to document the child's progress.

Problems with scheduling are possibly the greatest obstacle associated with the arena approach to assessment. Assembling all team members (including the family) for an assessment planning meeting, one or more assessment sessions, and a summary meeting can be difficult. However, the information this type of assessment process provides makes it well worth the effort.

Types of Information

The basic purpose of any assessment procedure is to collect information. What information is collected depends on the questions that are asked. Diagnosis and eligibility determination require different types of information than is required for planning intervention goals and outcomes. The questions are different in each case. The next section will highlight the questions asked and answered (a) when determining diagnosis and eligibility, and (b) when planning intervention goals and outcomes.

1. **Diagnosis and Eligibility.** Diagnostic assessment rarely provides either the quantity or the type of data needed for planning intervention. For example, a diagnosis of cerebral palsy or Down syndrome tells nothing about the child's abilities or intervention needs, because children with a particular etiological label differ from one another as much as children classified as "normal." The questions asked when assessment is for the purpose of *diagnosis* are: (a) Is there a delay or disability? (b) What is the nature of the child's problem(s)? and (c) What is the cause or causes of the delay or disability? Diagnostic information provides valuable data concerning specific health and medical conditions that may be contributing to the child's developmental problems or functioning, or to physical and sensory impairments.

The question being asked in *eligibility determination* is "Is this child entitled to services?" What procedures are used to answer this question depends on the specific eligibility definition. How eligibility for services is defined varies from one state to another. Recall that Part H makes reference to two groups of infants and toddlers who are eligible for early intervention services: (a) developmentally delayed, and (b) established conditions that typically result in developmental delays (such as infantile autism, Down syndrome, cerebral palsy, sensory impairments, or chronic illness). It is left to the discretion of individual states whether services will be provided for children at risk of becoming delayed or handicapped.

The law does not define developmental delay. The definition is left up to policymakers in each state or territory. One method for determining degree of delay is to establish a cutoff point. The cutoff point may be based on (a) percentage deviation of chronological age from developmental age, and/or (b) deviations in standard deviation units on standardized measures (Sheehan, 1989).

The first approach, using a percentage deviation of chronological age from developmental age, is fraught with difficulties. The major difficulty is that this approach requires a valid and reliable developmental age score. This requirement depends on the availability of instruments designed to yield developmental age scores or accurate percentage delay scores for children with disabilities. There are few measures capable of fulfilling this requirement. (See Bailey and Brochin [1989] for in-depth discussion of this issue.)

The second strategy relies on comparison of the child's standard score to the reported standard deviation of the test to determine divergence from normal performance. For example, an infant obtaining a score of 68 on the Bayley Scales of Infant Development (Bayley, 1969), which has a standard mean of 100 and a standard deviation of 16, would be rated as 2 standard deviations below the mean ($100 - 68 = 32$; $32/16 = 2$). This method also has problems in that it relies on norm-referenced tests. Reliance on traditional norm-referenced tests is problematic for two reasons: (a) there is a shortage of reliable and valid instruments for infants, particularly those who are at risk, developmentally delayed, or disabled; and (b) many delays are difficult to detect with traditional assessment instruments (Simeonsson & Bailey, 1989).

Harbin, Gallagher, and Terry (1991) suggest some ways to overcome the problems inherent in defining developmentally delayed. One approach is for state policy to provide for more than one way to establish eligibility for developmental delay. (Recall that definition of developmental delay is one of the 14 components that each state is required to include in its plan.) Because some types of delays and disabilities are difficult to detect and document using only standardized tests, state policy should allow for qualified professionals to use other documentation in addition to standardized tests to establish atypical development. The second recommendation is to require assessors to use whatever score the assessment instrument provides (or the instrument's procedures and tables for converting scores), rather than developing their own formulas or procedures for converting scores.

As noted, each state and territory decides whether infants and toddlers who are at risk of developmental delay are to be included in the definition of the eligible population. If at-risk children *are* included, "at risk" must also be defined. Determining eligibility for at-risk infants and toddlers is even more complicated than determining eligibility with a developmental delay definition. Harbin and colleagues (1991) analyzed at-risk criteria suggested by 27 states. They found (a) wide variability across states (a total of 69 different criteria across the 27 states); and (b) vague definitions that permitted any number of different interpretations.

Based on these findings, Harbin (1991) and the others recommend considering multiple risk factors when defining at-risk eligibility criteria. This is because risk factors multiply and their combined effect is greater than the sum of any group of factors. Since the literature is not definitive regarding the exact number of risk factors that should be used, states choosing to serve at-risk children should probably require at least three risk factors. These three risk factors may be all biological, all environmental, or a combination of the two. Examples of combinations of risk criteria include (a) birth weight less than 1500 grams, intraventricular hemorrhage, and ventilator assistance; or (b) documented parental substance abuse, maternal age less than 16, and low income.

Intervention Planning.   Assessment to identify specific intervention outcomes and procedures asks these questions: What are the child's skills relative to developmental and environmental expectations? Specifically, what are the child's strengths and specific abilities in the areas of cognitive development, physical development, communication development, social/emotional development, and adaptive development? (Adaptive development concerns center around the child's ability to participate in activities in natural environments.) Additionally, assessment should determine (a) how the child seems to learn best (to assist selection of materials and strategies that will maximize motivation and skill acquisition); (b) behavioral characteristics that will affect learning; and (c) sensory or motor impairments relevant to achievement and performance.

Assessment may use any combination of the procedures described earlier in the chapter: tests, observations, and interviews. The procedures may be unidimensional (focusing on a single domain), or they may be multidimensional (assessing behaviors in several domains).

Unidimensional procedures assess behavior in only one domain: cognitive development, physical development, language and communication development, social/emotional development, or adaptive development. We will provide a brief overview of the focus of assessment procedures in each of these areas.

Cognitive development subsumes development of basic sensorimotor skills (object permanence, causality, means-end behavior, spatial relationships, schemes for relating to objects, and imitation) and later symbolic structures (mental representation). Simply stated, *cognition* is the process through which knowledge is acquired and stored.

Basic sensory and motor behaviors become increasingly better integrated and refined during the period from birth to approximately 24 months. Problem solving during this period is not an internal activity, rather, it is what might be termed "motor thinking." It involves the external processes of perception and movement patterns. To get some sense of what this level of problem solving is like, try to describe the steps in tying a shoelace. You are exceptional if you are able to describe the steps without having to find a shoelace and actually go through the motions of tying. Most people have trouble visualizing the steps in the task. They find it necessary to problem solve by actually performing the behavior. This is an example of problem solving at a sensorimotor level rather than a mental level.

One reason that assessment of sensorimotor achievements is so important is that sensorimotor development is implicated in development of skills in other domains. Delay in sensorimotor achievement will affect developmental progress in language/communication, social development, and adaptive skills. The interrelatedness of skills in cognitive, social, and language/communication areas contributes to the importance of functional, developmentally appropriate cognitive goals.

The majority of instruments that assess sensorimotor development are based on a Piagetian framework. They generate information about the general level of development (at which of the six stages of sensorimotor development the infant is functioning) and progress in each of the six sensorimotor skill areas: (a) object permanence, (b) causality, (c) means-end behavior, (d) spatial relationships, (e) schemes for relating to objects, and (f) imitation.

The Ordinal Scales of Psychological Development (Uzgiris & Hunt, 1975), commonly referred to as the Uzgiris-Hunt Scales, is the most commonly used Piagetian assessment tool. This instrument assesses seven areas: means-ends relationships, visual pursuit and object permanence, causality, gestural imitation, vocal imitation, the construction of objects in space, and behaviors relating to objects. Dunst (1980) has provided a very helpful guide for using the Uzgiris-Hunt Scales.

Another commonly used instrument, currently being restandardized, is the Bayley Scales of Infant Development (BSID) (Bayley, 1969). The Bayley Scale of Mental Development (BSMD), one of the three scales of this instrument, provides an example of a traditional approach to assessment of cognitive development. While the BSMD is the most widely used standardized test of cognitive ability for infants and toddlers, it has some shortcomings. There is not a logical sequencing of items because it does not have an underlying theory of cognitive development (Garwood, 1982). Moreover, the BSID is not appropriate for children with severe cognitive, sensory, and communication impairments, as there are no provisions for adapting the items.

Physical development refers to the acquisition of postural control and the necessary movement patterns to produce functional motor acts. Unless there is a neuromotor disability (that is, central nervous system damage or dysfunction), achievement of motor milestones generally proceeds in a predictable sequence. What varies is the rate of acquisition of motor milestones—which is influenced by such variables as sex, stimulation, motivation, and genetic inheritance.

Physical and occupational therapists have major responsibility for assessing physical development skills when a child has an identified motor impairment. However, teachers and other team members (including parents) should observe and participate in the assessment process. This requires a basic knowledge of (a) the terminology of physical and occupational therapy and (b) the rationale for different elements of the process (Bailey & Wolery, 1989). Teachers and parents or caregivers should be able to:

1. Identify children in need of motor assessment,
2. Participate in planning physical intervention programs,
3. Integrate physical skill development in activities across curricular domains,
4. Document child progress and monitor the effectiveness of intervention strategies, and
5. Communicate effectively with occupational and physical therapists concerning specific physical impairments.

Motor assessment of infants and toddlers has four broad objectives: (a) observing and testing head control in varying body positions (supine, prone, and sitting), (b) determining how different body positions affect functional motor control, (c) describing the status of primitive reflexes and higher level automatic reactions, and (d) assessment of specific motor milestones (for example, rolling, sitting, standing, and walking) (Copeland and Kimmel, 1989). Ideally, both gross motor (large movements such as rolling and sitting) and fine motor (movements involving the hands, such as pointing and grasping) skills are evaluated in the natural environment within the context of functional activities such as eating, dressing, and play.

The first assessment concern, head control in varying body positions, can be assessed by observing the child's participation in functional activities. Because functional activities, such as play and eating, provide naturally motivating objects and events, there is an increased likelihood that the child will demonstrate optimal skill levels. Observing head control during functional activities also provides an opportunity to determine how adequate the child's skills are for the task at hand. For example, some children who cannot maintain head control for long periods of time in other circumstances, can demonstrate adequate head control to receive a spoonful of food or to make eye contact for a favorite play activity (like peek-a-boo). Head control should be assessed in prone, supine, side-lying (horizontal positions), and sitting and standing (antigravity positions). The following are guidelines for observing head control in horizontal and antigravity positions. (Keep in mind that normally developing children typically attain fairly good head control by 3 to 4 months of age.)

1. *Prone.* If the child does not prop on her forearms or extended arms, assess head control with her lying on her stomach and over a roll or wedge. Observe:
   - Does she turn her head to one side if her face is on the supporting surface?
   - Does she raise her head when lying on her stomach?
   - Does she prop on her forearms? Does she prop on extended arms?
   - What is the typical angle of her head relative to the floor?
   - Does she hyperextend her neck when raising or maintaining her head upright?
   - Does she rest her head between her shoulders, appearing almost to be shrugging her shoulders to help hold her head up?

- Does she maintain her head in midline to raise it, or does she turn it to one side when raising it?
- Does she maintain head control in a midline position?
- How long can she maintain her head upright?
- How well does she tolerate being in the prone position?
- How much effort does it take for her to raise her head?
- Does she raise her head while reaching for objects?

2. *Supine.* Observe:

- Does she maintain her head in midline while awake?
- Can she raise her head off the surface to look at an object or while reaching for an object?
- Can she turn her head from side to side and back to midline?
- When pulled to sit from supine, does her head drop back below her shoulders (head lag)?

3. *Side-lying.* Observe:

- Can she raise her head?
- Can she maintain her head in an upright position briefly?
- Does her head push back behind her shoulders (hyperextension of the neck), or can she maintain her head in alignment with her spine, or slightly forward?

4. *Sitting and standing.* The normal position of the head in upright postures is midline and slightly forward (chin tuck). Observe:

- Does she raise her head?
- What is the typical angle of her head relative to the floor?
- Does she hyperextend her neck when raising or maintaining her head upright?
- Does she rest her head between her shoulders, appearing to be shrugging her shoulders to help hold her head up?
- Does she maintain her head in midline to raise it, or does she turn it to one side when raising it?
- Does she maintain head control in the midline position?
- How long can she maintain her head upright?
- How much effort does it take for her to raise her head?
- Does she raise her head and maintain head control while reaching for objects?

The second assessment concern, determining how different body positions affect functional motor control, is evaluated by observing the child in horizontal positions (prone, supine, and side-lying) and antigravity positions (long-sitting, side-sitting, chair-sitting, kneeling, and standing) (Copeland & Kimmel, 1989). Copeland and Kimmel suggest asking these questions to assess functional control in each of the positions:

1. Is the head at midline and can the child visually focus on the desired target?
2. Is the trunk symmetrical and well-aligned with the rest of the body?

3. Are the lower extremities properly aligned? If seated, kneeling, or standing, are the lower extremities bearing weight equally?
4. Are the upper extremities properly aligned and in functional positions for weight bearing or manipulation of objects?
5. Does this position promote the development of tightness, contractures, deformity, or pressure sores? (p. 48)

The third major concern in assessing physical development is the status of primitive reflexes and higher-level automatic reactions. Primitive reflexes are the reflexes present in nondisabled newborns and infants, such as the suck, startle, and asymmetrical tonic neck reflexes. There is a "normal" time frame in which each reflex typically appears and then subsides as it is integrated into purposeful movement. Most are integrated by 4 to 6 months of age. Other reflexes, such as the startle and gag reflexes, persist through life. There are two concerns when describing the status of primitive reflexes: (a) whether they are appearing and being integrated within the expected time frame, and (b) whether they appear with the expected frequency, consistency, and strength. If reflexes are abnormal, their absence or presence will likely interfere with the progression of normal physical development.

The two higher automatic reactions are (a) *righting reactions* (postural reactions that seem to encourage upright antigravity and aligned postures), and (b) *equilibrium reactions* (balance). These reactions are essential for the development and functional use of physical skills. Several published assessments evaluate the status of primitive reflexes and higher automatic reactions (such as Barnes, Crutchfield & Heriza, 1978; Capute et al., 1978; Fiorentino, 1973; Kliewer, Bruce & Trembath, 1977).

The final major concern in assessing physical development is the status of specific developmental milestones. In addition to noting the presence or absence of specific skills, it is important to assess the qualitative aspects associated with their development. Two widely used standardized scales of gross and fine motor skills are the psychomotor scale of the BSID and the Peabody Developmental Motor Scales (Folio & Fewell, 1983). These two scales measure the acquisition of selected milestones. Qualitative aspects of the skills should be noted on the assessment forms.

Because the way a child is handled and positioned affects his or her posture and movement abilities, assessment of physical skills should be conducted prior to the assessment of skills in other domains. Assessment of oral motor functioning is particularly important because it is critical to eating, drinking, and development of speech. Among the myriad difficulties that interfere with normal eating and drinking patterns are problems with swallowing and breathing, choking, vomiting, and inability to maintain the head in an upright and midline position. Morris (1982) provides a detailed rating scale for assessing mealtime skills.

Language development and **communication development** are related but not identical achievements. *Language development* is acquisition of the symbolic code that the child's particular culture uses to express ideas and feelings. *Communication development* is acquisition of the skills to use that code in a socially accepted manner. While speech is the most common language/communication mode, there are a range of other options, such as pointing to pictures or symbols, gestures, and signs. Most important to recognize is that the development of language and communication skills can proceed regardless of whether the toddler is able to produce speech.

Language and communication skills are intimately related to and highly dependent on cognitive, social, and motor development. Among the social behaviors of concern for early communication are eye contact, touch, and attention-getting behaviors. Early cognitive attainments thought to contribute to language include object permanence, means-end behaviors, causality, and schemes for relating to objects. Development of oromuscular control is critical for speech production. Development of gross motor skills is equally important because the child who is not able to explore the environment may be delayed in constructing the meanings that give him or her something to talk *about.*

In the past decade, language and communication assessment, like assessment in other domains, has moved away from isolated and highly structured testing and therapy rooms to the natural environments where language and communication skills are actually used. As in other domains, it is critical to use a combination of direct testing (using both standardized and nonstandardized tests), observation, and interviews to get the best picture of the child's abilities.

There are a number of important decisions that need to be made when planning assessment of language and communication skills. One is the mode of communication. If the child is not producing speech or showing progress in babbling and production of early speech sounds, the behaviors (pointing, gesturing, switch activation) associated with use of alternative communication modes (for example, manual signing, a communication word board) should be elicited and assessed. Most important is to ensure that the child has a means with which to communicate, and not to penalize her because of an inability to produce speech or any other production problems caused by sensory and/or motor impairments.

Language/communication assessment with infants and very young children focuses on these questions (McCormick & Schiefelbusch, 1990):

> *How* does the child convey messages? For example, does the child use gestures, facial expressions, vocalization, words, or word combinations?
>
> *Where, when,* and *with whom* does the child communicate most often and most effectively? Are there some situations (or persons) where communication is more likely than others?
>
> *What* does the child communicate *about?* What are the child's interests and preferences?
>
> *Why* does the child communicate? What objects, activities, services does he request? How does he greet people? How does he indicate displeasure? Does the child know how to initiate interactions? Does he know how to take turns?

Finally, there also needs to be clarity as to whether assessment is considering comprehension or production or, as is often the case, both.

A language/communication sample is very often the best procedure for collecting the desired information about language and communication skills. A language/communication sample is an observation and record of a communicative exchange. It is most appropriate for toddlers who use some speech; the spontaneous language/communication sample may provide useful information about both language and communication abilities. Recording of a language sample is typically done when a familiar adult interacts with the child in a naturalistic context such as a playroom or at mealtime. Because the majority of infants and toddlers demonstrate their most sophisticated language and communication abilities with parents or caregivers in a familiar setting, the home is an ideal setting.

The goal is to get a representative sample of the child's language and communication behaviors on videotape, audiotape, or in written form. Videotaping has both advantages and disadvantages. Videotapes provide a great deal of information but taping can be intrusive and impractical (from the standpoint of requiring expensive equipment and a camera operator). Audiotapes with written notes about the context and the child's nonverbal behavior are a good choice if the child's verbal behavior is of the quantity that warrants such a record. In most cases, on-line recording (written narrative form) is a good option for infants and toddlers.

These are the specific considerations when arranging for a language/communication sample:

- Whether to take a broad look at the child's language/communication behavior or focus on a particular aspect of that behavior (for example, requesting);
- How long the session will last or how many child utterances are desired;
- What activities will be used (they should be age-appropriate and interesting);
- Where the sample will be collected;
- The communication partner; and
- Whether to try to elicit particular language behaviors (for example, ask open-ended questions) or simply record spontaneous productions.

Information generated by the language/communication sample may be supplemented with information from direct testing. Some scales that focus exclusively on language are:

- Environmental Prelanguage Battery (Horstmeier & MacDonald, 1978) with criterion norms for children between the ages of 1 and 2:6;
- Environmental Language Intervention Program (MacDonald, 1978) with criterion norms for children between the ages of 1 and 4:9;
- Receptive-Expressive Emergent Language Scale (Bzoch & League, 1971) for children functioning at 1 month to 3 years;
- Callier-Azusa Scale-H: Scales for the Assessment of Communicative Abilities (Stillman & Battle, 1985) is especially for infants who are deaf-blind and severely/profoundly handicapped.

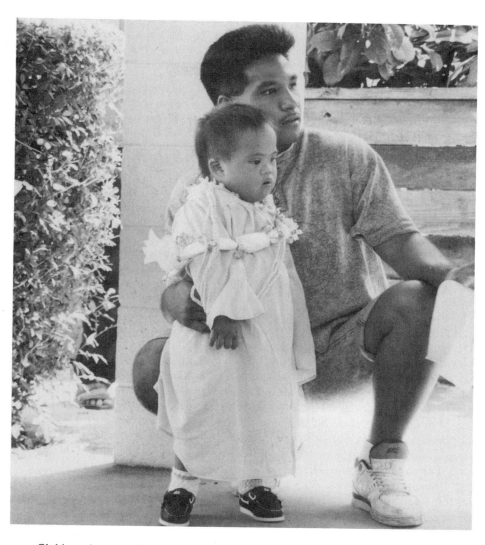

Children demonstrate attachment when they use a parent as a "secure base" for exploring the world.

Social and emotional development in infancy and early childhood hinges to a great extent on attachment. According to Ainsworth and Bell (1970), the quality of the infant's ability to use a parent attachment figure as a "secure base" to explore the world is the most sensitive index of the security of the infant's relationship with the caregiver. The attachment relationship forms very early, reaches a peak at 12–18 months, and subsequently develops and changes form in the preschool years. Thus, measures of parent-child interactions provide useful data for constructing a total picture of the child's social development. Unfortunately, there are very few valid and reliable interaction scales, and what few are available are difficult to locate (Farran, Clark & Ray, 1990).

There are no standardized tests that look specifically at the social interaction skills of very young children. Available nonstandardized procedures include (a) observation in natural settings, (b) interviews with parents or caregivers, (c) rating scales, and (d) multiple-domain criterion-referenced and norm-referenced tests. One very useful scale for systematic observation of social interaction behaviors is called the Systematic Anecdotal Assessment of Social Interaction (Odom, McConnell, Kohler & Strain, 1987). Appropriate for children of any age, this scale is part of Odom's (1988) social interaction curriculum.

Adaptive skill development is acquisition of the self-care skills (feeding, dressing, toileting) leading to independence. Self-care skills are complex skills comprised of many component skills. Their development is highly related to, and to varying degrees dependent on, development of motor, cognitive, language/communication, and social skills. For example, think about the skill of brushing one's teeth: it includes the fine motor skills of grasping and manipulation, gross motor skills of head control, trunk control in standing or sitting, and coordination, and the cognitive/communication skill of following directions.

Some instruments (such as the Brigance Diagnostic Inventory of Early Development and the Battelle Developmental Inventory) have items (or a separate section) assessing self-care behaviors. However, there are too few items in the various self-care areas to generate enough information for effective intervention planning for infants and toddlers, so direct observation and parent/caregiver interviews are important. One method to provide structure for observations is to locate or develop a checklist for the parent or caregiver to complete. Specific items on the checklist may derive from information about developmental milestones or task analysis. Figure 3-1 showed an example of a checklist based on normal development of dressing skills.

Development of a checklist from task analysis of the target skill is another option. Task analysis, the process of breaking a skill down into component subskills or steps, is discussed in Chapter 6. Task analysis of dressing would yield a list of the smaller units (or subskills or steps) leading to performance of the skill at whatever level the target child is functioning.

Another method of collecting information about adaptive skills is interviewing the parents or caregivers. Interviews can serve three functions: (a) generating information about child skills; (b) validating information collected through some other method, such as observation and testing; and (c) determining parents' values about the skills being assessed (Wolery & Smith, 1989). The last purpose is particularly important. Should it become apparent that the parents or caregivers do not place a great deal of value on the skill in question, they are not likely to be willing to expend much effort in teaching it.

In summary, this section has provided guidelines for assessment of infants and toddlers in the areas of cognitive development, physical development, language and communication development, social/emotional development, and adaptive skills development. The focus has been on assessment methods to generate information for planning intervention. Child behavioral states, temperament, and the environment are also important considerations when planning intervention.

Behavioral state assessment considers how alert, attentive, and active the infant is during a specified observation period. There are two reasons for assessing behavioral states. First, state influences performance: if an infant is drowsy, it is not the best time to assess cognitive development. The second reason for assessing behavioral state is that state organization is an indicator of dysfunction (Thoman, Denenberg, Sieval, Ziedner & Becker, 1981). Brazelton (1973) defines six states that can be distinguished through observations: deep (quiet) sleep, light (active) sleep, drowsy, quiet alert, active alert, and crying. These states can be assessed reliably with Brazelton's Neonatal Behavioral Assessment Scale (Brazelton, 1984).

Another scale that assesses states is the Carolina Record of Individual Behavior (CRIB) (Simeonsson, Huntington, Short & Ware, 1982). One component of the CRIB records the infant's predominant state as well as all the states observed during the proceding activity. The second component considers these eight behaviors: activity, reactivity, goal directedness, attention span, response to frustration, responsiveness to caregiver, tone of body, and responsiveness to examiner. The third part of the CRIB considers 23 specific behaviors (for example, exploratory patterns, communicative styles, and rhythmic habit patterns).

Temperament is behavioral style. Assessment of temperament is important for the same reasons that assessment of behavioral state is important. First, assessment of temperament is important because at least some of the differences in style that are apparent in infancy seem to be present in later personality. The second reason is that the infant's temperament characteristics may have an influence on the mutual adaptation of the infant and the family: different styles elicit different responses from caregivers (Sirignano & Lachman, 1985).

The most widely used categorization of temperament derives from the work of Chess and Thomas (1986). They identified three different constellations of temperament traits that seem to subsume all young children: the "easy" child, the "difficult" child, and the "slow-to-warm-up" child. Information about temperament characteristics can be obtained by interviewing caregivers or observing the infant or toddler. Temperament scales are another option. Among the most widely used standardized measures are the Infant Temperament Questionnaire (Carey & McDevitt, 1978) and the Toddler Temperament Scale (Fullard, McDevitt & Carey, 1978).

The *environment* where infants and toddlers spend the majority of time is the home environment. Failure to consider the home environment in the assessment process can mean loss of important information. Most basic when considering the home environment is sensitivity and respect for the family's values, their culture, and their right to privacy.

The most commonly used instrument to assess the home environment is the Home Observation and Measurement of the Environment (HOME) (Caldwell & Bradley, 1972). There are two versions of this scale: one rates homes of children ages 0 to 3, the other rates homes of children ages 3 to 6. The HOME is administered by a person who visits the home, observes the child's normal routine for about an hour, and interviews the caregiver or parent. The parent interview collects information about (a) trips out of the home and visitors to the home, (b) toys available to the child, (c) the daily routine, and (d) discipline.

This chapter provides an introduction to the important topic of assessment of infants and toddlers. There are a number of excellent books that deal exclusively with assessment. These include *Interdisciplinary Assessment of Infants* by Gibbs and Teti (1990), *Infant-Toddler Assessment* by Rossetti (1990), *Assessing Infants and Preschoolers with Handicaps* by Bailey and Wolery (1989), and *Assessing Young Children with Special Needs* by Susan M. Benner (1992).

 The IFSP Process

The purpose of the IFSP is to identify formal and informal resources and plan how they can be assembled to facilitate attainment of families' goals for their children and themselves. Recall from Chapter 1 that the law is very specific as to what the IFSP must contain. It must have:

1. A statement of the child's present levels of functioning in cognition development, communication development, social/emotional development, physical development, and adaptive development;
2. A statement of the family's resources, priorities, and concerns related to enhancing their child's development;
3. A statement of expected intervention outcomes (for infant or toddler and family), including criteria, procedures, and timelines;
4. A description of the specific early intervention services necessary to meet the unique needs of the child and family (see the following);
5. A statement of natural environments where early intervention services will be provided;
6. Projected dates for initiation of services and expected duration of services;
7. The name of the service coordinator who will carry out the responsibilities of the plan and coordinate with other agencies and persons; and
8. Procedures to ensure successful transition from infant services to a preschool program.

According to the legislation, early intervention services may include any one or all of the following:

◆ family training, counseling, and home visits;
◆ special instruction;
◆ speech pathology and audiology;
◆ occupational therapy;
◆ physical therapy;
◆ psychological services;
◆ service coordination services;

◆ medical services (for diagnostic or evaluation purposes);
◆ screening and assessment services;
◆ health services necessary to enable the infant or toddler to benefit from other; early intervention services;
◆ social work services;
◆ vision services;
◆ assistive technology devices and assistive technology services; and
◆ transportation costs.

The IFSP is not so much a document or a plan as it is an ongoing process (McGonigel, Kaufmann & Hurth, 1991). The form for the written IFSP is relatively unimportant. What is important is the process that is recorded and the interactions inherent in the process. The heart of the IFSP is the gathering, sharing, and exchange of information between families and early intervention professionals. The goal of the ongoing IFSP process is to enable families to make informed choices about what they want and need in the way of early intervention services for their children and themselves.

There is considerable variability in IFSP procedures across states. The individual needs and circumstances of each state, and various programs within each state, determine its policies and procedures. One place this is most evident is in the differences in IFSP forms. Figures 3-3 and 3-4 are examples of IFSP forms from different states. Figure 3-3 shows a form used in Hawaii. Figure 3-4 shows the form used by one program, the Western Carolina Center, in North Carolina. In both forms, it is common to have three to seven separate goals/outcomes pages.

There are some notable commonalities among states. Every state includes these key activities in the IFSP process:

1. Initial contacts;
2. Identification of assessment goals;
3. Child assessment;
4. Discussion of family concerns, priorities, and resources; and
5. Development of outcomes.

Two other activities that may be conceptualized as part of the IFSP process are development of the IFSP and formal and informal evaluation. Because these activities typically come under the rubric of service coordinator responsibilities, they were addressed in Chapter 2.

Initial Contacts

There are numerous possible sources of referrals to early intervention services. A family member may initiate the first contact, or it may be initiated by staff of the hospital neonatal intensive care unit (NICU), a local physician (or other primary care provider), a well-baby clinic (or other screening program), a social service or child protection program, or another early intervention program. From the standpoint of

Zero-to-Three Hawaii Project

Individual Family Support Plan

```
                                      ___ Interim
                                       X  Initial
                                      ___ Review
```

Child: Kalei Pumehana _____ DOB: 11/17/90 _____ Age: 14 mos. _____ Date: 1/21/92

Family: Anne Pumehana _____ Adjusted Age: _____

Address: 623 Kepahila Ave. _____ Phone: (H) 956-7890 _____ (W) 956-1670

Doctor: Bart Rogers _____ Phone: _____

Co-Care Coordinator: Kealoha Nakamura _____ Phone: 956-0066

INFORMATION ABOUT THE CHILD

Screening/(Evaluation) Tool: _____ Date: 1/7/92

Explanation/Notes: Comprehensive evaluation at Diamond Head Child Development Program. (Refer to attached reports of the transdisciplinary team's findings.) Kalei was tired and coming down with a cold so the family feels all results may not provide an accurate picture of Kalei's skills.

Hearing evaluation will be completed on 1/27/92 at Kapiolani Medical/Hearing Center. Neurological follow-up will be scheduled in the next few months with Dr. Higa. Other recommendations include referral to Feeding Clinic and therapy services (OT, PT, SLP) at the infant program.

My Child Kalei _____ has the following strengths, qualities & needs: [By parents]

Kalei knows my voice. He smiles and tries to reach out to me when I talk to him. He likes being in the living room with the family when we watch TV or talk story. He gets lots of attention in the family. He probably loves grandpa best. Kalei is very loving and he likes to be kissed and hugged. He likes music and the stories grandpa tells him.

Figure 3-3 Hawaii's Individual Family Support Plan (IFSP)

Zero-to-Three Hawaii Project

Child's Name: Kalei Pumehana

Family's Strengths and Concerns Related to Enhancing the Development of the Child (Optional):

Resources:

1. I live with my parents and they help me take care of the boys. They help me lots with Kalei's care.

2. My dad is great about playing and telling stories to the boys. Kalei loves it the most.

3. I'm having many for a car so I can take Kalei to his appointments. Now I catch the bus or Bruno Dad's or my brother's car.

4. Kalei's brothers (Sonny and Jimmy) help a lot. Sometimes I take them with me to Kalei's appointments and they help me get Kalei ready in the morning. They are really good kids and they really love Kalei.

5. My boss is great. He lets me off work to take Kalei to the doctor. I work only part time but he lets me have first choice each week when schedules are set.

Concerns and Priorities:

1. I feel bad that I have to rely on my parents so much to help with the boys.

2. My husband left me and he isn't helping with support for the boys, not even with Kalei's bills.

3. Kalei cannot even crawl. He can't hold a spoon and he chokes on food and even juice. He sometimes (often) wakes up at night and keeps everyone awake for hours. He is sick alot. His muscles are so stiff. I wonder if he will ever be able to do any of the things that other children do.

Figure 3-3—(continued)

(continued)

Individual Family Support Plan
Zero-to-Three Hawaii Project

Child's Name: Kalei Pumehana

I/We want:	Ways to get it:	Our resources and who can help:	Time it may take:
1 Kalei to eat like other children (with a spoon) and be able to eat with the family.	Get an appointment/help from the feeding clinic. See if the therapists will come to our house to show us what to do at mealtime.	Ellen will call the clinic and provide all background info (to save time). OT will coordinate a home visit.	1 week 1 week
2 To find out why Kalei isn't sleeping and what we can do.	Ask the doctor if he can think of any reason Kalei wakes up and won't go back to sleep. Check with VCP about his naps during the day. Ask therapists and feeding clinic staff for suggestions.	I can do this myself.	2 weeks
3 To find out why Kalei is sick so much and if there is anything I can do.	Ask the doctor and feeding clinic staff. Make a list of when he is sick, what kind of sickness, and what's happening at that time.	The nutritionist at the feeding clinic may be able to help. I will talk to the doctor.	2 weeks 3 weeks

Parent Signature ___Anne Pumehana___   Date _____

Figure 3-3—(continued)

Individual Family Support Plan
Zero-to-Three Hawaii Project

Child's Name: Kalei Pumehana

I/We want:	Ways to get it:	Our resources and who can help:	Time it may take:
4 To get Kalei's hearing checked because he always has ear infections and I want to know if Kalei will ever talk.	Make an appointment with the ENT who is next to the doctor's office so I can take him when I go to the doctor. Get the SLP to tell me about what to do to help Kalei learn to talk.	I can do this. SLP will schedule time to teach me what I need to do.	1 week 2 weeks
5 To know how my parents and Sonny and Jimmy can be informed and more involved with helping Kalei learn.	See if my parents want to come to the program with me. Ask the therapist and Allen and Keloha to give me suggestions on come to the house	Keloha will arrange a time when my parents can see what Kalei does at the program. Keloha will make arrangements for Sonny and Jimmy to come to Sibs Group.	2 weeks 1 week Ongoing
6 To have additional income so we can get our own face media my parents' and I don't have to depend on them.	Check with my boss regarding increasing my hours from 20 to 30 hours a week. Apply for respite services. Find out about job training so I can make more.	I will do this. Keloha will get the application. I will fill it out. Keloha will get me the information about job training.	2 weeks 1 week 2 weeks

Parent Signature _Anne Pumehana_　　Date _____

Figure 3-3—(continued)

Western Carolina Center
Family, Infant and Preschool Program
Individualized Family Support Plan

Background Information:

Child's Name: Tammy Natasha

Family's Name: Shook

No. OPD-0 2: 0000

Date of Birth: 8-19-88   Age: 12 mos

County: Cook

Family Member's Name:	Relationship to Child:
Sandy	Mom
Woody	Dad
Amy	Sister

Family Support Plan Team

Name	Title	Agency	Date
Sandy Shook	Parent		
Woody Shook	Parent		
Patricia Y. Bill, RN	Case coordinator	Family, Infant and Preschool Program	10-12-89
Jim Bush, MD	Pediatrician	Family, Infant and Preschool Program	10-12-89
Mary Lou O'Keefe	Physical therapist	Family, Infant and Preschool Program	10-12-89
Jean C. David	Speech-language therapist	Family, Infant and Preschool Program	10-12-89
Laurel Bernstein	Social worker	Family, Infant and Preschool Program	10-12-89
Donald Gilbert	Staff psychologist	Family, Infant and Preschool Program	10-12-89
Lynda Gram	Teacher	Family, Infant and Preschool Program	10-12-89
Marilyn Jakimivich	Family resource specialist	Family, Infant and Preschool Program	10-12-89

Team Review Dates

30 Days: 11-14-89   3 Months: 1-16-90   6 Months: 9 Months:

Figure 3-4 Western Carolina Center IFSP

SOURCE: The following IFSP forms are reprinted with permission of Dunst, C. J., & Deal, A. G., Family, Infant, & Preschool Program, Western Carolina Center, Morganton, N. C.

Child's Name: Tammy   OPD 0: 0000   Family's Name: Shook   FIPP Staff Member: P. Bell   IFSP# 1   Page# 1

Griffiths Scale of Mental Development

Domain	CA	Age Level/Range
Locomotor	12 mos	2.7 mos
Personal/Social	12 mos	2.3 mos
Hear/Speech	12 mos	4.6 mos

Child's Functioning Level

Domain	CA	Age Level/Range	Domain	CA	Age Level/Range
Eye/Hand	12 mos	2.3 mos	Gen. quot.		24.5
Performance	12 mos	2.7 mos	Mental age	12 mos	2.9 mos

Child's Strengths

— Vocalizes and makes sound imitations
— Sleeps through the night
— Enjoys being held
— More alert to surroundings

Family's Strengths

— Love one another
— Have good coping skills for dealing with stress
— Commitment to getting treatments for Tammy
— Take preventive measures with the children
— Advocate for children's needs

Formal Resources and Support Services	Dates Started	Dates Ended
Cook Co. DSS	8-88	
Cook Co. Mental Health	2-90	
Cook Co. Cluster	7-89	
FIPP Home-based serv.	6-89	
Social Security	7-89	
Cook Co. Health Dept.	8-88	
Private pediatricians	8-88	
Private PT	7-89	

Informal Resources and Support Services	Dates Started	Dates Ended
Maternal grandparents		
Pastor		
Contribution fund from church		
Friends Gail		
Tim		
Cousins Michele & Albert		

(continued)

Figure 3-4—(continued)

Child's Name: Tammy   OPD 0: 2-0000   Family's Name: Shook   FIPP Staff Member: P. Bell   IFSP# 1   Page# 1

Date	#	Need/Project Outcome Statement	Source of Support/Resource	Course of Action	Family's Evaluation Date	Rating
06-12-89	1	Parents will obtain information about FIPP in order to decide which resources are going to best meet their needs.	Parents—ability to process information and choose resources Case coord.—information on FIPP Social worker—information on FIPP	Case coord. & social worker will provide information about FIPP during home visit. Parents will review information, ask questions and decide if they wish to access FIPP resources. If FIPP resources are not chosen, other alternate resources will be explored.	07-12-89 08-08-89	4 7
06-22-89	2	Parents will obtain information on available financial resources in order to meet expenses related to Tammy's care.	Parents—abilities to gather information Case coord.—information Social security—information	Case coord. will share information about community financial resources during weekly home visit. Parents will contact social security and social services for eligibility information and gather family financial records.	07-12-89 08-07-89	3 6
07-12-89	3	Parents will obtain information on available physical therapists in order to obtain service for Tammy.	Parents—abilities to process information & schedule appointment with PT Case coord.—information PT—consultation	Case coord. will share names of PTs in the area during weekly home visit. Parents will contact PTs to ask about availability and schedule a consultation with PT of choice.	07-19-89 08-07-89 08-28-89	4 6 7
07-19-89	4	Woody will obtain counseling in order to learn ways to control his anger.	Woody—ability to schedule appointment and utilize counseling Family members—support & encouragement Case coord.—information & support DSS caseworker—information & support	DSS caseworker & case coord. will provide information to Woody on available counseling services during weekly home visit. Woody will make an appointment & attend counseling sessions. Family will give support & encouragement.	08-07-89 09-20-89 10-23-89 on hold	2 4 5

Family's Evaluations:

1 .... Situation changed, no longer a need
2 .... Situation unchanged; still a need, goal or project
3 .... Implementation begun; still a need, goal or project
4 .... Outcome partially attained or accomplished
5 .... Outcome accomplished or attained, but not to the family's satisfaction
6 .... Outcome mostly accomplished or attained to the family's satisfaction
7 .... Outcome completely accomplished or attained to the family's satisfaction

Figure 3-4—(continued)

Child's Name: Tammy   O.P.D.0.: 2-0000   Family's Name: Shook   FIPP Staff Member: P. Bell   IFSP#: 1   Page#: 2

Date / #	Need/Project Outcome Statement	Source of Support/ Resource	Course of Action	Family's Evaluation Date	Rating
08-01-89 / 5	Parents will participate in PT sessions in order to learn handling techniques for Tammy.	Parents—abilities to utilize PT suggestions & provide feedback on usefulness of techniques PT—evaluation of Tammy & information on handling techniques	Parents will schedule PT evaluation & share information about Tammy with PT. PT will evaluate Tammy's motor development & demonstrate handling techniques during weekly PT sessions held at local recreation department.	08-28-89 09-20-89 ongoing	4 7
08-21-89 / 6	Parents will identify their goals and priorities for Tammy in order to prepare for assessment and intervention planning day at FIPP.	Parents—ability to identify goals Case coord.—developmental screening of Tammy & provide information about assessment procedures	Case coord. will administer Griffiths during weekly home visit & discuss results with parents. Parents & case coord. will discuss family's goals & priorities for Tammy and decide on objectives for the assessment & IPD.	09-20-89 10-01-89 ongoing	3 7
09-20-89 / 7	Parents will use firm, deep pressure during physical contact with Tammy in order to increase her tolerance for touch.	Parents—abilities to use PT techniques PT—consultation on handling techniques Case coord.—support & feedback	Parents will schedule & participate in weekly PT sessions with Tammy. PT will demonstrate handling techniques. Case coord. will assist family in incorporating techniques into daily routines & give feedback on use of techniques.	09-27-89 10-05-89 ongoing	4 7
09-20-89 / 8	Parents will obtain as much information as possible about Tammy's medical history in order to have a better understanding of events that occurred during her hospitalization.	Parents—skill in generating questions Case coord.—medical information Family physician—information & consultation FIPP physician—consultation	Case coord. will obtain medical records and schedule meeting with FIPP physician. Parents will identify their questions and consult with physicians. Family physician & FIPP physician will interpret records & answer questions.	10-12-89 11-06-89 12-18-89	4 4 6

Family's Evaluations:
1 ...... Situation changed, no longer a need
2 ...... Situation unchanged, still a need, goal or project
3 ...... Implementation begun; still a need, goal or project
4 ...... Outcome partially attained or accomplished
5 ...... Outcome accomplished or attained, but not to the family's satisfaction
6 ...... Outcome mostly accomplished or attained to the family's satisfaction
7 ...... Outcome completely accomplished or attained to the family's satisfaction

Figure 3-4—(continued)

(continued)

Child's Name: Tammy   O.P.D.0: 2-0000   Family's Name: Shook   FIPP Staff Member: P. Bell   IFSP# 1   Page# 3

Date / #	Need/Project Outcome Statement	Source of Support/Resource	Course of Action	Family's Evaluation Date	Rating
09-20-89 / 9	Tammy will consistently hold her head up in order to work toward sitting independently.	Parents–abilities to use techniques to promote head control PT–consultation on techniques to promote head control Case coord.—support & information	Parents will attend PT consultation weekly and use suggested techniques with Tammy. PT will evaluate Tammy's motor abilities and suggest techniques for promoting head control. Case coord. will provide support to family in using techniques during weekly home visits.	10-12-89 11-06-89 12-11-89 See goal #18	3 4 4
10-12-89 / 10	Parents will take Tammy for an eye examination in order to determine her visual abilities.	Parents–abilities to schedule exam & understand results Private physician–information Eye doctor—evaluation & information Case coord.—support & information	Parents will obtain names of eye doctors from private physician and schedule eye evaluation. Parents will take Tammy for eye exam & consult with doctor. Case coord. will provide support & information related to eye evaluation during weekly home visits.	10-12-89 11-06-89	3 6
10-12-89 / 11	Tammy will use her hands to bring toys to her mouth in order to explore and become aware of her surroundings.	Case coord.—information Parents–abilities to use suggested techniques to promote hand use	Case coord. will demonstrate techniques for promoting hand use during weekly home visits. Parents will use techniques in daily routines with Tammy.	10-12-89 11-06-89 12-11-89 See goal #19	3 3 3
10-12-89 / 12	Tammy will tolerate being in water in order to make bathtime more relaxing.	Parents–skills in using suggested techniques for bathtime Case coord.—bathchair, information on use of chair & feedback on use of techniques	Case coord. will provide a bathchair on loan & demonstrate use during weekly home visits. Parents will use chair & other techniques such as keeping Tammy wrapped in towel until placed in the tub, gently placing her in warm water, having the bathroom warm, using gentle but firm motions & holding Tammy firmly.	11-13-89 12-11-89 01-22-90	4 4 7

Family's Evaluations:

1 ...... Situation changed, no longer a need
2 ...... Situation unchanged; still a need, goal or project
3 ...... Implementation begun; still a need, goal or project
4 ...... Outcome partially attained or accomplished
5 ...... Outcome accomplished or attained, but not to the family's satisfaction
6 ...... Outcome mostly accomplished or attained to the family's satisfaction
7 ...... Outcome completely accomplished or attained to the family's satisfaction

Figure 3-4—(continued)

Child's Name: Tammy   OPD.0: 2-0000   Family's Name: Shook   FIPP Staff Member: P. Bell   IFSP# 1   Page# 4

Date / #	Need/Project Outcome Statement	Source of Support/ Resource	Course of Action	Family's Evaluation Date	Rating
10-17-89 / 13	Parents will obtain information on respite options in order to make decisions on the best respite resources for their family.	Case coord.—information on formal respite programs—feedback & support Parents—ability to identify people they know for child care Grandmother—support & feedback	Case coord. will provide information on respite programs during weekly home visits. Parents will identify people they know (with Grandmother's help) who might provide respite. Parents will decide which options to pursue for respite.	10-30-89 11-06-89 12-11-89	3 6 7
10-17-89 / 14	Parents will gather information on preschool programs in their community in order to decide if attending preschool will further promote Tammy's development.	Case coord.—information on local preschools & feedback DSS—information on preschools Parents—ability to gather information & select services	Case coord. will provide information on available preschools & assist family in knowing what to look for in selecting a program, during weekly home visits. Will provide support to family as they consider programs. Parents will contact DSS for information on local programs and contact programs they choose to visit.	10-30-89 11-13-89 12-11-89 See goal #17	4 4 6
11-06-89 / 15	Parents will obtain a second neurological consultation in order to better understand the reasons for Tammy's delays.	Parents—ability to access community resources Physician—referral to neurologist Neurologist—evaluation of Tammy & interpretation of results Case coord.—emotional support & feedback	Parents will ask private physician for names of neurologists, schedule a neurological & ask their questions concerning Tammy's delays. Case coord. will assist the parents in listing their questions for the neurologist & provide emotional support during weekly home visits.	12-18-89 01-06-90 01-22-90	3 3 3
12-11-89 / 16	Woody will obtain information on local literacy programs in order to decide on enrolling in a program.	Woody—ability to get information & decide on enrolling Family—support & encouragement to Woody Case coord.—medical information Community college—information on enrollment	Case coord. will provide information on literacy programs during weekly home visits. Woody will contact community college for information. Other family members will provide encouragement to Woody in learning to read.	01-22-90 02-28-90 on hold	4 4

Family's Evaluations:
1 .... Situation changed, no longer a need
2 .... Situation unchanged, still a need, goal or project
3 .... Implementation begun; still a need, goal or project
4 .... Outcome partially attained or accomplished

5 .... Outcome accomplished or attained, but not to the family's satisfaction
6 .... Outcome mostly accomplished or attained to the family's satisfaction
7 .... Outcome completely accomplished or attained to the family's satisfaction

Figure 3-4—(continued)

(continued)

Child's Name: Tammy	OPD.0: 2-0000	Family's Name: Shook	FIPP Staff Member: P. Bell	IFSP# 1	Page# 5

Date	#	Need/Project Outcome Statement	Source of Support/ Resource	Course of Action	Family's Evaluation Date	Rating
12-11-89	17	Parents will complete application papers for Family Place in order for Tammy to be enrolled in the preschool program.	Parents—ability to complete application & provide information on their goals for Tammy Family Place staff—information on application process Case coord.—support & feedback for family	Parents will make appointment & meet with Family Place staff to complete application process & share their goals for Tammy. Case coord. will provide support to family in completing application process. Family Place staff will meet with Tammy's parents & keep them informed on enrollment process.	01-16-90 01-22-90 on hold	3 6
12-11-89	18	Tammy will consistently hold her head up for 30 seconds during playtime in order to develop skills for sitting independently.	Case coord.—support & information Parents—ability to use suggested techniques to promote head control PT—techniques for head control	Parents will take Tammy to weekly PT sessions & use suggested techniques with Tammy during playtimes. PT will demonstrate techniques during weekly sessions. Case coord. will provide feedback on use of techniques during weekly home visits.	01-22-90 02-28-90	3 4
12-11-89	19	Tammy will use her hands to bring her 6 oz. bottle with handles to her mouth in order to become more aware of hand use.	Case coord.—information Parents—ability to teach Tammy to hold her bottle	Case coord. will demonstrate ways to encourage Tammy to hold bottle during weekly home visits. Parents will talk to Tammy about what they are doing as they place the bottle in her hands and use prompts to encourage her to hold it.	01-22-90 02-28-90	3 6
12-11-89	20	Parents will explore financial resources in order for Amy to be able to attend Family Place.	Case coord.—information on resources DSS & Family Place—information on financial resources Parents—ability to access community resources	Case coord. will provide information on possible financial resources during weekly home visits. Parents will contact DSS & Family Place to inquire about other possible financial resources for funding daycare for Amy and pursue options they think are appropriate.	01-16-90 01-22-90 02-28-90	3 4 7

Family's Evaluations:

1 .... Situation changed, no longer a need
2 .... Situation unchanged, still a need, goal or project
3 .... Implementation begun; still a need, goal or project
4 .... Outcome partially attained or accomplished
5 .... Outcome accomplished or attained, but not to the family's satisfaction
6 .... Outcome mostly accomplished or attained to the family's satisfaction
7 .... Outcome completely accomplished or attained to the family's satisfaction

Figure 3-4—(continued)

Child's Name: Tammy   OPD 0: 2-0000   Family's Name: Shook   FIPP Staff Member: P. Bell   IFSP# 1   Page# 6

Date / #	Need/Project Outcome Statement	Source of Support/ Resource	Course of Action	Family's Evaluation Date	Rating
01-16-90 / 21	Parents will consult with physician in order to determine if Tammy may receive immunizations.	Case coord.—information on immunizations Parents—ability to access & share information with physician Physician—information & recommendations on immunizations	Case coord. will share information about importance of immunizations with parents during weekly home visits. Parents will consult with private physician about immunizations for Tammy & their plans to enroll her in daycare. If immunizations are not advised, parents will obtain statement from physician for Family Place.	01-22-90 02-28-90	3 3
01-22-90 / 22	Parents will gather information on housing options in Cook County in order to consider the possibilities of buying a house.	Case coord.—information & emotional support DSS, Housing Authority, & FHA—information on housing options Parents—ability to gather information & consider options	Case coord. will provide information on local housing agencies & provide emotional support during weekly home visits. Parents will contact local DSS, Housing Authority & FHA to gather information on options & provide information on their financial status.	02-28-90	4
01-22-90 / 23	Tammy will eat 2 or 3 mashed table foods in order to adjust to more texture in her food.	Case coord.—demonstration of ways to add texture to food & feeding techniques Parents & grandparents—abilities to teach Tammy to eat table foods	Case coord. will provide information on adding texture & suggestions on foods to try (bananas, cooked carrots, scrambled eggs, etc.) during weekly home visits. Parents & grandparents will give Tammy 1 or 2 bites of mashed foods as she will tolerate.	02-28-90	5
01-22-90 / 24	Parents will obtain a third neurological consultation in order to get another opinion on the reason for Tammy's delays.	Parents—abilities to access community health resources Case coord.—emotional support & feedback Neurologist—evaluation of Tammy & interpretation of results	Parents will select a neurologist from previously recommended list, make appointment & ask questions at neurological. Case coord. will assist family in reviewing their question list & provide emotional support during weekly home visits.	02-28-90	3

Family's Evaluations:

1 .... Situation changed, no longer a need
2 .... Situation unchanged, still a need, goal or project
3 .... Implementation begun; still a need, goal or project
4 .... Outcome partially attained or accomplished

5 .... Outcome accomplished or attained, but not to the family's satisfaction
6 .... Outcome mostly accomplished or attained to the family's satisfaction
7 .... Outcome completely accomplished or attained to the family's satisfaction

Figure 3-4—(continued)

(continued)

Child's Name: Tammy   OPD. 0   0000   Matrix # 1

IFSP Goal # / Date Started	Objectives	Mealtimes	Dressing & Diapering	Bathtime	Independent Playtime	Playtime with Others	Date Attained
#9 9-20-89	Tammy will consistently hold her head up in order to work toward independent sitting.	X	X	X			See #18
#11 10-12-89	Tammy will use her hands to bring toys to her mouth in order to explore and become more aware of her surroundings.				X	X	See #19
#12 10-12-89	Tammy will tolerate being in water in order to make bathtime more relaxing. (Use bathchair for support and put Tammy in the water slowly.)			X			1-22-90
#18 12-11-89	Tammy will consistently hold her head up for 30 seconds during playtime in order to work toward independent sitting.					X	2-28-90
#19 12-11-89	Tammy will use her hands to bring her 6 oz. bottle with handles to her mouth in order to become more aware of her hand use.	X					3-28-90
#23 1-22-90	Tammy will eat 2 or 3 mashed table foods in order to adjust to more texture in her food (start with one or 2 bites of the food).	X					2-28-90

Figure 3-4—(continued)

the early intervention program, the major goal of initial contacts is to learn about the family—specifically, their concerns and priorities related to their child's development. The key questions at this point in the process are: What does the family want in the way of early intervention services for their child? And how does the family want early intervention to become involved in family life (if at all)?

Some families who enter early intervention from other services are readily able to discuss their child's strengths and their own concerns, priorities, and resources related to their child's development. The topics suggested by Meisels and Provence (1989) provide an outline for an informal initial interview (or these topics could be used as the basis for a checklist that caregivers and professionals complete together). Table 3-1 was based on this list. These topics should not be viewed as a pre-conceived agenda. Rather, they are reminders of the type of information that is useful for planning intervention. Most important is to consider the concerns and priorities of the caregivers (and other family members) and make the interview a positive reciprocal interaction with sharing of information among all parties.

Figure 3-2 presented an example of a form to collect information during initial informal discussions with parents or caregivers. This particular form was developed by participants in the Hawaii Interdisciplinary Infant Specialization Training Program to be sensitive to the cultural differences in Hawaii. When it is used, this form is completed either by the parents or caregivers or the service coordinator during the course of initial information-sharing sessions. (The term in Hawaii for these information-sharing sessions is "talking story.")

In contrast to those families who are ready to discuss what they would like to get out of the program, there are other families who need time to familiarize themselves with the early intervention setting and personnel before they are ready to share concerns or discuss desired outcomes and expectations. This is more often the case when families were served in hospital units, where personnel did not see discussion of future intervention options as part of their role, or when parents have only recently learned that their infant or toddler needs early intervention services. Also, the family's cultural style, values, and structure affect how soon (if at all) they are ready to discuss their concerns, priorities, and desired outcomes. The existence of so many cultures, values, and alternative lifestyles in American society makes it imperative to allow each family to define itself. (The definition of family has been greatly expanded over the past several decades to include single parents with babies, gay and lesbian couples with children, and grandparents raising their children's children.)

The family focus of Part H has contributed to a heightened awareness among professionals of cultural differences in views concerning medicine and health care, childrearing practices, and disabilities (Hanson, Lynch & Wayman, 1990). Entering into interactions with a family whose language, customs, signs, and values are very different from your own requires early interventionists with great sensitivity, patience, and—above all—caring and respect. To be effective, early intervention-ists must take cultural differences into account and meet the special needs of the child in a manner that is culturally acceptable to the family. Whether a family's cultural identification is strong or weak, their cultural values will affect all aspects of their participation with the early intervention program. This is unavoidable. The cultural values will affect the family's willingness to seek help in the first place, their communication styles with professionals, the amount and type of participation, the goals/outcomes they select for their child, and the family members who will participate in intervention activities (Hanson et al., 1990). Similarly, professionals must recognize that their own cultural identities, beliefs, and values will affect their participation in the process. This too is unavoidable.

The way questions are asked during initial contacts is as important as the type of questions. There is no excuse for intimidating or embarrassing a family member. Questions should be very carefully screened: no questions should be asked that cannot be fully justified and explained. The family should be told the reason for each question and that they need not answer any questions that make them uncomfortable. It may not be clear to families why certain personal information (for example, pregnancy history) is being sought. Family members will also have questions of their own that they should be encouraged to ask during initial contacts.

Identification of Assessment Goals

If the family and staff decide that there is a need for services and the family indicates a desire to move into the next phase of the IFSP process, then planning for assessment activities begins. A temporary service coordinator may be appointed at this time (if one has not already been selected) to ensure that the planning moves along in a timely and sensitive manner. The IFSP team, composed of the family, the service coordinator, and other relevant program staff, continues the exchange of information begun during initial contacts. However, now there is a specific focus: to determine what child assessment measures and procedures will be needed and appropriate.

As discussed earlier in this chapter, the traditional approach to child assessment typically took the form of individual evaluations by professionals of relevant disciplines. When all assessments were finished there would be a meeting, called a *case conference,* to provide an opportunity for the evaluators to share their findings with one another and arrive at a synthesis. Finally, a condensation of the synthesis was shared with family members. This has all changed. Assessment is now family-guided and family-centered: It is responsive to the family's agenda. Ideally, the family decides (a) which professional disciplines will be involved on the assessment team (and even the particular individuals who will represent these disciplines); (b) what the family's role on the assessment team will be; (c) what kinds of assessment measures will be used; and (d) when and how assessment information will be synthesized and shared.

Part H requires that a child referred for services must receive a multidisciplinary assessment within 45 days. It further specifies that the assessment procedures must be conducted by a multidisciplinary team composed of persons with training in appropriate methods and procedures. The multidisciplinary assessment process has two objectives: (1) assessment of the unique strengths and needs of the infant or toddler and identification of services appropriate to meet these needs, and (2) consideration of the family's resources, priorities, and concerns, and identification of supports and services to enhance the family's ability to meet the needs of their child.

The typical first step is to review pertinent records related to the child's current health status and medical history. Then the child's present functioning is assessed in these areas: (a) cognitive development, (b) communication development, (c) social or emotional development, (d) physical development (including vision and hearing), and (e) adaptive development.

Child Assessment

The assessment process includes three related activities: (a) identification and sharing of the family's perceptions regarding the child's strengths and needs; (b) identification and sharing of the professional's perceptions regarding the child's strengths and needs; and (c) sharing, discussing, and interpreting assessment results (Turnbull, 1991). Parents or caregivers are encouraged to share what they see as their child's strengths with other team members, and professional team members share assessment information and results with parents/caregivers.

Family Resources, Priorities, and Concerns

Recall that the original Part H regulations required assessment of family strengths and needs. The 1991 reauthorization altered this requirement to read that what is needed is a statement of the family's resources, priorities, and concerns. The Part H regulations stating that family members can be designated recipients of services remains, however. The issue is how to determine what services to provide for parents. As discussed in Chapter 2, many in early intervention are not comfortable with the idea of assessing and intervening with parents.

Slentz and Bricker (1992) present some of the problems associated with family assessment. One problem is the lack of appropriate instruments. Most of the currently available instruments have been adapted from clinical family research projects. They were not designed for (and therefore should not be used to) assess families for early intervention services. When assessment instruments are used for purposes other than those for which they were designed, whatever data they yield are likely to be invalid and misleading. Those few instruments that have been developed specifically for family assessment in early intervention programs may not be used properly or they may not be appropriate for the particular families with whom they are used.

A second major problem with family assessment is that it tends to interfere with efforts to establish the type of parent-professional relationship that is basic to effective early intervention services. As Slentz and Bricker point out, it sends the wrong messages. When parents are asked to respond to questions about family interactions, functioning, and feelings, there is an implicit assumption that one of the objectives of the early intervention program is to affect these broad family functioning variables. This is *not* the purpose of early intervention services. The second wrong message that family assessment can send is that the IFSP will address the needs of all family members. Lack of personnel and other resources make it impossible to meet this expectation. The resulting disappointment and resentment on the part of families when all their needs are not met to their satisfaction is detrimental to parent–professional–agency relationships.

The third and most serious wrong message is the implicit suggestion that where there is a child with special needs there must be a dysfunctional family—or at least a family with many problems that need to be carefully scrutinized. How can professionals expect to establish equal partnerships with family members when the sharing of intimate information is a one-way activity?

Finally, family assessment sends the message that early interventionists are family therapists. This wrong message not only misleads families—it can contribute to difficulties with interagency and interdisciplinary coordination. Comprehensive family assessment and therapy are the exclusive province of specially trained family therapists.

The best way to find out what families are comfortable with when it comes to sharing information is to ask them. That is what Summers and colleagues (1990) did. These researchers convened parent groups in four states to ask parents for their preferences concerning methods and procedures for identifying family strengths and needs. Parents expressed a strong and consistent preference for informal approaches and open-ended conversations rather than structured interviews. Some pointed out that even open-ended interviews can be too structured. Terms that came up frequently in the family members' comments were "conversations" and "stories." They liked informality and nonintrusive questions. They wanted professionals to be willing to invest whatever time is necessary to develop rapport and friendships. One mother said that she was put at ease by the fact that the home visitor always wore jeans and a T-shirt. Emphasizing the importance of taking the time to develop a genuine friendship and build trust, another mother said that professionals should "Just come and get acquainted. Just hold my hand and say 'I have some things for you when you are ready'" (Summers et al., p. 87).

Other parents stressed the importance of keen listening skills. They noted that professionals should learn to listen better, because very often statements are not phrased exactly as expected. Professionals need to be sensitive to needs that may be expressed in indirect statements. For example, rather than "I need this" or "I need that," there may be statements like "I didn't get much sleep last night," or "I haven't had time to take my older children for their school clothes."

Another area in which there was broad consensus among the parents was that only family strengths or needs clearly relevant to the child's specific IFSP objectives should be discussed. Family members were emphatically clear that *they* should be the ones to identify family strengths and needs, not professionals (except in the case of child abuse or neglect). Similarly, parents insisted that they should be the ones to say precisely what would appear in writing on the IFSP. They made it clear that they wanted to be able to share some confidences with program staff and trust that statements referring to these particular comments would not appear in the IFSP.

What comes through in all discussions of the IFSP process and other joint parent-professional activities is that parents want program staff to be supportive, accepting, and nonjudgmental. Parents resent any suggestions that they must share sensitive and personal family information in order to receive early intervention services. They want respect, trust, commitment, and honest communication, and they want to feel that they are being heard. Families define emotional support as giving positive feedback, being flexible and responsive to rapid changes in the family circumstances, and making home visits to make the family comfortable (Summers et al., 1990). They want the focus of assessment and intervention to remain primarily on the child. They emphasize that interactions with families should take place in an unhurried atmosphere and that family concerns should be addressed if and when they arise—not as a precondition to receiving help for their child.

Development of Outcomes

During this final phase of the IFSP process, the team reviews the assembled information, prioritizes possible objectives, and decides what actions need to occur and what to anticipate as a consequence of these actions. These positive expectations are phrased as *outcome statements.*

It cannot be overemphasized that the IFSP and the process that generates the IFSP belongs to the family. Both family outcomes and child outcomes reflect the changes that family members want to see occur for their child and themselves. Outcomes may focus on areas of child development or family life that family members consider to be related to their ability to enhance the child's development. Ideally, they are stated in terms of the process (actions that need to occur) and the product (consequences of these actions). Refer to the IFSPs in Figures 3-3 and 3-4 for examples of outcomes.

Outcomes are written with the family's wording, not in the words of professionals. Here is an example of a family outcome phrased as an "in order to" statement—that is, Action A will be accomplished (or implemented) *in order to* attain Outcome B (Deal, Dunst & Trivette, 1989).

> Norma will find a daycare program that will enroll both Jennifer and Taylor in order to free her up to go to school full-time.

Development of outcomes is the point in the IFSP process at which there is the greatest potential for conflict. If this occurs, the best way to proceed is to openly acknowledge a difference of opinion. Most people will readily acknowledge that differences of opinion are "normal"—that they sometimes even disagree with the views of their closest family members or friends.

Team members (including parents or caregivers) should assume that there will be differences in their values, perspectives, and priorities. Even those individuals who are closest to one another, such as sisters, have some differences in values, perspectives, and priorities. What is important is negotiation and resolution of differences in priorities and expectations. Of course, if they cannot be resolved through collaborative team processes, then the wishes of the family must take precedence. *IFSP outcomes must reflect the family's priorities, not those of the program staff.*

After outcomes have been identified, the team is ready to consider what activities to initiate in order to achieve the specified outcomes. These activities will include establishing necessary linkages with other programs, services, and persons, so as to achieve the desired outcomes. Again, there will be significant differences among families. Some families need relatively little input when selecting strategies and activities to achieve the outcomes they want for their child and themselves. They have a clear idea of the available resources (physical therapy, insurance or other financial help, family assistance) and how to access these resources. Other families need help identifying sources of help and support, and creative ways to use existing resources.

There should be criteria and timelines for each outcome so that they can be evaluated. One suggestion for outcome evaluation is this seven-point scale suggested by Deal, Dunst, and Trivette (1989):

RATING	CRITERIA
1	Situation changed—no longer a need
2	Situation unchanged—still a need, goal, or project
3	Implementation begun—still a need, goal, or project
4	Outcome partially attained/accomplished, but not to the family's satisfaction
5	Outcome attained/accomplished, but not to the family's satisfaction
6	Outcome mostly attained/accomplished to the family's satisfaction
7	Outcome completely attained/accomplished to the family's satisfaction

The legislation specifies that the IFSP must be evaluated once a year and reviewed at least every 6 months. However, IFSP outcomes and strategies should be informally reviewed more often and at the family's request.

 Summary

This chapter stresses that the IFSP is a process, not a product. It is the ongoing supportive planning process that is important, not the document. The IFSP can be continually modified as programming progresses.

This chapter also stresses the importance of viewing families as guides as well as participants in both the assessment and the intervention processes. These guidelines, suggested by Bennett, Lingerfelt, and Nelson (1990) summarize the perspective we have tried to present in this chapter:

1. Family-identified concerns, needs, and aspirations should receive the most weight in the IFSP process. Help the family identify and prioritize their

concerns, needs, and aspirations and specific projects on which they want to work.

2. Help the family to identify and use their existing strengths and resources. Use the family's own abilities to solve problems and obtain needed resources.

3. Help the family develop a strong informal social network to promote development and well-being of the family unit. Work to identify and maintain all sources of informal social support already available to the family.

4. Expand the family's repertoire of skills and competencies. Create opportunities for the family to develop valuable new skills and capabilities (Bennett, Lingerfelt & Nelson, 1990).

Most basic for early interventionists in the IFSP process is to establish a healthy and productive working relationship with the family. Service providers must respect, and truly want to hear, what family members have to say and what they want.

Finally, there are a number of excellent books that deal almost exclusively with the IFSP process. One is *Guidelines and Recommended Practices for the Individualized Family Service Plan (Second Edition),* edited by McGonigel, Kaufmann, and Johnson (1991). This excellent volume provides a wealth of sample materials and straightforward guidelines. Another excellent resource is the text *Enabling and Empowering Families: Principles and Guidelines for Practice* by Dunst, Trivette, and Deal (1988).

Activities

1. Locate as many of the tests in this chapter as you can. Review and categorize instruments as norm-referenced, criterion-referenced, or curriculum-referenced. Determine whether each test is standardized and describe standardization procedures. Most important, describe the type of information that each instrument yields.

2. Secure a copy of an IFSP form used in your community or state. Determine how and by whom it was developed and compare it with the forms provided in this chapter.

3. Adapt/modify the Na Lei Kamili'i information form of Figure 3-2 to be appropriate for your community or region.

4. Ask some parents or caregivers of young children (with or without disabilities) what they would be comfortable with when it comes to sharing information about their family strengths and needs. Compare their answers with the preferences generated by the Summers et al. (1990) study.

Review Questions

1. State the Part H requirements related to assessment and development of the IFSP.
2. Describe the type of information that, according to best practices, the assessment process should generate.
3. Differentiate the three basic methods for collecting assessment information in terms of how information is collected and the type of information collected with each method.
4. Differentiate the three major categories of tests and give an example of at least one instrument for infants/toddlers in each category.
5. Compare arena assessment procedures with traditional assessment in terms of the processes and the products.
6. Contrast information needs for diagnosis and eligibility with those for intervention planning.
7. Discuss the primary focus of assessment (the questions being asked) in each of the developmental domains: cognitive development, physical development, language and communication, social/emotional development, and adaptive development.
8. Describe the major activities in the IFSP process.
9. Discuss the problems associated with family assessment (specifically, the wrong messages that it can send).

IEP Development

1. *Discuss general concerns related to assessment at the preschool level.*

2. *Describe assessment of social behavior, speech, language, and communication skills, cognitive behaviors, motor behaviors, self-care skills, and ecological information.*

3. *Describe procedures for IEP development.*

A ssessment of preschoolers uses the same basic procedures (tests, observation, and interviews) as assessment of infants and toddlers and the same broad categories of tests (norm-referenced, criterion-referenced, curriculum-referenced). Moreover, the broad purposes for assessment at the preschool level are the same: diagnosis and eligibility determination and intervention planning.

 ## Preschool Assessment Concerns

We begin with a brief discussion of some concerns related to assessment at the preschool level: (a) eligibility criteria, (b) misuse of test results, (c) psychometric problems, (d) judgment-based procedures, and (e) assessment modifications.

Eligibility Criteria

In a perfect world, eligibility for special services would not be an issue. All children and families would be eligible for and receive whatever service they want and need. However, despite continuing concerns about the potentially harmful effects of labeling, in the "real world" children with special needs must be determined to be eligible for services (and labeled) before they can be served.

As discussed in Chapter 1, Part B–Section 619 of the Individuals with Disabilities Education Act (IDEA) gives children ages 3 through 5 the same special education and related services as provided children and youth who are ages 6 through 21. The eligibility categories used with older children have been extended to the preschool-age group (mentally retarded, learning disabled, speech/language impaired, visually handicapped, hard of hearing/deaf, emotionally disturbed, orthopedically impaired, other health impaired, multihandicapped, traumatic brain injury or autism, and deaf/blind). The one difference is that states have some flexibility where preschoolers are concerned. They can choose not to label and report preschool children by category. Instead, they can use a generic category such as "developmentally disabled" in addition to or in place of the eleven eligibility categories listed above. Consequently, eligibility criteria for preschool children vary widely among the states and territories (Harbin, Danaher, Bailey & Eller, 1991). Some states have adopted broadly inclusive noncategorical criteria, while others maintain the same categories used with school-age students.

Further complicating eligibility is the fact that states have considerable flexibility in determining eligibility for the birth to 3-year-old population. In practice this has several implications. One is that infants and toddlers may be eligible for services in some states (those with broad at-risk eligibility criteria) but not in others. Another implication of the flexibility is that, in some states, children may be eligible for service prior to but not after age 3 because of differences in eligibility between Part H (infant/toddlers) programs and Part B (preschool) programs.

2 Misuse of Tests Results

When tests are developed they are intended for a specific purpose, such as screening, diagnosis, or intervention planning. As emphasized in Chapter 3, they should only be used for the purpose for which they were intended. An example of misuse would be using a scale with developmental pinpoints to generate intervention objectives. The items on developmental scales are typically drawn from standardized tests designed to differentiate children who are not developing at an expected rate; they are not intended as a means of identifying developmental or functional skills needs for intervention (Gaussin, 1984; Keogh & Sheehan, 1981).

A related concern is overreliance on test results to the exclusion of information from other sources. It is not appropriate to rely exclusively on test results for the information needed to formulate goals and objectives or to design instruction (Bailey, 1989).

The limitations associated with the instruments themselves are compounded by the myriad problems associated with testing young children. There are many variables affecting the performance of a young child during a formal assessment session. Young children tire easily; they are highly susceptible to distractions; they are frequently inconsistent in their responses. It is especially difficult to get a clear picture of the abilities of young children with sensory and/or motor impairments. Even the most patient, experienced, and skilled assessment team may not elicit the child's optimal performance. The only solution, because there is always the potential for inaccurate conclusions, is to continually verify test results with multiple sources, such as observations, and parent reports.

3 Psychometric Problems

Many of the assessment instruments that are used with preschool-age children with disabilities have serious psychometric limitations (Bailey, 1989). These include: (a) technical problems (they lack reliability and validity for children with disabilities); (b) sampling problems (some instruments suggest interpreting their results as developmental age scores when they were not standardized with a representative sample of children); (c) narrow focus (many measures ignore generic learning behaviors such as attending, goal-directedness, or persistence); and (d) rigidity (many instruments fail to consider the specialized assessment needs of young children with disabilities).

Just because an instrument has instructions for adapting its items for children with sensory and/or physical impairments does not make it appropriate for use with children with disabilities. It should also have norms derived from children with sensory and/or physical disabilities. It is deceiving and unfair to compare the performance of a child with severe sensory and/or physical impairments with a set of norms derived wholly from children who have no disabilities.

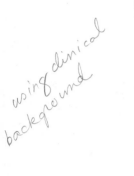

4. ## Judgment-Based Assessment

Judgment-based assessment (JBA) is defined as "the formal use of structured, quantified judgment to (a) complement norm- and curriculum-based measures, (b) measure ambiguous child characteristics, and (c) serve as a vehicle for team decision making" (Neisworth & Fewell, 1990, p. ix). Judgment-based assessment gives credence to and uses *clinical judgment*—the insights and perceptions of those who know a child best (parents, teachers and early intervention staff, and peers). JBA measures are a valuable supplement for data from traditional assessment sources.

JBA has only recently begun to receive the attention it deserves as a source of valuable information. In fact, in 1990 an entire issue of the journal *Topics in Early Childhood Special Education* (Fall 1990) was devoted to examination of qualitative assessment and the use of judgment.

JBA data provide a clear and sensitive picture of the child as he or she behaves in different contexts, permitting examination of aspects of the child's behavior that might not be seen if assessment is limited to use of standardized procedures in a single setting. The most commonly used JBA methods are rating scales, structured interviews, questionnaires, and inventories.

5. ## Assessment Modifications

With some children with disabilities (particularly children with sensory deficits and neuromotor impairment), it is necessary to modify assessment instruments and strategies. Langley (1991) suggests the following as options for modification:

1. Adapt the manner in which the test stimuli are presented. For example, hold the pictures closer to the child's eyes.
2. Modify the administration procedures. For example, allow more time for timed tasks.
3. Alter the test stimuli. For example, provide larger pictures or speak more slowly.
4. Alter the response requirements. For example, permit the child to look at the desired response (called "eye pointing") rather than pointing manually.
5. Incorporate additional aids, equipment, and management procedures. For example, permit the child to use a head pointer or communication board.

Remember that using any of these modifications threatens the validity and reliability of the instrument. They should be used only when assessment is for the purpose of collecting information for program planning. In that situation, scores are not important and should not be calculated.

In conclusion, this section has highlighted five concerns in assessment of preschoolers: (a) eligibility criteria, (b) misuse of tests, (c) psychometric problems, (d) judgment-based procedures, and (e) assessment modifications. There is one other major concern in preschool assessment. That is the overriding concern for ensuring direct linkages between assessment findings and intervention goals and practices. This topic is covered in the final section of the chapter as part of the discussion of the IEP.

Assessment Procedures

The broad goal of assessment for intervention planning is to generate an accurate and comprehensive picture of the child's functional skills and the conditions in which the child will be most likely to perform and expand upon these skills. More specifically, the objectives of assessment in the naturalistic curriculum model are (a) to identify tasks and activities the child needs in order to function in the environment, (b) to specify skills that will enable performance of these tasks and activities, and (c) to determine the best arrangements for teaching and supporting skill acquisition. Assessment typically uses a combination of strategies to establish the child's baseline functioning, generate intervention goals and objectives, and plan the steps and appropriate procedures for intervention.

This section outlines assessment procedures for 3-, 4-, and 5-year-old children. While the developmental domains (social, language, cognitive, motor, and self-care) are each discussed separately, we emphasize their interrelatedness and interdependence. The overlapping nature of development makes it difficult (and perhaps inappropriate) to assess (or attempt to facilitate and remediate) any one domain in isolation. For example, try to imagine assessment of the dressing skills of a 4-year-old without also considering the child's cognitive level and motor abilities. Similarly, it would not be appropriate to assess the language competence of a 3-year-old without also considering the child's cognitive, social, and motor skills.

Assessing Social Behavior

The development of meaningful and productive relationships with one's peers, what is termed *social competence,* is one of the essential tasks of early childhood. By age 3, social interactions with peers are becoming more frequent and complex (Hartup, 1983) and friendships are becoming increasingly important. Children are beginning to learn essential social skills, such as how to gain the cooperation of others, how to refuse to participate in a group activity, and how to deal with conflict. They are making the transition from playing alone (but in close proximity to peers) to interactive and, finally, cooperative play.

Early intervention programs place heavy emphasis on peer-related social competence. One reason is related to the requirements of integration. There is recognition that social competence contributes to successful integration *and vice versa* (participation in mainstreamed settings facilitates social competence) (Guralnick, 1990b). A second reason for stressing peer-related social development is more future-oriented. Research suggests that there is a relationship between

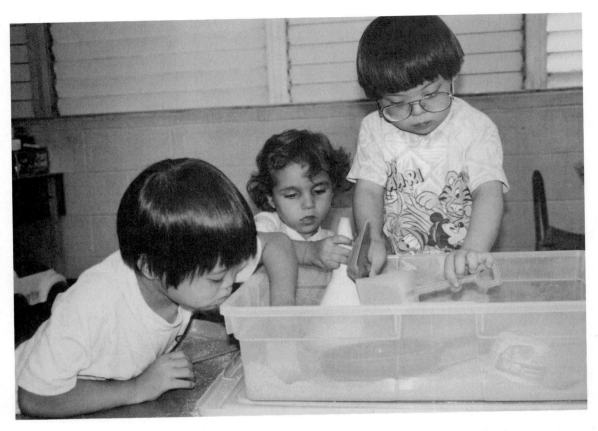

Preschoolers are beginning to learn the social skills for participating in group activities.

adjustment problems in later life and peer relations in early childhood (Parker & Asher, 1987).

Use of multiple sources and multiple measures is important in all domains, but it is particularly important in assessment of social behaviors. The three types of information that are relevant to the development and evaluation of social skill interventions for preschool-aged children are (a) information about the target child's social behavior; (b) information about the social behaviors of peers (to help determine which additional children and interactive behaviors should be involved in intervention for the target child); and (c) information about the interactions of "normal" children. The reason for collecting information about the social behaviors of normally developing peers is to assist identification of interaction behaviors that are typical for the particular setting and the age group (but lacking in the target child).

Methods for assessing social skills development of young children include (a) anecdotal reports, (b) direct observation, (c) rating scales, (d) sociometric nominations or ratings by peers, and (e) tests (Odom & McConnell, 1989).

A. **Anecdotal Notes.** The data recorded through such procedures as anecdotal notes, diaries, and logs assist in formulating goals and objectives and planning intervention strategies. To be maximally useful, anecdotal notes should be written at the time or immediately after the behavior occurs, but may be recorded later in the day. Everything that occurs in a specific time period or setting—all of the target child's social behavior and the reactions of others to the behavior—should be described in an objective and concise manner. The best anecdotal notes include details of the context (time, activity, materials, and persons present), and they clearly differentiate descriptions of what actually occurred from interpretations and judgments.

B. **Direct Observations.** Direct observations differ from anecdotal reporting methods in that the focus is on recording occurrences of a particular predefined behavior (or behaviors) *while the behavior is actually occurring*. The most representative samples of child social behaviors will come from observing the child in natural environments such as the home, the playground, and the preschool, with familiar persons such as teachers, peers, caregivers, and other family members. Direct observations of social skills will answer these questions:

1. Does the child need social skills training?
2. Which social skills should be taught?
3. Who would be the best social skills teacher for the child?
4. How should social skills be taught to this child?
5. When (and where) should social skills be taught?

After intervention has been implemented, systematic observations will provide information concerning generalization of behavior change in nontraining settings and whether the new behaviors have been maintained over time. Direct observation procedures can also provide information about peer interactions—specifically, how peers respond to the social behaviors of the target child.

The four most commonly used direct observation recording systems are event recording, interval recording, duration recording, and time sampling. *Event recording* (also called *frequency recording*) is counting the number of times a behavior occurs during a specified time period. This method is appropriate for recording discrete social behaviors of short duration with easily discernible beginnings and endings. A sample data sheet is presented in Figure 4-1. (Note that rate per minute is easily computed when frequency and time data are available.) Event recording is also appropriate when assessment is concerned with the sequence of social initiations and responses (as well as frequency): it can show the social behavior chain.

Duration recording is recording the number of seconds or minutes from initiation to termination of a behavior. It is used when the length of time a behavior

Name: _____ Date: _____

Definition of behavior 1 (B^1): _____

_____

Definition of behavior 2 (B^2): _____

_____

Start time: _____ Stop time: _____ Observer: _____

B^1 | | | | | | | | | | | | | | | | | | | | | | | | | |

B^2 | | | | | | | | | | | | | | | | | | | | | | | | | |

B^1 Total occurrences: _____

B^2 Total occurrences: _____

Total observation time: _____

$B^1 \dfrac{\text{Total occurrences}}{\text{Total minutes}}$ = _____ (Rate per minute)

$B^2 \dfrac{\text{Total occurrences}}{\text{Total minutes}}$ = _____ (Rate per minute)

Comments:

Figure 4-1 Sample data form for event recording

occurs is of interest. Duration recording is most appropriate for behaviors that occur at a very high rate, behaviors that occur for extended periods of time, and behaviors that are variable in length (for example, play episodes).

There are three ways to analyze and report duration data: (a) average duration per occurrence, (b) percent of total session, and (c) total duration. Average duration per occurrence (or episode) requires recording of the duration of each occurrence and number of occurrences. Episode times are then summed and the total time is divided by the number of episodes. Percent of total session is computed by dividing the total time engaged in the behavior during the session by the total length of the observation session and multiplying by 100. Total duration is the total amount of time the child is engaged in the target behavior during the observation session. Figure 4-2 shows a data sheet for recording duration data.

Name: _____ Date: _____

Definition/description of behavior: _____

_____

Observation   Observation   Total
start time: _____   stop time: _____   observation time: _____

Occurrences/episodes	Start	Stop	Total time
1.			
2.			
3.			
4.			
5.			

Total occurrences/episodes: _____

Total duration of target behavior: _____

Average duration per episode: _____

Comments:

Figure 4-2 Sample data form for duration recording

Interval recording is a data collection procedure for documenting the occurrence or nonoccurrence of one or more target behaviors within short, prespecified intervals. It is not as sensitive a measure as duration or frequency. The advantage of interval recording is that it permits an estimate of duration and frequency when they are otherwise difficult to measure (for example, when a behavior occurs too quickly to count). The observation period is divided into equal intervals (usually from 5 to 50 seconds in length) depending on the average frequency and duration of the target behavior. Regardless of the number of times the target behavior occurs during an interval, it is scored only once per interval. Interval recording can be used to record more than one behavior at a time or the behavior of more than one child. Figure 4-3 shows an example of a data sheet for interval recording.

Time sampling is similar to interval recording in that the observation period is divided into equal intervals. However, rather than scoring the target behavior *during* the interval, both observation and scoring are done at the end of the interval. This method is something like taking quick snapshots of the child at intervals throughout a specified observation period. Because it does not require

Name: _____ Date: _____

Behaviors: 1. _____

2. _____

Start time: _____ Stop time: _____ Total observation time: _____

Observer: _____

	1 2 3 4	1 2 3 4	1 2 3 4	1 2 3 4	1 2 3 4	
B¹						5 minutes
B²						

	1 2 3 4	1 2 3 4	1 2 3 4	1 2 3 4	1 2 3 4	
B¹						5 minutes
B²						

	1 2 3 4	1 2 3 4	1 2 3 4	1 2 3 4	1 2 3 4	
B¹						5 minutes
B²						

Total intervals observed:_____

Total B¹:_____   Total % intervals:_____

Total B²:_____   Total % intervals:_____

Comments:

Figure 4-3 Sample data form for interval recording

an observer's undivided attention, time sampling may be a more practical option than interval recording in many settings. Figure 4-4 shows a data sheet for time sampling recording.

Scanning is a variation of time sampling where data are collected simultaneously on a number of children (possibly even a whole class). With scanning, the observer records behaviors for one child, then moves on to the next child and repeats the process, and so on. When data for the last child have been recorded, the observer begins again with the first child. An alternative is to observe each child for a prespecified period before moving to the next child.

Name: _____ Date: _____

Behavior description: _____

_____

Week beginning: _____   0 = nonoccurrence
                                            + = occurrence
                                            X = no observation

	8:15	8:20	8:25	8:30	8:35	8:40	8:45	8:50	8:55	9:00	9:05	9:10
Mon.												
Tues.												
Wed.												
Thur.												
Fri.												

Total observations: _____

Total occurrences: _____   Total nonoccurrences: _____

Comments:

Figure 4-4   Sample data sheet for time sampling recording

Rating Scales.   Rating scales require adults to record their judgments concerning the child's behaviors based on their observations and experience with the child over some period of time. There are two basic types of social behavior rating scales. One type lists specific social behaviors, each with a precise description and a continuum for rating the degree of the behavior demonstrated (or not demonstrated). There are also procedures for summarizing the ratings and computing either subscale scores or a total score. The second type of rating scale lists social behaviors and asks the adult to indicate with a yes or no response whether the child demonstrated the behavior(s) during a particular observation period.

Sociometric Nominations.   Sociometric nominations are procedures that ask peers to provide general information concerning the social acceptance or likeability of other children. These procedures are mentioned here because they are widely used to assess children's peer relations and to evaluate the outcome of social skills. However, they have limitations that are serious enough that Strain and Kohler (1988) have recommended against their use with preschool-age children. One limitation is that there are a range of variables (physical attractiveness, sex) *other than* social behaviors that influence children's peer nominations. Thus a low score may not necessarily indicate the need for facilitation of social skills. A second limitation is the very poor test-retest reliability when sociometric procedures are used with preschoolers (Asher, Singleton, Tinsley & Hymel, 1979). The third limitation has to do with the tendency of preschoolers with special needs to respond in a stereotypic manner. It is not unusual to find that, when asked to generate peer nominations or provide some type of peer rating, they give everyone in the class the same rating (Odom & DuBose, 1981). The fourth limitation of sociometric nominations and ratings is that some preschoolers simply are not able to understand what they are being asked to do.

E .   **Tests.**   Recall from Chapter 3 that criterion-referenced and curriculum-referenced instruments measure a child's performance against a set of previously established skills or curriculum objectives. Criterion-referenced tests (also called content-, or objective-referenced tests) measure the child's performance against some prespecified criteria (most often developmental criteria). They typically list items in a developmental sequence with an indication of the average age at which the skill should be accomplished. Criterion-referenced tests may provide curriculum suggestions. The items on curriculum-referenced tests (also called curriculum-based assessment) come directly from the concepts and skills that make up the curriculum. Curriculum-referenced assessment has been described as a test-teach-test approach wherein children are assessed on objectives from the curriculum, provided with instruction on those they have not yet attained, and then again assessed to evaluate achievement of the objectives (Bagnato, Neisworth & Capone, 1986). Both approaches differ from norm-referenced procedures in that they do not compare a child's skills with those of a normative sample population.

There are a number of criterion-referenced scales that have subscales for assessing social skills. Examples include the *Battelle Developmental Inventory* (BDI) (Newborg, Stock, Wnck, Guidubaldi, & Svinicki, 1984) and the *Portage Guide to Early Education* (Bluma, Shearer, Frohman & Hilliard, 1976). (The BDI is among the few instruments that are both criterion-referenced and norm-referenced.)

Odom and McConnell (1989) suggest some characteristics to look for in selecting criterion-referenced measures: (a) ecological validity, (b) compatibility with intervention, (c) focus on discrete skills, (d) the basis for item sequencing, and (e) sensitivity to small changes in behavior. The criterion of ecological validity is particularly important where social behavior is concerned. To have ecological validity, the instrument must allow for assessment (ideally, direct observations) of the child's social behavior across the range of the child's natural environments. If the focus of assessment is not compatible with intervention possibilities, it is unlikely to yield the specific type of information that teachers need and will use for programming.

What is needed are data concerning the child's performance of the discrete skills essential to effective social interactions (for example, making positive verbal bids to peers, looking at peer when spoken to). A global score from a criterion-referenced instrument is no more useful for planning intervention targets and strategies than a global score from a norm-referenced test.

Criterion-referenced instruments typically arrange skills in a normal development sequence or a hierarchy based on task analysis. Either way, what is important is for users to be conscious of the basis for the sequencing of items when formulating intervention objectives from the findings. Finally, Odom and McConnell (1989) emphasize the importance of selecting a criterion-referenced instrument that is sensitive to small changes in behavior so it can be used to monitor progress.

Norm-referenced tests to assess the social interaction skills and social competence of preschool-age children rely primarily on parent ratings. The exception is the *Battelle Developmental Inventory* (BDI) mentioned above. The *Personal-Social Subscale* of the BDI can be completed either by direct observation or by interviewing the child's primary caregiver. The only norm-referenced teacher rating scale is the *California Preschool Social Competency Scale* developed in 1969 (Levine, Elsey & Lewis).

The *Vineland Scales*, designed for use with children from birth to age 18, provide scores in four domains, including socialization. The socialization domain has three subdomains: interpersonal relations, play and leisure time, and coping skills. Two of the three versions of the current edition of the *Vineland Adaptive Behavior Scales* (Sparrow, Balla & Cicchetti, 1984) use parents (or other informed adults) as primary sources of data.

In summary, this section has provided an overview of methods for assessing the social development of young children with special needs. Sociometric nominations is the only method that is used exclusively for assessment of social skills, but it is not recommended for preschoolers. The other methods are also represented in procedures to assess performance in other developmental domains.

Assessing Speech, Language, and Communication Skills

To be active participants in the assessment process, all team members need an understanding of the relevant dimensions of speech, language, and communication skills and available measurement procedures. Table 4-1 provides a summary of these three separate but interrelated dimensions. The discussion that follows provides an introduction to the types of problems experienced by children who are having language and communication difficulties.

Types of Speech, Language, and Communication Problems. The three major categories of speech disorders are articulation disorders, voice disorders, and fluency disorders. *Articulation disorders* are characterized by nonstandard or defective speech sounds. They may be caused by structural defects, neuromotor deficits, or hearing impairment. *Voice disorders* are deviations of voice pitch, loudness, or quality. Possible causes include physiological causes (for example, growths within the larynx), voice abuse (for example, excessive crying), and hearing impairment. The most common *fluency disorder* is stuttering. The cause or causes of stuttering have not been established.

TABLE 4-1
Definition of Speech, Language, and Communication Dimensions

Speech: the verbal mode for expressing language. Because it is dependent on precise coordination of breathing, sound production, and articulation, speech is more difficult than other language modes for most children (i.e., manual signing, writing).

Language: knowledge and systematic use of a symbolic code and rule-governed combinations of symbols to represent and share ideas and intentions. Language has five components, each with its own rule system:

Phonology: rules for structuring, distributing, and sequencing speech sounds into words. Phonological development tends to follow a predictable sequence.

Morphology: rules for how basic meaningful units (morphemes) of a language can be combined into words. First morphemes are evident at around 13 months and morphological development continues until around age 5.

Syntax: rules specifying how words are strung together to express intended meanings, what sentences are acceptable in a language, and how to transform sentences into other sentences. By about age 3, preschoolers have begun to learn and use complex sentences.

Semantics: content or meaning associated with words and word combinations. The developmental order of acquisition of semantic relationships tends to reflect cognitive development. Children learn words to be able to talk about the things they know.

Pragmatics: knowledge and skills related to using language to accomplish desired goals and functions (including social interactions). To be competent communicators, children must learn (a) to adapt their language to the social context, (b) to take listeners' prior knowledge into account when formulating messages, and (c) rules for cooperative exchanges (conversational postulates).

Communication: the exchange of ideas and messages between a speaker and a listener. For an exchange to be properly termed communication, a message must be conveyed and it must also be received intact with its intended meaning preserved.

If screening indicates an articulation problem, the speech-language pathologist (SLP) collects case history information and administers one or another of the commercially available articulation tests (or uses clinician-made materials) to determine the nature of the problem. Articulation tests sample articulation with picture-naming responses. (Pictures are of items that can be named with a single word.) They typically test each consonant in initial, medial, and final position. The SLP tests for stimulability by providing a model for the child to imitate. This is to see if the child has the phonetic ability to produce the sounds. Children who can imitate their error sounds correctly are thought to present the most favorable prognosis.

In-depth assessment is implemented to specifically define and describe the problem and outline a remediation program. (There may be a decision to delay referral if the SLP thinks there is a strong likelihood that the young child will self-correct the errors.) In the process of assessing speech and language, the SLP is constantly alert to possible voice problems (problems in voice quality, resonance, pitch, and loudness) and stuttering. In these areas, the SLP's trained ear is the most useful assessment tool.

Preschool children with problems related to language present a wide variety of characteristics. Some are described as language delayed, meaning that they are acquiring language skills similar to those of their same-age peers but at a slower rate. (Their language may be almost exactly like the language of a younger child.) Others may be described as language disordered, meaning that there are discrepancies in the pattern of development. An example is the 4-year-old child whose phonological development is that of a 3-year-old, morphological and syntax skills are similar to those of a child 2½ years old, and pragmatic skills are only minimally delayed. Children with *specific language impairment* are those whose problems are exclusively with language. Their performance is within normal limits in all other areas (Leonard, 1990).

Assessment Processes and Procedures. There are a limited number of standardized instruments available for assessing 3- through 5-year-olds. Those that are available vary considerably with respect to technical adequacy. This further strengthens arguments for a combined use of standardized and nonstandardized measures, with emphasis on informal observations (for example, Miller, 1981; Muma, 1978). Standardized tests consider about the same language dimensions as nonstandardized procedures and use many of the same types of tasks. Nonstandardized procedures do not permit comparison of the child's performance with that of age peers, but they have the advantage of providing more detailed information about specific skills, particularly pragmatic skills. Selection of instruments will depend on initial screening or referral information—whether the SLP suspects a delay or disorder in phonology, morphology and syntax (typically assessed together), semantics, or pragmatics.

Children who fail to produce the sounds anticipated for their age group are assessed to determine their specific phonological problems. Phonological errors result from the patterns of simplifications adopted when learning words (called phonological processes) (McReynolds, 1986). Children with phonological disorders often demonstrate a capability of producing the correct sounds but they do not always do so when called for. They may misarticulate a given sound in one word and then subsequently produce that sound correctly in another word (where another sound may be misarticulated).

Children who use shorter and less complex sentences than same-age peers may have syntactic difficulties. Assessment for these children focuses on describing the type and frequency of their complex sentences. Assessment considers both comprehension of morphological and syntactic forms and production of these forms.

Assessment of semantic abilities typically focuses on determining the child's receptive and expressive vocabularies. Word comprehension is assessed by having the child point to a picture corresponds to the word presented by the SLP. Comprehension of longer utterances is assessed by having the child follow simple directions. Productive vocabulary is assessed by having the young child name pictures or objects.

There are a few tests to determine the preschool child's ability to use language effectively in social communication contexts. These include the *Preschool Language Assessment Instrument* (Blank, Rose & Berlin, 1978) and the *Test of Pragmatic Skills* (Shulman, 1986). The *Test of Pragmatic Skills* is a standardized test that provides information on how the young child (3 to 8 years) uses language to accomplish various functions such as naming/labeling, requesting, denying, and reasoning. The test also permits assessment of the child's ability to use conversational intent to organize discourse. This test provides an alternative to the language sample as a way to collect information about the child's pragmatic skills as actually used in social exchanges.

Assessment and diagnosis of communication disorders is even more difficult than assessment of language disorders because communication disorder is a relative concept (Taylor, 1990). Communicative competence depends on communication rules and expectations, and these differ drastically among cultural groups. A communication disorder can only be determined in the context of the rules and expectations of the particular language community. The conundrum facing the SLP is distinguishing between a communication *difference* and a communication *disorder*. This determines the type of assistance needed (whether the child needs language intervention or second language instruction).

The initial diagnostic assessment of a preschool child who has been referred as possibly having a speech, language, or communication problem typically includes a case history, a hearing screening, examination of the oral peripheral mechanism, an articulation test, language assessment, and perhaps a test of auditory discrimination. The parents and teacher(s) are asked to describe communication behaviors that the child now uses or is learning to use to request objects, actions, or attention. Specifically, they are asked to describe how the child requests desired objects and activities and how other language intentions are expressed (with gestures, facial expressions, speech or nonspeech sounds, words, or manual signs) and the contexts where these communicative functions are used. Assessment for the purpose of intervention planning will then establish (a) baseline functioning in the area or areas where the child is delayed, (b) how the child learns best, and (c) optimal intervention materials and contexts.

Assessment procedures include tests (standardized and nonstandardized), rating scales, direct observation, and language sampling. These procedures are similar to assessment procedures in the social developmental domain. The only assessment procedure unique to language/communication is language sampling, which was discussed in Chapter 3.

Language sampling is a type of direct observation in which the objective is to collect a representative sample of the child's language and communication skills. The length of time required to collect a sample of 50 to 100 different spontaneous utterances varies. With preschoolers it is often necessary to present open-ended questions or requests to increase the likelihood of getting a sufficient number of utterances to constitute a representative sample. While language sampling is time consuming, it is worth the time and effort because the information that a language sample (or better still, several language samples) yields is extremely valuable— especially for describing language pragmatic abilities.

In summary, when children have been screened as having problems related to expressing or understanding ideas and intentions, the SLP will first pinpoint whether the difficulty is related to speech, language, or communication abilities. Then some combination of assessment strategies (language sampling, informant interview scales, tests, and naturalistic observations) will be used to determine specific skill deficits and delays and generate intervention goals and strategies.

Assessing Cognitive Behaviors

In this section the terms *cognition* and *intellectual ability* will be used interchangeably to refer to all mental activities by which sensory input is used (perceiving, learning, remembering, categorizing, organizing) and the products of these activities (thoughts, concepts, cognitions, knowledge, solutions to problems). The concept of cognition (or intelligence) is multifaceted and enormously complex. A good illustration of this is the insightful description of the stages professionals go through in learning about intelligence testing that has been provided by Patton, Beirne-Smith, and Payne (1990). They identify these stages as (a) ignorance, (b) fascination, (c) disillusionment, and (d) appreciation. In the initial stage, ignorance, intelligence testing is viewed as "a mysterious process by which an IQ is extracted from a child's head" (p. 96). At this stage many professionals seem to view learning and intelligence as separate constructs. They may never have actually seen the contents of an intelligence testing kit. In the second stage, fascination, there is a growing appreciation of the construct of intelligence as having theoretical underpinnings. At this stage, many find themselves captivated by the contents of an intelligence test kit. "How marvelous that someone could think to pose such provocative questions!"

The third stage is disillusionment. Professionals begin to learn about psychometric inadequacies and other limitations of intelligence tests (standard error, poor sampling conditions, cultural biases) and the many questions about intelligence that remain unanswered. Finally, in the last stage, there is appreciation and more realistic appraisal of the value of intelligence testing. There is recognition that it is "neither good nor bad, perfect nor imperfect, but only a tool—a tool to be used while constantly remembering that it is the child who is important, not the testing tool" (p. 96). The important point is: *assessment of intelligence requires a realistic perspective concerning the strengths and limitations of the constructs of intelligence and intelligence testing.*

Most items on preschool measures of cognitive development come from one or another of three theories of cognition: (a) Piagetian theory, (b) social learning theory, or (c) information processing theory. Table 4-2 provides an overview of the major tenets of these theories. Both standardized and nonstandardized tests draw from these theories and their respective description of normal development.

Assessment Processes and Procedures. Psychologists and teachers are typically the professionals responsible for assessing cognitive development. Among the standardized tests most widely used to make diagnosis or placement decisions for preschoolers are the

> Wechsler Preschool and Primary Scale of Intelligence (WPPSI) (Wechsler, 1967)
> Stanford-Binet (Thorndike, Hagen & Sattler, 1986)
> Kaufman Assessment Battery for Children (K-ABC) (Kaufman & Kaufman, 1983)
> McCarthy Scales of Children's Ability (McCarthy, 1972)

It is important to keep in mind that the global scores from these instruments reflect only a very limited sample of the young child's cognitive abilities. These tests have limited usefulness for intervention planning because they are not designed to provide this type of information. However, a skilled professional can arrive at some conclusions about a child's cognitive skills and deficits or delays from careful analysis of the specific tasks that are passed and failed.

Tests used for intervention planning contain one or another of two types of tasks (or, in some cases, both): (a) tasks referenced against normal development of specific constructs (e.g., conservation) and/or processes (e.g., recall memory); and (b) preacademic tasks (e.g., differentiation of sounds and phonemes, letters, and sound-letter associations). These cognitive and preacademic tasks are typically included in subscales of broad-based developmental instruments such as the

> Brigance Inventory of Early Development (Brigance, 1978)
> Arizona Basic Assessment and Curriculum Utilization System (ABACUS) (McCarthy, Bos, Lund, Glatke & Vaughan, 1984)

Some tests look specifically at concept development. The *Boehm Test of Basic Concepts–Preschool Version* (Boehm, 1986) is one such test. It measures the preschool child's grasp of a range of concepts and situations (and requires only a pointing response). The *Bracken Concept Development Series* (Bracken, 1986) is another. It includes a basic concept scale (for ages 2½ to 8) and a concept development program.

In summary, cognitive assessment is similar to assessment in the other developmental domains in that (a) it is essential to use multiple sources of information, and (b) there is substantial interrelationship and interdependence of

TABLE 4-2

Sources for Items on Preschool Cognitive Measures

Piagetian Theory (Piaget, 1950):

Labels the years from ages 2 to 7 as the preoperational period with two substages: the preconceptual period (ages 2 to 4) and the intuitive period (ages 4 to 7). Views the emergence of symbolic thought as the most notable achievement of the preconceptual period.

In the intuitive period, children become less egocentric and more capable of classifying objects on the basis of shared perceptual attributes (i.e., size, shape, and color). The best illustration of intuitive reasoning comes from watching the child try to solve a conservation problem. Ask the child to adjust the volumes of liquid in two identical tall containers until each has "exactly the same amount." Then pour the liquid from one container into a short, broad container and ask the child whether the two containers have the same amount of liquid. Until children are 6 or 7 they typically respond that the tall, thin container has more liquid. Their thinking centers on a single perceptual feature — in this case, the relative height of the liquids in the two containers. They do not understand that certain properties of objects remain unchanged despite the appearance of having been altered.

Social Learning Theory (c.f., Bandura, 1986):

Considers observational learning to be the key process in cognitive development. Maintains that children learn new behaviors by observing the behavior of a model, remembering what they see, and then using the mental representations to reproduce the model's behavior at a future time. Children do not have to be reinforced or even respond in order to learn. All they need to do is pay close attention to the model's behavior and store the information about the observed behavior so that it can be retrieved at a later date.

Observational learning permits young children to acquire new responses in a variety of settings. Their "models" are not necessarily aware of being teachers but are simply pursuing their own interests.

Information Processing Theory (c.f., Newell & Simon, 1972):

Concerned with growth of specific cognitive skills, such as attending, perceiving, thinking, learning, and remembering. Compares the mind to a computer to explain how children of different ages process information about objects and events to "construct" knowledge and solve problems. As the brain and nervous system mature, children adopt more sophisticated strategies for attending, interpreting, and remembering what they experience. Information processing theory explains the problem-solving failures of preschool children as stemming from memory deficiencies that prevent them from gathering, storing, and simultaneously comparing the many pieces of information needed to arrive at a correct solution. The processing skills thought to have the greatest influence on cognitive development are (a) attention, (b) memory, and (c) problem solving.

cognitive skills and skills in other development domains. When assessing cognitive development, remember that cognition in young children changes very rapidly, often in uneven patterns.

Assessing Motor Behaviors

Motor development follows fairly regular sequences with early skills prerequisite to later responses. As is the case with speech and language skills, all team members need to be knowledgeable concerning both the nature and the sequence of motor development processes and assessment procedures. As stressed in Chapter 3, it is extremely important to recognize the effect of a motor delay or disability on development in other domains.

Motor skills are skills related to the development and use of muscles and limbs. As discussed in Chapter 3, assessment of physical development includes assessment of postural tone, primitive reflexes and automatic reactions, posture and movement patterns, and oral motor functioning.

Assessment Processes and Procedures. Comprehensive motor assessment considers attainment of both fine motor and gross motor developmental milestones. Ideally, the product of the assessment process will be a clear description of the child's functional motor skills, developmental progress, and specific data for formulating intervention goals and procedures.

The term *functional motor skills* refers to the child's ability to perform necessary daily activities. In functional assessment approaches, the emphasis is on functional motor independence rather than on normal motor functioning (Haley, Hallenborg & Gans, 1989). The focus on the function of a skill rather than its form or quality does not mean using abnormal movement patterns and postures in order to achieve functional independence. It simply underscores the importance of functional skills that are fundamental to activities and routines in present and future natural environments. A comprehensive functional assessment considers (a) the functional aspects of mobility and self-care, (b) how much assistance the child needs, (c) generalizability of the performance, (d) the amount of time needed to accomplish the functional tasks, (e) the technical complexity of necessary specialized equipment and devices, and (f) the technique and approach used for functional tasks (Haley et al., 1989).

Traditional developmental tests in the areas of gross and fine motor development assess skills considered to reflect developmental maturity—that is, creeping, cruising, kneeling, jumping, skipping, ball throwing, reaching and grasping, and building a tower with blocks. Scores are typically based on either pass or fail ratings.

Assessment (whether functional or developmental) may use norm-referenced or criterion-referenced tests in addition to direct observations. Sometimes a test fits into both categories. The *Peabody Developmental Motor Scales* (Folio & Fewell, 1983) is an example of a norm-referenced test that can also be used as a criterion-referenced test, depending on the purpose of the testing and interpretations of the child's responses.

In order to generate intervention-relevant information, motor assessment must consider both quantitative and qualitative aspects of the child's motor skills (Campbell & Stewart, 1986). Quantitative data indicate how many skills, or which portions of various skills, the child can perform; qualitative data describe aspects of movement such as postural tone, primitive reflexes, automatic reactions, symmetry and alignment, and muscle strength.

The lack of tests appropriate for young children with motor disabilities has led to dependence on the direct observation skills of occupational and physical therapists to assess children with movement disorders. However, there are a number of instruments that can be used to document functional motor skills (for intervention planning purposes). Most of the multidimensional standardized instruments listed in Chapter 3 and in this chapter, (such as the *Battelle Developmental Inventory* and *Bayley Scales of Infant Development*, have subscales for assessing motor development. In the absence of a therapist, teachers and other professionals can administer these tests.

Observation guidelines such as those provided in the *Transdisciplinary Play-Based Assessment* (TPBA) (Linder, 1990) are also very useful. The TPBA provides observation guidelines for collecting information on (a) mobility in sitting and standing, (b) jumping, (c) standing, (d) ball-playing skills, (e) grasp, and (f) manipulative prehension.

The *Carolina Curriculum for Preschoolers with Special Needs* (CCPSN) (Johnson-Martin, Attermeier & Hacker, 1990) is a curriculum-referenced assessment with an excellent motor assessment section. Assessment items are organized according to logical teaching sequences (rather than by mean ages of skill emergence). Assessment is designed to be conducted during daily routine activities using common materials. The child is observed alone or engaging in social interactions (over a period of several days, if necessary). There are an assessment log, a developmental progress chart, and teaching activities. General guidelines are provided for development of the IEP, daily data collection, and activity planning. A special feature of the CCPSN is a set of instructions for implementing group and individual activities in home, preschool, and daycare settings.

Assessing Self-Care Skills

All cultures have the expectation that normally developing children will eventually become competent in the self-care skills of self-feeding, dressing and undressing, toileting, and grooming—as these skills are critical to independent functioning. However, there are many differences among cultures as to the value placed on these skills and expectations for when they should be acquired (Peterson & Haring, 1989). The importance placed on these skills at differing ages and how they are facilitated varies even among families within every culture. Acquisition of these skills is deeply embedded in family's unique preferences and expectations. Some parents want their children to be proficient in self-care skills at a very early age. Eating skills are an example of the variability among families. In some families children are encouraged to use their fingers; others insist that children use conventional silverware or chopsticks. Some families prefer to assist their child's eating long after the child actually needs assistance.

Whatever the family or cultural differences, by age 3 most children can hold and drink from a glass, serve themselves from a serving bowl, and spread jam (or other spreadables) with a knife. By age 4 they are able to pass serving bowls, cut food with a fork, and help set the table.

Most 3-year-olds are competent at basic dressing skills. By the time they start school at age 5, most have learned to perform more difficult dressing skills involving a variety of closures, such as zippers, buttons, snaps, laces, and buckles.

Three-year-olds typically manage their own toileting needs during the daytime, though some may continue to have accidents in the preschool years. While most sleep through the night without wetting the bed, there may be periods when they lapse into bedwetting.

Children gradually become aware of the importance of personal grooming because of parental reminders. By age 3 they do a fair job of washing themselves in the bathtub. Four-year-olds do an even better job, including brushing teeth. By age 5, most bathe independently (though they may need some help getting started).

Assessment Processes and Procedures.   The only instrument that is concerned exclusively with self-care skills is the *Balthazar Scales of Adaptive Behavior* (BSAB) (Balthazar, 1976). It has a ten-item toileting questionnaire, an eating scale that considers dependent feeding, finger foods, spoon usage, fork usage, and drinking, and a dressing scale.

The primary method for assessing self-care skills is direct observation (typically using checklists of developmental milestones). Some checklists referenced on the criterion of normal development milestones include the *Learning Accomplishments Profile* (LAP) (LeMay, Griffin & Sanford, 1977) and the *Battelle Developmental Inventory* (Newborg, Stock, Wnek, Guidubaldi & Svinicki, 1984). Another criterion-referenced measure with a subscale considering self-help skills is the *Brigance Inventory of Early Development*. Unfortunately, most of the self-care items on these checklists have yes/no scoring, which may not provide useful information for developing instruction.

The most intervention-relevant information comes from a task analysis of the component behaviors (steps) of the skills that a child has not yet mastered. The task analysis is scored indicating which steps have been mastered and notes are recorded as to the level of assistance needed for steps not performed independently.

Caregiver interviews are another important source of information concerning self-care skills because, as noted, the young child's acquisition of self-care skills is embedded in the family's routines and their expectations. In addition to providing valuable information, caregiver interviews can validate information collected from other sources. Caregiver interviews are especially valuable, in that they provide an opportunity for parents to indicate the self-care skills they consider to be instructional priorities.

Ecological Information

Throughout this chapter we have stressed the important role that parents/caregivers play as members of the assessment team and the significance of the information they provide through responses to questionnaires, rating scales, and interviews. The reliability of parents as sources of information concerning their own children has been well documented (Vincent, Laten, Salisbury, Brown & Baumgart, 1981). Family members know the child best because they spend the most time with the child and thus have opportunities to observe the child's behavior in the greatest number and variety of situations.

While there has been some discussion of assessment for diagnosis and placement, the primary focus of this chapter has been on collecting information that will assist programming decisions—specifically, the child's functional skills and developmental abilities. The child's achievements are only part of the picture that needs to be assembled. Intervention planning requires information about (a) the child's unique likes and dislikes, and (b) what significant adults in the child's environment want the child to know and be able to do. This type of information is called *ecological information.*

The best source of ecological information is a parent interview, preferably a structured interview. Falvey (1986) and Savage (1983) provide examples of forms that can be used or adapted for this purpose. However, the printed form is not important. (Programs or teams can develop their own formats.) What is important are the types of information that will be collected. The following types of information are useful for planning intervention. The team needs information about:

1. The child's favorite and least favorite activities
2. The child's favorite and least favorite objects and toys
3. The child's favorite and least favorite foods (and allergies, if any)
4. Who the child plays with (children *and* adults) and what they play
5. How the child indicates preferences (how the child lets others know what things are favored and what are not)
6. When the child is most cooperative
7. How the child assists/participates in self-care (feeding, dressing, toileting, bathing)
8. What frightens the child
9. The caregivers' perspectives on how the child seems to learn best
10. What present activities or routines the family would like the child to participate in and the level of independence they would consider appropriate
11. What future activities and settings the family would like the child to be able to participate in and the level of independence they would like to achieve
12. What specific goals and objectives the family would like included in the IEP.

One way to help parents or caregivers think about present family activities and routines is to talk about weekday and weekend routines. Encourage parents/

caregivers to share the details of routine activities and the child's participation in these activities.

Considerations related to the child's next educational environment, as discussed in Chapter 13, are also important. Some parents/caregivers are ready at the initial assessment sessions to discuss their child's future educational options. Others are not. The important thing is to be sensitive to parent/caregiver readiness and concerns. It is certainly appropriate to introduce the concept of kindergarten survival skills at the IEP meeting in the course of discussing goals and objectives. (*Kindergarten survival skills*—those skills that will help the child be successful in kindergarten—are discussed in Chapter 13.)

In summary, this section has described procedures for assessment of social behavior, speech, language, and communication, skills, cognitive behaviors, motor behaviors, self-care skills, and the ecology. The remainder of the chapter describes how to use information about the child's developmental and functional strengths and needs and ecological information to generate intervention goals and objectives and procedures. Intervention planning culminates with a mutually agreed upon Individualized Education Program.

 # The Individualized Education Program (IEP)

One of the major provisions of the IDEA is the requirement that each eligible child must have an Individualized Education Program (IEP). The IEP is a written record of decisions that the parents and school personnel agree on for the special education program for the eligible child. The law is very specific that this written document must include:

The child's present levels of educational performance;
Annual goals and short-term instructional objectives in all areas where the child need specially designed instruction;
A statement of the specific educational services needed;
Extent of regular classroom participation;
Projected date for initiation of services and anticipated duration of services;
Criteria, evaluation procedures, and schedules for determining (at least once a year) whether instructional objectives are being met.

The IEP must be developed by a committee that includes *at least* the parents (or a guardian), the child's teachers, and a representative of the school district, such as a principal or special education coordinator. When the child is evaluated for the first time, there must also be a member of the assessment team on the IEP committee.

Figure 4-5 provides an example of an IEP. This Hawaii IEP form recently underwent revisions to better reflect the importance of parent/caregiver information and concerns. Comparison of the IEP with the IFSPs in Chapter 3 highlights the differences between the two documents. What is not so readily apparent are the

STATE OF HAWAII
DEPARTMENT OF EDUCATION

Individualized Educational Program: Total Service Plan

(Print)
1. Student's Name *Aloha*   *Jesse*   2. School Code ___ ___ ___
                        Last   First

3. Birthdate 12/29/88   4. Grade Pre-   5. Receiving School Name *Oahu*

6. Student's I.D. Number ___ ___ ___/___ ___ ___/___ ___ ___ ___   7. IEP Conference Date 9/5/92

8. IEP Anniversary Date 9/5/93   9. Class Index No. ___ ___ ___ ___

10. Type of Placement (check one):
    X 1. In special education class on regular school campus
    ___ 2. In special education school
    ___ 3. In regular class with itinerant services
    ___ 4. In contracted school
    ___ 5. Home/hospital instruction

11. Educational Arrangement (check one):
    X 1. Full-time self-contained
    ___ 2. Integrated self-contained
    ___ 3. Resource services
    ___ 4. Itinerant services
    ___ 5. Support services

13. Graduation Option: N.A.
    ___ 1. Certificate   ___ 2. Diploma

12. Related Service
    X 1. Transportation
    X 2. Speech/language therapy
    ___ 3. Occupational therapy
    X 4. Physical therapy
    ___ 5. School counselor services
    ___ 6. Mental health services
    ___ 7. Other: _____

14. Eligible for Extended School Year
    X 1. Yes   ___ 2. No

15. Identified as SLEP
    ___ 1. Yes   X 2. No

16. Reeval Date ___/___/___

Conference Participants
Name Ms. Barbara Williamson   Position Administrator/Designee
Name Ms. Judy Aloha   Position Mother
Name Mr. Henry Flores   Position Grandfather
Name Ms. Joanne Yamamoto   Position Teacher
Name Ms. Cheryl Kelly   Position Speech/language path.
Name Mrs. Nathan Pang   Position Occupational therapist
     Ms. Ann Akamine   Head Start coordinator

Record of Contact for IEP Conference:

Telephone Call Date(s) _____

047 Date(s) _____ RRR _____ PD _____

Personal Contact _____

Other _____

Figure 4-5   State of Hawaii's IEP forms

(continued)

Special Education/Related Support Services for Student

Services to Be Delivered	Implementation Date Reg. sch. yr. Summer prog.	Hours/Week Reg. sch. yr. Summer prog.	Anticipated Completion Date Reg. sch.yr. Summer prog.
Special Education			
Speech/Language Therapy			
Physical Therapy			
Transportation			

Extent of Student Participation in Regular Education Program: *Beginning August 1992, Jesse will spend mornings in a fully self-contained SPED classroom and afternoons in the Head Start Program (which has both morning and afternoon sessions on the school campus).*

Adaptations required for regular education classes: (if applicable)

None

Nature and extent of SLEP services:

None

Extended school year information:

Yes **X**   No _____   The standard for an extended school year has been applied, and the student (DOES)/DOES NOT meet the criteria for the extended school year.

Yes	No	
	NA	I have discussed graduation options and chosen: Diploma/IPP
X		I have been informed of my due process rights.
X		I agree with the IEP.
X		I would like to have a copy of the IEP.
X		Student attends the school he/she would attend if not disabled.
		(If NO justify: _____)
	NA	ITP developed (for students grade 9 or age 15 and above).
	NA	For terminal year students only: I understand that the receipt of a diploma will terminate special education services.

Judy Aloha   9/5/92   _____
Parent Signature (Optional)   Date   Student Signature (Optional)   Date

Figure 4-5—(continued)

Student's Name _Jesse Aloha_ _____ Date _____

Person(s) Responsible _____ Position _____

_____   _____

_____   _____

Present Levels of Performance
(only current data!)
(I. Achievement levels,   II. Speech/language,   III. Behavioral data,
IV. Learning style,   V. Medical data,   VI. Social/family information)

I. Achievement levels:

Cognitive development: Able to point to four body parts and circle and square when named. Sorts and matches objects by color (but not size or function). Follows directions for "in," "on," and "out." Understands same and different and big and little. Enjoys stories and finger-play songs. Demonstrates emerging understanding of one-to-one correspondence with three or four objects.

Functional motor skills: Sits alone with wide base of support (legs extended) and some swayback (lordosis). Shows good balance (equilibrium) reactions to all sides (front, sides, and back), and is able to use his hands freely in play. Moves in and out of standing independently and walks with a wide gait (sometimes "locking" or hyperextending knees) with arms raised for balance ("high guard"). Equilibrium reactions are not fully demonstrated in standing and sitting. Fine pincer grasp is demonstrated in play and finger feeding. Holds and marks with a crayon using an ulnar-palmer grasp. Hand preference is not evident.

Self-care skills: Feeds self with fingers. Just beginning to learn to handle a spoon. Good control of a cup or glass. He is not toilet trained but does let his parents or the teacher know when his diaper is soiled. Washes and dries his hands and face. Mother reports that he is beginning to try to wash himself when she is bathing him. Takes off his own shoes, socks, pants, and shirt but has not learned any dressing skills.

The Individualized Education Program is a statement of the services needed and of the anticipated goals and objectives. Unless your child requires summer programming as part of a free and appropriate public education, the Individualized Education Program will be in effect during the regular school year.

Figure 4-5—(continued)   _(continued)_

Present levels of performance (cont.)

II. Speech/language: Vocal quality, pitch, and volume are within normal levels. His speech is 80 to 90% intelligible. Language skills are delayed. He is able to name family members, favorite foods (cookie, juice, fries, pop [for popsicle]), some toys (turt [turtle], tuck [truck], ball, Batman), two animals (doggie, kitty), and function words (more, bye-bye, eat, all gone). Total expressive vocabulary is about 15 words. Receptive vocabulary is much larger. He responds to his name and follows one-step directions. He answers yes/no questions with a smile or a nod. No evidence of combining words, though he is using word-gesture combination—e.g., "more" said while holding out his cup, "bye-bye" while trying to turn the doorknob. Most verbalization is in response to a model or a question.

III. Behavioral data: Shows affection for familiar persons: hugs, smiles, etc. Generally plays alone but is beginning to watch other children play. Willing to share food and toys with a familiar adult but not with peers. Childcare teacher reports very little social interaction with peers; he is sometimes even actively resistant to activities that involve several other children.

IV. Learning style: Jesse adapts well to new situations (and new adults). When engaged in an activity of his choice, he does not seem to be distracted by other activities, sounds, or people. Personal choice of activity and adult attention appear to maximize his attention span. Jesse frequently imitates both peers and adults. He follows one-step verbal directions.

V. Medical data: Jesse has Down Syndrome. His only hospitalization since birth was at 8 months for pneumonia. With the exception of a mild heart defect and occasional ear infections, he is in good health.

VI. Social/family information: Jesse lives with both parents and a younger brother (16 months old). Both parents work.

2

Figure 4-5—(continued)

Individualized Education Program
Annual Goal/Progress Report

Name ___Jesse Aloha___

Date _____

Person(s) Responsible:

_____

_____

_____

Annual Goal # __1__   ESY Goal # ____

INCREASE GENERAL CONCEPT DEVELOPMENT.

_____

_____

_____

EVALUATION CODE:
NP- No Progress: No gains or improvements
P - Progress: Shows gains in learning the objectives
M - Mastered: Has learned the skills for objective
NA- Not Applicable: Objectives not yet covered

METHOD OF EVALUATION:
1 - Tests
2 - Observation, records
3 - Daily work
4 - Other _____

Short-Term Objectives:	Method of Evaluation	Progress Report				
		Q1	Q2	Q3	Q4	ESY
When given an example of what belongs in each group, Jesse will sort 10 or more familiar (functional) objects into 5 groups according to color.	2					
When given an example of what belongs in each group, Jesse will sort 10 or more familiar objects in 3 groups according to function.	2					
When given groups of objects of different colors, Jesse will indicate red, blue, and yellow objects.	2					
When given a direction, Jesse will demonstrate an understanding of **up, down, top,** and **bottom.**	2					
When given at least 3 different size objects, Jesse will select **big** or **little** objects on request, without errors.	2					

Comments:

Figure 4-5—(continued)

(continued)

Individualized Education Program
Annual Goal/Progress Report

Name _Jesse Aloha_

Date _____

Person(s) Responsible: _____

Annual Goal # **2**   ESY Goal # ____

INCREASE BALANCE IN STANDING AND WALKING.

_____

_____

EVALUATION CODE:
NP- No Progress: No gains or improvements
P - Progress: Shows gains in learning the objectives
M - Mastered: Has learned the skills for objective
NA- Not Applicable: Objectives not yet covered

METHOD OF EVALUATION:
1 - Tests
2 - Observation, records
3 - Daily work
4 - Other _____

Short-Term Objectives:	Method of Evaluation	Progress Report				
		Q1	Q2	Q3	Q4	ESY
Jesse will demonstrate walking balance when (a) walking backward at least 5 feet, and (b) walking forward on an uneven surface without falling.	2					
Jesse will demonstrate standing balance standing on one leg while putting on shoes or pants and walking up and down stairs without a rail.	2					
Jesse will demonstrate dynamic balance by kicking a ball at least 3 feet.	2					

Comments:

DISTRIBUTION: WHITE-File Copy; BLUE-1st Qtr.; GREEN-2nd Qtr.; CANARY-3rd Qtr. PINK-4th Qtr.; GOLDENROD-ESY   RS 91-0378

Figure 4-5—(continued)

Individualized Education Program
Annual Goal/Progress Report

Name _Jesse Aloha_   Person(s) Responsible:

Date _____

Annual Goal # _3_   ESY Goal # ____

INCREASE INDEPENDENT SELF-CARE SKILLS.

_____

_____

EVALUATION CODE:
NP - No Progress: No gains or improvements
P - Progress: Shows gains in learning the objectives
M - Mastered: Has learned the skills for objective
NA - Not Applicable: Objectives not yet covered

METHOD OF EVALUATION:
1 - Tests
2 - Observation, records
3 - Daily work
4 - Other _____

Short-Term Objectives:	Method of Evaluation	Progress Report				
		Q1	Q2	Q3	Q4	ESY
Jesse will independently eat an entire meal with a spoon (with minimal spilling).	2					
Jesse will pour liquid from a small pitcher into a cup (with minimal spilling).	2					
Jesse will independently put on his pants, T-shirt, sweater, socks, and shoes (without fasteners).	2					
Jesse will consistently indicate the need to toilet.	2					

Comments:

DISTRIBUTION: WHITE-File Copy; BLUE-1st Qtr.; GREEN-2nd Qtr.; CANARY-3rd Qtr. PINK-4th Qtr.; GOLDENROD-ESY   RS 91-0378

Figure 4-5—(continued)   *(continued)*

Individualized Education Program
Annual Goal/Progress Report

Name _Jesse Aloha_____ Person(s) Responsible:

Date _____ _____

_____

_____

Annual Goal # _4_   ESY Goal # ____

INCREASE LANGUAGE AND COMMUNICATION

SKILLS.

EVALUATION CODE:
NP- No Progress: No gains or improvements
P - Progress: Shows gains in learning the objectives
M - Mastered: Has learned the skills for objective
NA- Not Applicable: Objectives not yet covered

METHOD OF EVALUATION:
1 - Tests
2 - Observation, records
3 - Daily work
4 - Other _____

Short-Term Objectives:	Method of Evaluation	Progress Report				
		Q1	Q2	Q3	Q4	ESY
Jesse will use at least 50 words spontaneously (without a model or question).	2					
When asked "What is that?" Jesse will name at least 10 pictures in a familiar age-appropriate picture book.	2					
Jesse will use two-word combinations when requesting desired actions (e.g., "go bye-bye") or objects (e.g., "more juice").	2					
Jesse will ask at least 3 simple questions (e.g., "What doing?") a day.	2					
Jesse will use two-word combinations to indicate possession (e.g., "my truck") and nonexistence (e.g., "no juice").	2					

Comments:

DISTRIBUTION: WHITE-File Copy; BLUE-1st Qtr.; GREEN-2nd Qtr.; CANARY-3rd Qtr. PINK-4th Qtr.; GOLDENROD-ESY   RS 91-0378

Figure 4-5—(continued)

Individualized Education Program
Annual Goal/Progress Report

Name _Jesse Aloha_

Date _____

Person(s) Responsible:

_____

_____

_____

Annual Goal # _5_   ESY Goal # ____

DEVELOP PEER-RELATED SOCIAL SKILLS.

_____

_____

_____

EVALUATION CODE:
  NP - No Progress: No gains or improvements
  P - Progress: Shows gains in learning the objectives
  M - Mastered: Has learned the skills for objective
  NA - Not Applicable: Objectives not yet covered

METHOD OF EVALUATION:
  1 - Tests
  2 - Observation, records
  3 - Daily work
  4 - Other _____

Short-Term Objectives:	Method of Evaluation	Progress Report				
		Q1	Q2	Q3	Q4	ESY
Jesse will share food or toys (either spontaneously or when asked) with peers on at least three occasions.	2					
Jesse will take turns with peers when requested.	2					
Jesse will participate in small-group activities with peers.	2					
Jesse will consistently play alongside peers (using the same or similar play materials).	2					

Comments:

DISTRIBUTION: WHITE-File Copy; BLUE-1st Qtr.; GREEN-2nd Qtr.; CANARY-3rd Qtr. PINK-4th Qtr.; GOLDENROD-ESY   RS 91-0378

Figure 4-5—(continued)

differences in procedures associated with the different plans. One difference (not necessarily a desirable one) is that the IEP tends to be a more static document because it must be completed before programming can officially begin. Thus, the IEP seems more like a product than a continuous process. Another difference is that there is no requirement that the IEP address the strengths and resources of the family: the focus is exclusively on the child. Also there is no requirement that a service coordinator be designated and there are no specific regulatory requirements related to inclusion of transition planning (except at the secondary level).

Formulating Goals and Objectives

The most challenging task facing the IEP committee is drafting annual goals and short-term objectives. First, all of the assessment information must be assembled, summarized, and interpreted. The focus is not on scores or the child's developmental age, but rather on what the child knows and can do and how the child learns best. For preschoolers, it is important to describe (a) specific skills that are mastered in each domain, (b) skills that are in the process of being acquired, and (c) needed skills. Here is an example of a present level of performance statement in speech, language and communication for Brendyn, a 3-year-old with severe disabilities:

> Brendyn communicates primarily with facial expressions (smiling or frowning), crying or laughing, looking or looking away, and pointing with his whole hand. There are three occasions when Brendyn *may* vocalize: (a) when someone is talking to him, (b) when trying to get someone's attention, or (c) when asked to say his name. Brendyn communicates clearly when he wants to terminate an interaction—he looks away, cries or frowns.
>
> Brendyn's receptive vocabulary is between 30 and 45 words. He knows family members, three primary colors, teachers, his own first and last names, names of favorite foods, and objects used in routine activities at home and in his preschool classroom.
>
> Oral-motor assessment indicates that Brendyn has little head control: He is unable to hold his head in midline for more than 5 seconds. His respiration is labored. He keeps his tongue to the back of his mouth, obstructing his airways.

If caregivers and other family members have not been active participants in the assessment process, this is the time to elicit their observations and insights concerning their child's skills, motivators, and interests. They should be encouraged to talk about what they see as important skill needs and what they observe to be their child's strengths.

Collaborative Goal-Setting.   Too often in the past, caregivers and sometimes even the receiving teacher walked into the IEP meeting to find that considerable time had already been committed to drafting goals and objectives. This is unfortunate, and counter to the intent of PL 94-142. Fortunately, this practice is becoming less common. The task of formulating goals and objectives should have the maximum participation of the family and both sending and receiving teachers. The term for parents, teachers, and other team members jointly determining intervention goals and strategies is *collaborative goal setting* (Bailey, 1987). The concept is applicable to goal setting for both the IFSP and the IEP.

for school age ch. as well?

Goals and objectives, particularly those on a child's first IEP, are hypotheses (McCormick, 1990b). They are educated guesses (based on as much data as can be collected in the available time) about what the child can and cannot do, and what appear to be the child's most critical needs in order to participate in present and future environments.

There are two ways to generate goals and objectives from assessment findings: a top-down approach and a bottom-up approach (Snell, 1987). The bottom-up approach uses information about the child's present performance in each developmental area to generate goals and objectives. Goals will typically be the next skills in whatever sequence is used (either a task analysis or a list of developmental milestones). The top-down approach uses information concerning the skill requirements of activities and expectations in present and future environments to generate goals and objectives. With this approach, goals and objectives are selected on the basis of their functionality and their ability to maximize participation in ongoing tasks.

The bottom-up and top-down approaches both have value; they can complement one another. The top-down approach may be used to identify the activities (circle time, snack time, cooking in the preschool classroom) the child needs to learn in order to participate in important natural environments such as the home and the preschool. A task or activity analysis is then completed with these activities and the bottom-up approach is used to determine the child's status and needs relative to the skills required to increase participation in the activities. Goals and objectives for the child reflect those skills on the task analysis the child needs to master. Table 4-3 provides some guidelines to help in developing goals and objectives.

Goals and objectives differ in their specificity. Goals tend to be very broad. They identify the skill area that will be the focus of instruction. Consider this example:

> Susannah is a 4-year-old with Down syndrome. Despite very obvious enjoyment of interactions with adults, she seems to avoid peer encounters. She initiates interactions and expresses her wants and needs to adults (primarily with gestures and one- or two-word utterances) but does not approach peers. Staff of the childcare center where Susannah goes after preschool and the preschool staff completed an informal social behavior rating scale that indicates she always plays alone or stands watching on the outskirts of an activity. Her parents also report concern that she never plays with other children (and in fact, runs away when children approach her at Sunday School and other settings). The parents and other members of the team decide that increasing social interactions with peers is a priority

---

TABLE 4-3

Guidelines for Developing Goals and Objectives

---

1. **Begin by identifying skills that are partially acquired or skills that are demonstrated in some contexts but not others.**
   Target mastery of these skills and provide practice in all natural environments.

2. **Identify skills that will permit the child to participate in routine daily activities with nonhandicapped peers.**
   If the child's disability prevents mastery of skills for full participation, target adaptations or alternative skills for full participation or partial participation.

3. **Determine skills that would be instrumental in accomplishing the greatest number of other skills or functional tasks.**
   These are tool skills which, while they may not be immediately functional, will yield results over time.

4. **Identify skills the child is highly motivated to learn.**
   Look for evidence of interest. The motivation for learning is there if the child is interested in particular topics or activities. For example, if the child always watches peers on the jungle gym or using the computer, or if the child always heads straight for the crafts table, consider ways to provide instruction in these activity contexts.

5. **Identify skills that will increase opportunities for interactions with nondisabled peers.**
   Target behaviors (social, communication, motor, or self-care) that will result in the child's being viewed more positively by peers and thus increase positive interactions with peers.

6. **Identify skills that will increase participation in future environments.**
   Target skills that will increase options for participation in future environments.

---

for Susannah, not only because of the importance of social competence but also because peer social interactions are an important context for language learning.

It is clear that one of the goals on Susannah's IEP should be *increased appropriate interactions with peers.* The next step, then, is to formulate instructional objectives for this goal.

Writing Instructional Objectives.   Instructional objectives (also called behavioral objectives or short-term objectives) are more specific than goals. Instructional objectives should have three components: (a) a *definition* or *description* of the target behavior, (b) a specification of the *conditions* under which the desired behavior will occur, and (c) the *criterion* or *standard* for judging the adequacy of the behavior once it is performed (Mager, 1962). Criteria may be expressed as quantity (how much of the behavior will be required) or quality (how well the behavior is to be performed).

What constitutes a good objective? Wolery, Bailey, and Sugai (1988) say it should be *appropriate* and it should have good *form*. They note that an objective is appropriate if it is (a) functional and realistic, (b) directed toward generalization, and (c) socially and educationally valid. To be functional and socially and educationally valid, an objective must be directed to improving the child's functioning in present environments and facilitating transition to and participation in age-appropriate future environments (Voeltz & Evans, 1983; Wolf, 1978).

To have good form an objective must have the requisite three components (conditions, behavior, and criterion), describe a subskill of the goals (rather than simply restating the goal), state the conditions as exact circumstances under which the desired behavior will occur, describe the desired behavior in observable terms, and state a precise performance standard that addresses the relevant dimension of the behavior. Here are the objectives that accompany Susannah's goal of increased appropriate interactions with peers:

> Susannah will initiate at least two verbal requests to join an ongoing activity during the preschool free play or recess periods.
> Susannah will play cooperatively with a peer at recess for at least 5 minutes on three consecutive days.
> Susannah will take turns and share materials with a peer during at least five consecutive snack preparation sessions.

The next step is to decide what strategies, procedures, and materials will help Susannah achieve the instructional objectives and how progress will be monitored. These tasks are the responsibility of the transdisciplinary intervention team, which is typically composed of one or more teachers, parents, and appropriate related services personnel. Specifically, the intervention team decides (a) what to teach in order to attain the stated objectives; (b) how to modify or adapt curriculum content, materials, and procedures; (c) how to arrange the environment to facilitate skill acquisition; and (d) how to ensure generalization. These decisions are discussed in subsequent chapters.

Summary

Effective planning incorporates information about the child and conditions in the child's various natural environments (preschool classroom, childcare setting, home) that have the potential to facilitate skill development and maintenance. This chapter has dealt with two broad areas: preschool assessment and developing the IEP. Guidelines were provided to assist in developing goals and objectives.

Activities

1. Contact your state Department of Education for a copy of the eligibility criteria for preschool children. Compare eligibility for the birth-to-3 population in your state with eligibility criteria for services for 3- and 4-year-olds.

2. Contact at least three school districts in your state for copies of their IEP forms. Compare the forms as to information requirements, ease of completion, and sensitivity to family participation.

3. Talk with at least two professionals (teachers or therapists) who routinely assess young children for the purpose of planning intervention goals. List the types of procedures (tests, observations, interviews) and what specific instruments they find most useful.

4. Develop a "family-friendly" form (similar to Na Lei Kamali'i in Chapter 3) for collecting the type of information from parents that is delineated in the "Ecological Information" section of the chapter.

Review Questions

1. Discuss the following issues related to assessment: (a) criteria for eligibility for services at the preschool level, (b) misuse of test results, (c) psychometric problems, (d) judgment-based assessment, and (e) assessment modifications.

2. State the objectives for assessment for intervention planning in the naturalistic curriculum model.

3. Describe procedures for assessment in each area: social, speech, language and communication, cognitive, motor, self-care, and ecological.

4. Differentiate and provide an example of the four most commonly used direct observation recording systems.

5. State the key components of the IEP.

6. Contrast the top-down and the bottom-up approaches for generating goals and objectives and suggest how to reconcile the two.

7. Describe how goals and objectives are formulated and specify criteria for what constitutes good objectives.

Naturalistic Curriculum Model

1. *Describe and compare the traditional curriculum models in early intervention.*

2. *Discuss naturalistic trends in early intervention curricula.*

3. *Describe the content, instructional methods, and evaluation methods of the naturalistic curriculum model.*

4. *Discuss the requirements that the content of the naturalistic curriculum model be age appropriate and reflect developmentally appropriate practice.*

5. *Identify and describe the eight steps in implementing the naturalistic curriculum model.*

C urriculum can be defined in at least three ways. Most often, curriculum is defined as an organized and sequenced set of *content* to be taught: It is the "what to teach" (Bailey et al., 1983; Hanson & Lynch, 1989). In the second approach to defining curriculum, the *instructional techniques,* or the "how to teach," is added to the first definition: curriculum is defined as content and teaching techniques ("what and how to teach"). And third, sometimes content is not specified and curriculum is defined by the *process* for deriving content and planning instruction, rather than specific content and procedures. In this chapter, curriculum includes all three definitions: the instructional content, instructional techniques, and the process for deriving content and planning instruction.

The curriculum models that have characterized early intervention for infants and young children with special needs are (a) the developmental model, (b) the developmental-cognitive model, and (c) the behavioral model (Bailey, Jens & Johnson, 1983; Hanson & Lynch, 1989). These models are continually evolving and being modified to be more immediately relevant to the needs of young children and their families. The most recent modifications focus on the infant/young child interacting with the social and physical environment—naturalistic considerations. This chapter briefly reviews traditional curriculum models. The naturalistic components of the models are then synthesized and presented as a naturalistic curriculum model for early intervention. Finally, this chapter provides recommendations for implementation of a naturalistic curriculum model.

Traditional Curriculum Models

The *developmental curriculum model* is the original early intervention curriculum model. It was borrowed from the enrichment models of programs serving disadvantaged children in the 1960s (for example, Head Start and the Portage Project). It is sometimes referred to as an enrichment model because early childhood programs for disadvantaged children attempted to enhance or "enrich" the experiences of children living in poverty, and thereby give them an experiential foundation similar to their peers living in more economically privileged circumstances. In early intervention, the goal of the developmental model is to assist infants and young children with disabilities to progress through the normal sequences of development.

The developmental model is primarily a content model. The content consists of sequences of physical development (gross motor and fine motor), adaptive development (self-help and daily living skills), social development, and communication development based on child growth and maturation studies (cf. Gesell & Amatruda, 1947). Instructional strategies attempt to simulate activities engaged in by nondisabled infants, toddlers, and preschoolers. The activities provide opportunities for demonstrating or encouraging the targeted milestones (Furuno et al., 1979; Johnson, Jens & Attermeier, 1979).

The *developmental-cognitive model* is a theory-driven model based on the work of Jean Piaget. The Piagetian model is constructivist (biological and environmental interactionist). Piaget theorized that cognitive development occurs as a result of physiological growth and the child's interaction with the environment.

The developmental-cognitive model is defined by content and instructional technique. The content is similar to the developmental model but emphasizes the domain of cognitive skills. The cognitive domain consists of skill sequences derived from Piaget's description of the sensorimotor period of intellectual development (birth through age 2) (Piaget, 1952; 1954). Assessment and selection of cognitive goals typically rely on the *Scales of Psychological Development* (Uzgiris & Hunt, 1975). The scales address five separate areas of early cognitive development: object permanence (learning that objects exist even when they are not in sight), means for obtaining environmental ends (learning to use objects or activities as tools to accomplish a goal), causality (learning that people or mechanics can make things happen), imitation (learning to model verbal and gestural behavior), and schemes (learning to manipulate or interact with objects appropriate to the nature of the objects).

Instructional techniques emphasize Piaget's constructivist theory: tasks that are "challenging" are presented to create a state of "disequilibrium." Organization and adaptation occur as the child attempts to resolve the challenge that the task produces ("equilibration"). In the seventies, this model was applied to early intervention by the Brickers (Bricker & Bricker, 1976) and to compensatory education (Weikart, Rogers, Adcock & McClelland, 1971).

The *behavioral curriculum model* is primarily an instructional techniques model. It is based on the learning principles of behavioral psychology. Behaviorists such as B. F. Skinner, Sidney Bijou, and Donald Baer describe human development and learning as resulting from environmental interactions that allow individuals to experience the relationships among stimuli, actions, and the consequences of actions (reinforcement or punishment). Direct instruction procedures of prompting, shaping, or reinforcing are implemented in a precise and consistent fashion. Skill acquisition is monitored through frequent data collection, and program modifications are made based on the evaluation of child progress data. Instead of following developmental sequences for curricular content, behavioral interventionists apply remedial (or "functional") logic to the selection of skills, criteria that require targeted skills to be age-appropriate, meaningful, and immediately useful (Guess & Noonan, 1982).

Professionals who are familiar with the three curriculum models will realize that these descriptions are oversimplified. Today all three models are evolving toward a naturalistic focus.

Naturalistic Trends

Specific naturalistic trends are evident with each of the traditional curriculum models. The developmentalists have broadened their focus to include an emphasis on child/caregiver interaction. Infant and early childhood behaviors are interpreted in the context of cyclical interactions with the caregiver—infant behavior affects caregiver behavior, which in turn affects infant behavior, and the cycle continues. As a cyclical process, infant/child *and* parent behaviors are considered as the appropriate unit of focus for assessment and instruction. The shift of the developmentalists to a more naturalistic perspective is philosophically compatible with the recent conceptualization of early intervention as "family-focused." Goals and instruction involve the infant and the caregivers/family within the family system, not only the infant.

The developmental-cognitive model has broadened to include a strong social development component. This perspective is based largely on the work of Jerome Bruner, a psycholinguist (Bruner, 1975; 1977; Ratner & Bruner, 1978). Bruner describes early social skills as "social-cognitive" behaviors that serve a prelinguistic function. Such skills include following an adult's line of regard (the infant's gaze shifts to look where the adult is looking), joint attention (adult and infant demonstrate concurrent sustained attention to the same object/activity), and turn taking.

The developmental-cognitive model now also includes a concern for environmental control (Beckman, Robinson, Jackson & Rosenberg, 1986; Dunst et al., 1987; McCollum & Stayton, 1985). Environmental control is response-contingent learning: infants and young children learn that their behavior has a predictable effect on their social and physical environments. Environmental control is significant because it decreases children's dependency on adults to identify and meet their needs. Instruction to teach environmental control teaches parents to attend to their infant/child's subtle ways of responding to environmental stimuli and reinforce behaviors that might serve an environmental control function. For example, if an infant winces when a spoon of food is presented, the parent might withdraw the food saying, "Oh, you don't want any more of that right now," and give the child some milk instead. Thus, the child learns that expressing displeasure by wincing controls the environment: the unwanted food is withdrawn.

For the behavioral model, the shift to a naturalistic perspective in early intervention is evident in goal selection and instructional procedures. Goal selection is referenced to environmental demands or expectations. One method to determine environmental demands is a parent interview that asks parents or caregivers and other family members to describe family routines, the child's participation in these routines, and what they would like the child to learn to better participate in family routines (Falvey, 1989; Kilgo, Richard & Noonan, 1989).

Instructional techniques in the behavioral model are gradually shifting from a focus on teacher-directed discrete skill training to more naturalistic procedures. Rather than teaching skills in isolation, they are taught in sequence with other skills as they would typically occur (Sailor & Guess, 1983), at the times when they are needed (Hart & Risley, 1978), using natural stimuli and consequences (Falvey, Brown, Lyon, Baumgart & Schroeder, 1980), and with strategies that promote independent, child-initiated behaviors (Halle, 1982). For example, instead of teaching a preschooler to use two-word phrases by looking at picture cards and describing them, two-word phrases are taught throughout the day in free play, snack time, circle time, and story time when the child initiates speech.

The shift to a generalization focus in the behavioral model has resulted in planning for generalization when new skills are initially taught. Instructional procedures referred to as "general case" methods facilitate generalization by targeting generalization in the objective, and providing instruction in several situations where the skill is needed (Horner & McDonald, 1982; Horner, Sprague & Wilcox, 1982). For example, the toddler who has difficulty with finger feeding because of poor fine motor skills has an objective to improve grasping (not just finger feeding), and is taught to grasp many small objects of various weights and shapes.

As the developmental, developmental-cognitive, and behavioral models gradually shift to a naturalistic perspective, each model is incorporating some of the naturalistic strategies and perspectives of the other models. The boundaries that differentiate these models are becoming blurred. The next section describes what might be termed a composite naturalistic model.

A Naturalistic Model

In addition to the naturalistic modifications occurring in early intervention curricula, there are other indications that the field is moving toward more environmentally focused early intervention. In a 1988 article on best practices in early intervention, McDonnell & Hardman recommended the following:

1. Reference curriculum to the unique needs and lifestyle of the child, family, peers, and community;
2. Plan instruction that can be implemented naturally in daily family routines;
3. Emphasize skills that are functional now and in the future.

The first recommendation of referencing curriculum to the child, family, peers, and community addresses the social aspects of the environment. Each child's social environment is unique: an individually tailored curriculum is responsive to the characteristics/needs associated with that social environment. The second recommendation is that instruction be conducted during the daily activities in natural settings. Instruction within daily activities eliminates the need to transfer newly acquired skills from an artificial teaching setting (such as the infant program center) to the home and community settings where the skill is actually needed (a difficulty for many youngsters with special needs). Bricker (1989) calls this *activity-based instruction*. The third recommendation, emphasis on skills with present and future utility, expands the early intervention curricular focus to include skills that facilitate participation in current and future environments. These three best practices are inherent in the naturalistic curriculum model.

The major goal of the naturalistic curriculum model is to increase the infant/young child's control, participation, and interaction in natural social and physical environments. The naturalistic model is primarily a process model, with content and instructional techniques derived through environmental analysis. The instructional techniques are based largely on naturalistic behavioral techniques. The remainder of this chapter describes the major components of instruction in the naturalistic curriculum model: content, context, methods, and evaluation.

Content of Instruction

In the naturalistic curriculum, goals for each infant/young child are developed on an individual basis, reflecting the skill demands of natural, age-appropriate environments. The content "grows with the child" and is responsive to the requirements of the increasing number of environments that infants/young children participate in as they get older.

Age-Appropriate Skills. Content that is age appropriate features skills and activities typically engaged in by infants and young children who are not disabled. In traditional curriculum models, only the behavioral model emphasizes the age appropriateness of content; the developmental and developmental-cognitive models prescribe content that corresponds to the developmental level of the infant/young child, regardless of the child's age.

The naturalistic model encourages participation and interaction across the full range of family routines and activities. Specific routines and activities are of particular importance at certain ages during the early childhood years. For neonates, the most important aspect of the environment is parent-infant interactions. During interactions, infants monitor input and learn selective responsiveness. Infants "control" their environment through behavior that effects the quality and quantity of incoming stimulation. This is one of the first ways infants learn to affect their environments.

The work of Brazelton has been particularly influential in highlighting infant control of the environment (Als, Lester & Brazelton, 1979; Brazelton, 1982). Brazelton describes how the newborn engages in a neurological and physiological system of interaction, disorganization, reorganization, and then, a return to interaction. As infants attend to and interact with the environment, they eventually become overstimulated. This overstimulation causes neuromotor and physiological disorganization. When disorganization occurs, the infant may fuss or cry and withdraw from the environment by looking away or falling asleep. Withdrawing from the environment allows the infant to reorganize neurologically and physiologically and reestablish homeostasis and energy/drive for subsequent environmental input when desired.

Parents must learn to recognize their infant's signals and determine when their interactions are appropriate and when the infant has received adequate stimulation and needs to rest. Infant specialists may observe the infant/caregiver dyad and provide feedback or reinforcement when the parent or caregiver shows sensitivity or responsiveness to the infant's behavior and effectively obtains or maintains the infant's attention. In this way, parents learn to become responsive to their infant, and the infant learns age-appropriate social interaction skills.

A successful parent-infant interaction is one in which there is mutual responsiveness, with the parent and infant each responding in accordance to the signals of the other. For example, when the parent coos at the infant, the infant stops moving and stares at the parent. The parent pauses, and coos again; the infant again shows intent interest. The cycle is repeated several times. Then the infant looks away and wiggles a bit. The parent recognizes these behaviors as signals that the baby has tired of the game and needs a rest from interaction, ceases the interaction, and rocks and cuddles the baby gently.

As an infant gets a bit older, there is increased interaction with the physical environment, and the social environment expands beyond parents to include siblings, relatives, and family friends. Environmentally referenced curriculum will include a wider range of behaviors to accomplish environmental interaction and control, with many in the interrelated domains of social, cognitive, and communication skills. For example, the infant may demonstrate environmental control by crying when a sibling takes a toy away, which results in the parent returning the toy to the infant.

During the infant's first year, the infant learns the turn-taking and signaling skills that form the basis of later social and communication interactions. Like the other sensorimotor behaviors in Piaget's model, social-cognitive skills develop in a progression leading to mental representation (thinking) and the establishment of the symbolic function—that is, the ability to use words to represent thoughts and actions (Seibert & Hogan, 1982; Seibert, Hogan & Mundy, 1982; 1987). When parents respond to an infant's vocalizations as a request to repeat a playful episode, they are teaching the infant that the vocalization is a signal to communicate "do it again." For example, the parents' pause after a playful episode, the infant's communicative signal, and the repetition of the play is a turn-taking routine, much like the turn taking involved in conversation. Typical play behaviors of infants also involve environmental interaction and control. As an infant explores a wide variety of objects and toys, the infant learns how to make the objects work and thus learns the function and mechanical properties of objects.

During the toddler years, the young child's play expands in sophistication, and the child begins to show an interest in the play of other children. Toddlers participate increasingly in the routines of other family members, sometimes as play (for example, sweeping with a toy broom as the father sweeps the kitchen floor), and sometimes as a contributing member of the family (as when the young child carries a dish to the table, or takes a turn rolling a ball with a sibling). Much of a toddler's participation in routines and activities in the home involves adaptive development activities, such as dressing or bathing. Initially, participation may be in the form of cooperation: lying still while having a diaper changed, or raising arms as a T-shirt is removed. Toddlers begin to learn the survival skills that will allow them to participate in preschool, many of which are group participation skills (following simple directions, sharing, attending to a task or speaker). And finally, during the preschool and kindergarten years, play, self-help, and survival skills take on even greater importance.

The current emphasis in early childhood curriculum for infants/young children who are not disabled is a model referred to as *developmentally appropriate practice* (DAP) (Bredekamp, 1987). There are two components to DAP: age appropriateness and individualization. Early childhood programs that ascribe to developmentally appropriate practice emphasize a child-centered curriculum characterized by individual choice making and exploratory play, rather than a teacher-directed, structured curriculum with a specific set of objectives identified for all children. The DAP model is based on the assumption that, if children are allowed to explore their interests, their interests will guide them to choose and learn content that they are developmentally "ready" to learn.

Infants and young children with severe disabilities, however, will not always be "ready" to learn the same activities as their nondisabled or mildly disabled age peers. To support the integration of disabled and nondisabled infants and young children, however, curricular activities should be age appropriate, even when the activities do not correspond to readiness levels. The activities should serve as a context for instruction. Specific objectives, or the way in which children with disabilities participate in activities, are individualized to address unique needs. Allowing for different types and levels of participation in the early childhood curriculum is consistent with the basic tenents of DAP: curriculum should be age appropriate *and* individualized. For example, a preschool child who is disabled selects a puzzle during morning free play and hands the pieces one at a time to a peer who puts the puzzle together. She has chosen an age-appropriate activity that is also of interest to her nondisabled friend. Although not able to assemble the puzzle, she is able to select puzzle pieces and to play cooperatively with a peer. Chapters 10 and 11 provide numerous strategies and examples for promoting peer interaction and independence in age-appropriate activities and integrated settings.

In summary, the age-appropriate content of the naturalistic curriculum model includes the skills needed by the infant and young child to participate in natural social and physical environments. These environments expand as the infant grows and develops, and the content of the naturalistic curriculum model expands accordingly to address the increasing range of behaviors needed for control, participation, and interaction. When a discrepancy exists between age appropriateness and readiness level, adapt the age-appropriate content to the child's abilities and needs.

Skills for Participating in Present and Future Environments.   In the developmental and developmental-cognitive models, content is identified by assessing the infant/young child against developmental skill sequences; instruction begins where the infant/young child fails to demonstrate a skill in the normal sequences of development. The behaviorists identify curricular content by selecting skills that are age appropriate, necessary, and useful for immediate functioning. There is no organized system for selecting the content in the behavioral model. The naturalistic model selects curricular content by identifying and analyzing the routines and activities of natural environments.

There are a number of ways to approach the identification and analysis of routines and activities. One method is an interview with parents or caregivers (sometimes referred to as an *ecological inventory*). They are asked to describe their daily routines and activities and the infant's or young child's present participation in these routines and activities. Potential goals and objectives are formulated as each routine and activity is discussed. The parent interview approach to curriculum development was first described in the Individualized Critical Skills Model, a community-based curriculum model for students with severe disabilities (Savage, 1983).

The parent interview approach to developing individualized curricular content is child-, family-, and cultural-specific. The routines and activities identified in the interview will reflect a child's capabilities, interests, and temperament. For example, a child recovering from a hospital stay may play for short periods of time only, and may play only with one or two other children to avoid roughhousing. In contrast, another child may enjoy roughhousing and show the greatest amount of participation with large groups of children.

The uniqueness of each family is reflected in the parent interview and thereby influences the content derived through this process. Routines and activities will vary from one family to another depending on such factors as family members present in the home, work and/or school responsibilities, social/recreational interests and preferences, interpersonal needs and strengths, and so on. Finally, culture will be reflected in the family's lifestyle, and likewise reflected in the daily routines and activities from which curricular content is derived. For example, culture might influence family member roles (who does what chores), arrangements for mealtimes and sleeping, and the extent and nature of participation in social or religious activities.

A second approach to identifying content referenced to the demands of the environment is the survival skills approach. Survival skills assessments and curricula are based on skills that early childhood educators expect or require of young children in childcare, preschool, or kindergarten settings (McCormick & Kawate, 1982; Murphy & Vincent, 1989; Noonan et al., 1992; Vincent et al., 1980). These assessments and curricula provide guidelines as to what skills are likely to be important in the "next environment" (Vincent et al., 1980). The survival skills studies employed in the development of these assessments and curricula are significant because the skills found to be critical for success in subsequent early childhood environments are mostly social and adaptive skills, rather than the preacademic skills previously thought to be necessary for success. For infants, the focus of survival skills is on childcare or preschool survival skills; for toddlers, survival skills focus on skills needed for preschool; and for preschoolers, kindergarten skills are the focus.

As discussed in Chapter 13, survival skills are not a complete curriculum. They are a portion of a naturalistic curriculum that focuses on facilitating success in

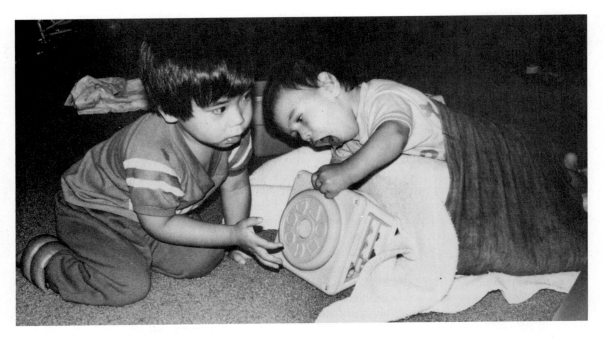

Family interactions are included in a naturalistic curriculum.

early childhood childcare or education settings that typically serve infants and young children who do not have special needs. As a portion of a naturalistic curriculum, survival skills should be considered in conjunction with naturalistic curriculum procedures that are more comprehensive in scope (for example, the parent interview).

The naturalistic model includes early intervention goals derived from the developmental and developmental-cognitive curriculum models. Developmental goals are included in early childhood assessment and curriculum development if they serve as appropriate evaluation measures and result in meaningful, age-appropriate objectives. These conditions would often be met in providing services to infants/young children who are at risk or who have mild delays/disabilities, the majority of children served in most early intervention programs. Developmental assessments may not be appropriate as evaluation measures or curriculum assessments for infants/young children with severe or multiple disabilities because meaningful changes in performance often will not involve the achievement of milestones, nor are developmental sequences necessarily the most efficient sequences for instruction (Baer, 1970). Instead, skill adaptations may be more practical goals for achieving age-appropriate and functional skills for these children.

Context for Instruction

Context is an element of the naturalistic model that differentiates it from other early intervention curriculum models. The naturalistic model focuses on *natural contexts* (social and physical environments) for determining the content of instruction, selecting and implementing the instructional methods, and evaluating child progress. In contrast, the developmental and developmental-cognitive models match curriculum to the present functioning levels of infants and young children. Only minimal consideration is given to the relationship between child goals and the environment. While the behavioral model requires that goals be functional and needed in the natural environment, the model lacks scope and sequence. Instead, it relies on the developmental scope and sequence, selecting goals that are functional or that can be recast into functional goals.

In the naturalistic model, curricular content is identified by assessing the skill requirements of relevant environments (for example, home, neighborhood, and childcare). Thus, the environment is the source of content. Once curricular goals are identified, the infant/young child's functioning relative to each goal is assessed in the natural environments. The environment is the assessment site. Finally, following goal identification and assessment, natural environments for teaching the skill are specified for the objective, instruction, and ongoing evaluation.

As an example of the importance of the environment in the naturalistic curriculum model, consider a 2-year-old named Missy who attends an early intervention toddler group once a week. The toddler group usually consists of five 2-year-olds who participate together in circle time, a physical development activity, and a snack. Missy plays with the other children and follows the simple rules of the activities, such as passing toys and taking turns. Observation in the home and reports from the family, however, indicate that Missy is usually on the sidelines watching as her two sisters (ages 4 and 5) play. Missy's parents would like her to play with her sisters. Note that the home environment provides very different information than the intervention program environment regarding Missy's social and play skills. An instructional plan is designed to reflect the characteristics of the home environment. Given that the home environment includes Missy's 4- and 5-year-old siblings, the instructional plan is directed at the play behavior of the siblings as well as Missy: Missy's sisters are taught to invite Missy to play with them and are shown various ways that Missy can join in, even when she doesn't know how to play their games; and Missy is taught to crawl close to her sisters when she wants to play with them. The success of instruction is evaluated in the home, during after-school hours, and on the weekends when the sisters typically play together. In all phases of this instruction—goal selection, instruction, and evaluation—the context has a significant influence.

For newborns, the most important environment is probably the home environment where most of their social interactions occur. As the infant develops beyond the first few months of life, the infant increasingly attends to environmental stimuli, including objects. The social interaction context of the family also expands and begins to include the extended family and friends. In the toddler and preschool years, the physical environment broadens to include a wide range of environments in and outside the home, such as the neighborhood, playgrounds and parks, and shopping centers. Young children interact extensively with objects in their environment and are becoming more and more independent in their interactions. Their social sphere now includes peers, as well as neighbors and family members of all ages.

To summarize, the context for instruction in the naturalistic curriculum model is the natural environment. Natural environments are the source of curricular content, as well as the instructional environments. The number and variety of natural environments expand as infants and young children grow.

Instructional Methods

The traditional curriculum models are characterized by instructional methods that are adult-directed and artificial in appearance. The developmental model provides activities appropriate to the child's developmental level. Assistance is given as needed, and the infant/young child is guided through activities. In the developmental-cognitive model, activities are again provided that are appropriate to the child's level of development. If the infant/young child needs assistance, the infant specialist or teacher demonstrates how the child might begin playing with the materials or attempts to arouse the child's curiosity and thereby motivate the child to interact with the materials. The purpose of the developmental-cognitive activities is to solve the "problem" presented by the materials, so direct guidance is not usually provided. Neither the developmental nor the developmental-cognitive curriculum models include strategies to promote skill generalization beyond the instructional environment.

In contrast, procedures to promote generalization are emphasized in the naturalistic curriculum model. The naturalistic model uses instructional methods that are minimally intrusive—that is, instruction that looks like naturally occurring events. Etzel and LeBlanc (1979) describe these instructional procedures as following the *principle of parsimony*. The principle of parsimony states that instruction should be no more complex than necessary to be effective.

Instructional Procedures for Newborns.   During the neonatal period, while curricular content focuses on parent-infant interaction, the primary instructional procedure is to observe parent-infant interaction and provide positive and descriptive feedback when the parent responds appropriately to the infant's signals. For example, a father holds his 1-month-old infant son on his lap and speaks to him. His son stares intently at him for several minutes. Then the infant looks away and begins to wiggle. The father interprets these behaviors as signals that his son is tired of the interaction. He stops talking to his son, picks him up, and carries him around the room to soothe him. The infant specialist praises the father for responding immediately to his son's signals, noting that parent behaviors such as these are instructional for the neonate, reinforcing the neonate's attempts to control the environment.

Instructional Procedures for Infants. For infants beyond the first few months, a number of early interventionists suggest instructional techniques similar to Brazelton's (Als, Lester & Brazelton, 1979; Brazelton, 1982), but focused on a larger repertoire of interactions, compatible with broadening social experiences (Beckman, Robinson, Jackson & Rosenberg, 1986; Dunst et al., 1987; McCollum & Stayton, 1985). For example, Dunst and colleagues (1987) suggest the following instructional procedures to assist the infant in gaining control over the environment and to teach parents to be more effective in participating and encouraging social interactions:

1. Sensitivity to the child's behavior,
2. Reading the child's behavior as intents to interact,
3. Responsiveness to the child's initiations,
4. Encouraging ongoing initiations,
5. Supporting and encouraging competence.

These procedures are operationalized through methods such as (a) guided learning, (b) violations of expectations, (c) introduction of novelty (Dunst, 1981), and (d) incidental teaching (Hart & Risley, 1978).

In *guided learning,* play or instructional situations are carefully arranged so that the situation attracts the infant's attention, appears highly motivating, and is at a level of difficulty that is optimally challenging. An example of guided learning is to present a 10-month old, who explores objects by banging them, with a variety of objects (such as a wooden spoon, metal spoon or whisk broom) and a variety of surfaces for banging (for example, a metal tray, wicker basket, or magazine). The situation is enticing to the infant because she enjoys banging objects, and the availability of several objects and surfaces is challenging. The environmental arrangement of the task guides learning. It also reflects sensitivity to the infant's present levels of performance, encourages the infant to initiate and participate in the activity without adult instruction, and supports and encourages competence.

The procedure of *violating expectations* requires that a predictable and repetitive play sequence be established. The sequence is then altered without warning. Violations of expectations surprise the infant, often increasing the infant's attention and curiosity (motivation), and stimulating a communicative response (a quizzical look at the adult, a vocalization or laugh), as if to say "What happened?" An adult who covers and uncovers her smiling face repeatedly with a cloth in a game of peek-a-boo violates the infant's expectations if she uncovers her face and is suddenly not smiling or has her eyes closed. The infant will usually respond to such a violation with a communicative response, and the adult should respond to any communication by the infant as a request to reestablish the expected sequence.

Using novelty is a minimally intrusive technique that can motivate exploratory behavior. For example, rather than placing all of the infant's toys around her, give her only one or two toys a day. Change the toys from day to day. The toys will appear novel each day and will encourage play because they seem more interesting. This technique encourages infant-initiated behaviors and supports and encourages competence.

Incidental teaching refers to a group of instructional techniques in which the infant's behavior serves to identify occasions for instruction. In response to a specific type of behavior (for example, the infant reaches for a toy out of reach), instruction is conducted to encourage more developmentally sophisticated behavior (the desired response is modeled or prompted "Tell me what you want"). Like most of the described procedures, incidental teaching is responsive and sensitive to infant-initiated behaviors. Incidental teaching is a strategy that is well suited to respond to the infant's behavior as intents to interact, and thus may shape social interaction behaviors. Incidental teaching is discussed at length in later chapters.

Instructional Procedures for 2- to 5-Year-Olds.   Incidental teaching methods are important instructional procedures for 2- to 5-year-olds. As noted, incidental teaching procedures support independent and child-initiated behaviors. Systematic instructional procedures that involve more intrusive adult-directed instruction are also included in the naturalistic curriculum model, but only in conjunction with specific techniques to facilitate generalization. For example, the general case instructional procedure (Horner & McDonald, 1982; Horner, Sprague & Wilcox, 1982) is teacher-directed and more tightly structured than incidental teaching procedures, but it is effective in promoting generalization.

General case instruction uses two generalization strategies: objectives are described as generalized skills rather than discrete skills ("child will grasp raisins or small candies, T-shirt bottom, and cup" rather than "child will grasp raisins"), and generalized skills are taught across a variety of situations with a variety of materials (for example, at breakfast, when getting dressed in the morning, and after recess). In selecting situations or materials, choose those that represent the range of characteristics of situations or materials that the skill is intended to generalize to. Stokes and Baer (1977) refer to teaching generalized skills as "training to generalize," and teaching across a variety of situations or materials as "training sufficient exemplars." Both of these techniques are a part of general case instruction.

Instructional procedures within the naturalistic model emphasize instruction that is as subtle as possible (while still being effective), promotes generalization, and fits into the natural settings, routines, and activities of the infant/young child and the family. The more naturalistic the instruction, the greater the likelihood that new skills learned will be used in the natural situations where they are needed.

Evaluation Methods

The primary focus of evaluation in the naturalistic curriculum model is generalized outcomes in natural settings. As previously noted, traditional curriculum models give little consideration to generalization. When the infant/young child acquires a new skill, generalization to natural settings is assumed. In the naturalistic model, generalization is not assumed, it is planned for.

Generalization is assessed in settings that are similar to the instructional settings, but settings where instruction has not occurred. For example, a 4-year-old is taught to ask for a turn at play rather than grabbing objects from his sister and the children next door. Generalization is assessed in natural noninstructional settings, including the daycare program and the park on Saturdays. The assessment is conducted under natural conditions in which the skill is expected, rather than in clinical or contrived settings typical of traditional assessments.

Implementing a Naturalistic Curriculum

The following eight steps provide a guide to implementing a naturalistic curriculum. These steps include descriptions of how content and strategies from the traditional models and related services can be included with the naturalistic curriculum approach.

Step 1: Ecological Assessment

Determine Needs Referenced to Current and Future Natural Environments. Meet with the infant/young child's family or caretakers to gather information about abilities, needs, and participation in family activities. If the family is comfortable about it, the home is the preferred setting for this meeting because it allows the interventionist to observe the child's natural setting. Many elements of the home setting are pertinent or useful for developing realistic and potentially effective instructional plans. Relevant elements of the home setting that may be observed in this meeting include, but are not limited to, the number of adults and children interacting in the home, social interactions that include the infant/young child with special needs, family routines and lifestyles (eating at a dinner table versus family members eating separately; rules such as no TV after dinner), furniture and home architecture (relevant to physical positioning and mobility considerations), and availability of toys and other materials and equipment. Some families, however, may consider this information part of their private lives and feel that it is too personal to share with the infant specialist or teacher. Families have a right to determine the extent to which they share their personal lives, and interventionists have an ethical obligation to respect their right to privacy. If parents do not want to meet in their home, a meeting can be scheduled in a neutral place such as a restaurant or, if they wish, the infant program or preschool setting.

Conduct the interview following the format of an ecological inventory such as that presented in Figure 5-1. The first portion of the inventory asks for identifying information, such as names and birthdates. In the second part, the interviewer notes observations about the neighborhood and home that would be relevant to

Date of Interview ___2/14/92___   Interviewer ___Maile___

I. Family Information

Child's name ___Casey Joseph___   Birthdate ___2/1/91___

Family member's names and relationships:

Kimo - father	Corey - 3 yr. old brother
Cinda - mother	Grandma Flo and Grandpa Jack

Names of other people significant in the child's life:

Auntie Jo, Tina (babysitter), Tommy & Patrick (neighbor children - 3 & 4 years old)

EMERGENCY INFORMATION:

Family phone numbers: 922-1234 (home)

922-5678 (mom - work)   922-3579 (work)

Physician and Hospital phone numbers:

Dr. Cheung 488-8888

II. Home and Community Observations

Neighborhood & community observations (Busy streets? Parks and playgrounds? Neighborhood children playing? Nearby daycares or preschools? Shops and community services? Availability of public transportation? etc.):

Quiet neighborhood (side street); Neighbors ages 2 & 3; Park with playground equipment

at end of street; beach is 2 blocks away; Home is 1 block from the bus.

Home observations (Yard for play? Accessibility concerns? Play area inside the house? Eating arrangements? Sleeping arrangements? Therapeutic uses for furniture and available materials? Play materials and/or toys? etc.)

Large front yard; carpeted family room (great play area for Casey & Corey); large

kitchen—room to play on kitchen floor when parents or grandparents are

working/socializing in kitchen; "Overstuffed" family room couch & chair could

be used for positioning; Bean bag chair in Casey's bedroom; Corey's old high chair

might be of use for Casey with some adaptations.

Figure 5-1 Early intervention ecological inventory

III. Developmental and Medical Information

Significant occurrences in birth history:

Breach birth position—emergency C-section when fetal monitors indicated

distress; On respirator for 36 hours.

Significant occurrences in medical history:

Pneumonia at 3 months.

Current medical concerns (including medications & dosages):

Chronic ear infections; is being monitored by ENT specialist.

Developmental accomplishments and needs:

Gross motor: Rolled prone to supine at 8 months; props on forearms in

prone for up to 10 minutes with some head control.

Fine motor: Beginning to swipe at objects with right hand in supine and

when propping on forearms in prone.

Social/behavioral: Knows all family members and many close family friends;

fusses when ignored for more than 10 or 15 minutes; easy to comfort

by talking to him or picking him up.

Communication: crying, smiling, watching intently, laughing

Cognitive: Loves turn-taking games & laughs expectantly when routine

stops.

Figure 5-1—(continued)

(continued)

IV. Daily Routines

Typical weekday schedule:

Time	Activity	What child does	What others do	Potential outcome/goal
5:30	Wake-up	Casey fusses but doesn't really cry	Mom & Dad take turns getting Casey. They bring him into their bed until 6:00 am	Call out for Mom and Dad
			Diaper change if needed	Pull to sit after diaper change
6:00	Mom, Dad, & Casey get up	Smiles & cuddles	Diaper change if needed	Pull to sit after diaper change
			Mom or Dad places Casey in infant seat on kitchen table	Lift arms to be picked up Vocalize to initiate interactions
	Breakfast preparation	Watches Mom & Dad	Dad makes coffee	Vocalize to initiate interactions
		Plays with toys attached to infant seat	Mom makes & eats breakfast	
			Mom prepares Casey's breakfast	Point to indicate preference for cereal or yogurt
6:30	Breakfast	Eats cereal or yogurt from spoon & drinks bottle	Dad feeds Casey	Play with spoon during feeding
			Corey eats breakfast at table	Maintain grasp on spoon while being fed
				Vocalize to request more cereal/yogurt
				Point to indicate preference for cereal/ yogurt or bottle
				Vocalize to initiate interactions with Corey
7:00	Dressing	Casey lies on back & stomach	Mom changes diaper if needed	
			Mom dresses Casey	Pull to sit after dressing
				Roll front to back
Etc.				

Figure 5-1—(continued)

Typical weekend schedule:

Time	Activity	What child does	What others do	Potential outcome/goal
5:30-7:30	Wake-up Breakfast Dressing	Same as weekday schedule . . . sometimes Mom, Dad, & Casey stay in bed until 7:00 or 7:30—depending on when Corey wakes up.		
7:30/ 8:00-9:30	TV Cartoons w/Corey	Sits in infant seat or lies on stomach	Corey turns on TV & changes channels Corey sometimes plays with Casey (rattle toys) or "reads" to Casey	Roll front to back when tired of propping on forearms Vocalize to initiate interactions with Corey Point to indicate toy or book Vocalize to request more play Maintains grasp on toy Call out to Mom or Dad when tired or bored with TV Lift arms to be picked up when cartoons are finished
9:30	Diaper change		Mom or Dad changes Casey	Pull to sit after diaper change
9:30-11:00	Grocery shopping w/family	Sits in infant seat placed in shopping cart	Mom or Dad push cart (Corey helps sometimes) Mom and Dad select & pay for items Corey selects cereal, fruit, & cookies	Point to indicate preference for cookies/crackers
Etc.				

Figure 5-1—(continued)   *(continued)*

V. Intervention Ideas and Priorities

Future outcomes or needs (ask family to consider activities not presently in their lifestyle or their child's lifestyle that they'd like to prepare for; consider needs related to environments child might be participating in 6 months from now and 1 year from now, etc.):

Play at park (Casey can't sit in swings or use slide)

Play with neighborhood peers

Attend daycare (concern that Casey is difficult to feed)

List potential outcomes/goals (based on entire interview):
Put an * next to family priorities and identify first and second priority

#1 *Identify potential daycare programs near Mom or Dad's work

  Point to indicate preference at mealtimes & play

#2 *Call out for Mom or Dad

  *Lift arms to be picked up

  Pull to sit after diaper change

  Vocalize to initiate interactions

  Maintain grasp on spoon while being fed

  Play with spoon during feeding

  *Maintain grasp on toy

  Vocalize to request more food/play

Figure 5-1—(continued)

instruction: Does the family live on a busy street where traffic is a hazard? Are there neighborhood children playing outdoors? Does the home have stairs? Is there a room for play? The third section of the inventory asks information about the child's history, such as difficulties at birth, behavior (strengths and weaknesses), development (physical development, communication development), and medical concerns, such as allergies and medications. This section is likely to cover most of the information that would be obtained through developmental assessment instruments, such as the *Hawaii Early Learning Profile* (Furuno et al., 1979) or the

Battelle Developmental Inventory (Newborg, Stock, Wnek, Guidubaldi & Svinicki, 1984) mentioned in earlier chapters. If the interviewer is not satisfied that complete developmental information has been obtained, the interview may be supplemented with a developmental assessment.

The fourth section of the inventory is the main portion of the ecological inventory and requires that the interviewer obtain a detailed description of typical activities that occur each day, the nature of the child's participation in each activity, and potential goals associated with each activity. *This portion of the interview is the primary source for identifying environmentally referenced goals in the naturalistic curriculum model.* The last sections of the inventory guide the interviewer in asking parents to select priorities for instruction.

Child needs and strengths associated with the "next environment" (childcare, preschool, or kindergarten) should also be discussed in the interview and may be followed up with an assessment of the child's performance on survival skills. Survival skills assessment may be conducted in several ways. One option is to complete a published survival skills assessment (for example, The Hawaii Kindergarten Survival Skills, McCormick & Kawate, 1982; the PIP Assessment, Noonan et al., 1992) indicating the child's present level of performance on each survival skill. The PIP Assessment and the Hawaii Kindergarten Survival Skills appear in Chapter 13. Presently available validation data suggest that these skills will be important to most preschool and kindergarten settings. A second option is to interview the teachers/childcare staff at the potential next setting and ask them to indicate the importance of each skill on the relevant survival skills assessment. This will provide a modified list of skills that can then be used to assess the child's present levels of performance on skills that are important for selected early childhood settings. A third option is to conduct a try-out in the potential next setting to determine the child's needs relative to the particular setting (Vincent et al., 1980). This is also a more specific assessment approach than the ready-made survival skills assessments, but it has the problem of trying to evaluate the child's abilities and needs in a setting with children that are at least several months older.

To summarize, naturalistic assessment begins with the collection of environmental and developmental information through parent interview and survival skills assessment strategies. A developmental assessment may also be administered if the interventionist does not feel that complete developmental information was obtained through the interview. Potential goals from these assessments should be listed in preparation for Step 2.

Step 2: Establishment of Priorities

Determine Instructional Goals. The naturalistic targets goals across all environmental domains: home, community, play/recreation, and early intervention/ early childhood program. A basic skills domain may also be included if separate goals are to be formulated to address communication, cognitive, or physical development. In most cases developmental needs will be incorporated in the goals within the environmental domains, and separate basic skill goals will not be needed. For example, the outcome/goal of "grasping" may be incorporated in several skills in the home domain (as in brushing teeth, brushing hair, and dressing) and in the play/recreation domain (as in passing toys to peer, manipulating toys).

Step 1 assessment procedures are likely to yield far too many potential goals for instruction. Therefore, the next step is for the transdisciplinary team (including the parents) to review all of the child's needs and potential goals and establish priorities that will provide direction for more detailed, in-depth assessment and a more reasonable list of goals. Priorities are established by asking families to identify their greatest concerns or preferences for their child.

Family concerns and preferences should *always* be prioritized and addressed to the greatest extent possible. When family priorities conflict with the professional priorities for the child (for example, professional thinks family is being unrealistic in expecting their child to walk, or professional thinks family is being overprotective by not wanting their child to attend a regular daycare program to meet their respite needs), professionals will find themselves in a dilemma: Do they "give in" to the family and do something that they feel is inappropriate, or do they try to persuade the family to see their point of view? If we truly respect families as the rightful decision makers for their children, and we wish to support and empower families, then we must follow the families' wishes and accept their priorities. Professionals can express their opinions and should provide rationales for their opinions. This gives families the same information as professionals and allows them to be knowledgable as decision makers. Professionals should strive to provide the information in a manner that informs but does not communicate an intent to persuade or coerce. The decisions in identifying priorities must be made by the families.

Sometimes families will have difficulty identifying their priorities. When this occurs, professionals can assist by asking them questions, such as "If we could write only one goal, what would it be?" or "If your child could pick one skill to learn, what do you think it would be?" Other questions to help families think about what is most important to them are:

◆ Are there skills that would enable your child to participate in family activities?
◆ Are there skills that would make your home life easier?
◆ Are there skills that your child has almost learned?
◆ Are there skills that would greatly increase the number of activities your child can participate in?

It is difficult to recommend an ideal number of goals because each child's situation relative to the amount of time that instruction can be implemented will vary considerably. Furthermore, different goals will require instruction that involves different amounts of adult involvement and time. What is important is that the type and amount of instruction associated with prioritized goals actually can be implemented—child goals must be realistic. Typically, 5 to 20 instructional goals are identified for an infant or young child with disabilities.

Step 3: Present Levels of Performance

Conduct In-Depth Assessment of Each Priority.   Once instructional goals have been prioritized, present levels of performance for each goal must be determined. Only the prioritized goals are assessed in this phase of the curriculum process; to conduct in-depth assessment on all potential goals is unnecessary because only a portion of them will actually be targeted for instruction. Present levels of performance are determined through selected assessment procedures appropriate to the nature of each goal. For basic skills, domain-specific developmental checklists or criterion-referenced assessment procedures may be used (refer to Chapters 3 and 4). For example, for a goal to develop self-feeding skills, physical development (fine and gross motor) scales (such as *Learning Accomplishment Profile*, LeMay, Griffin & Sanford, 1977) and an oral-motor assessment (for example, *Pre-Speech Assessment Scale*, Morris, 1984) may be conducted to provide a more thorough evaluation of the infant/young child's strengths and weaknesses related to feeding.

Potential goals in the environmental domains are likely to be activities rather than basic skills. Present levels of performance on activity goals are assessed with a task analysis procedure (Snell, 1987; also referred to as a discrepancy analysis or student repertoire inventory by Falvey, 1989). In this assessment procedure, the activity goal is task analyzed. As the infant or young child attempts the task, each step of the task analysis is scored indicating the infant or young child's performance. Comments are also made relative to potential instructional strategies, basic skill needs, and possible adaptations for each step of the task analysis. Determining the current level of performance provides essential information for formulating individualized objectives.

Step 4: Instructional Objectives

Formulate Generalized Instructional Objectives.   Use the information obtained from the assessment of prioritized goals to formulate instructional objectives. As discussed in Chapter 3, objectives have three essential components:

1. The conditions under which the skill is to be performed are specified. For example, *Given a small spoon with a built-up handle;* or *When Timmy wakes up after a nap.*
2. The skill is stated in observable, measurable terms: *Jeannie will scoop thick pureed or sticky foods and raise the spoon to her mouth;* or *Timmy will vocalize any sound.*
3. Performance criterion is specified. For example, *with half or more of the food remaining on the spoon, for 5 of 6 scoops, for two consecutive meals;* or *such that the sounds are audible outside the room where he has been sleeping, 8 of 12 consecutive opportunities.*

As discussed in previous chapters, instructional objectives are developed through a team process, with parents included as team members. By this point, the team has amassed considerable data (from parent interviews, observations, formal assessments, review of medical records). The team process continues and the assessment information is integrated across content domains. For example, in developing an objective for playing with an older sibling (a parent's high priority), a reach and grasp component of the skill may be included, addressing a fine motor skill need. The social/communication need to develop turn taking may be integrated in a play objective, with "playing" defined as manipulating a toy for 5 to 30 seconds and passing it to the sibling. A successful team process will result in objectives that address basic skill and therapeutic needs in the context of meaningful activities.

In addition to developing objectives relevant to meaningful activities, the naturalistic model emphasizes *generalized* outcomes. Until recently, generalization was a concern *after* initial skill acquisition. Now "general case" objectives are developed. They specify the instructional target as a generalized skill (for example, scooping a variety of sticky foods, rather than scooping one type of food; or maintaining grasp on a spoon, bottle, and toy, rather than maintaining grasp on only one item). The skill required to scoop different types of foods or to maintain grasp on a variety of objects varies slightly. Thus, as the infant/young child learns to scoop or grasp, a general case skill is being acquired.

In the naturalistic model, objectives are established with criteria that are meaningful and relevant to natural contexts. The primary question that must be addressed is "How well must the infant/young child perform the skill in order for the skill to have a meaningful and reliable effect?" How frequently must a child pass a toy to another child in order to sustain a play interaction? How much food must reach the child's mouth to motivate subsequent attempts at self-feeding, or to accomplish the meal in a reasonable amount of time?

To summarize, in addition to the three essential components of instructional objectives, objectives in the naturalistic model have the following characteristics:

1. Basic skill and therapeutic needs are integrated in functional, age-appropriate activities (that may themselves be objectives derived from the parent interview);
2. The context(s) for instruction is specified;
3. Instructional targets are stated as general case objectives; and
4. A functional criterion is included.

The following objective illustrates these four characteristics:

At snack and lunch at preschool, and at dinner at home *(context specified; generalized across settings and adults),* given a small spoon with a built-up handle, Jeannie will grasp the spoon *(basic skill of grasping is integrated)* and scoop thick pureed or sticky foods (mashed potatoes, pureed vegetables, or pudding; *generalized across food types)* and raise the spoon to her mouth with half or more of the food remaining on the spoon, maintaining grasp until she has the food in her mouth *(functional criteria)*, for five of six scoops, for five consecutive meals.

Step 5: Instructional Plans

Develop Individual Instructional Plans and Monitoring Systems.

Individual instructional plans are formulated for each goal. In addition to identifying information, such as date, name of infant or child, goal, all instructional plans should include six components (see Figure 5-2):

1. *Contexts or occasions for instruction:* When and in what situations will the instructional plan be implemented?

2. *Physical positioning or materials arrangement:* Does the infant/young child require any special positioning in order to perform the target skill? How or where are the materials presented? Are any specialized materials needed?

3. *Instructional techniques:* What techniques will be used to *teach* the skill and increase the likelihood of the infant/young child demonstrating the skill correctly?

4. *Infant/child response:* In operational terms, what is the specific response expected? Will any approximations or variations of the skill be accepted as correct?

5. *Consequences for correct response:* How will the infant/young child be reinforced for a correct response? Is the natural reinforcer obvious, or can it be made more obvious? Will any additional instruction be provided if the infant/young child responds correctly?

6. *Corrections for incorrect response:* What instructional techniques will be implemented if the infant/young child does not respond or makes an incorrect response? If the infant/young child makes a correct response following the correction procedure, is reinforcement provided?

Chapter 6 focuses on the development of instructional plans and provides detailed descriptions of each of these instructional components.

Because most instruction will be implemented across more than one situation, and because objectives are developed as general case objectives, instructional plans are designed as general case plans (Horner, Sprague & Wilcox, 1982). In general case instruction, two generalization strategies are incorporated into each plan. *Train sufficient exemplars* is incorporated into the contexts/occasions, materials, or instructional techniques sections of the plan. Approximately three exemplars are chosen to represent the stimulus class targeted for generalization. Each time the instructional plan is implemented, a different one of the three exemplars is used. For example, a child may be taught to share toys in three different situations: when his sibling comes home after school, during freeplay at preschool, and with neighbor children at the park.

Train to generalize is the second generalization technique that is incorporated into general case instructional plans. Training to generalize is accomplished by formulating the instructional goal as a generalized skill (as in general case goals) and implementing instructional procedures to teach the generalized skill when the child

General Case Intervention Plan

Infant/child: *Fia Corrado*   Interventionist(s): *Lani Smith,*   Date: *1/25/92*
                                    Mom, Dad, & Kimo

Outcome/goal: *When Fia wakes up in the morning or after a nap, Fia will vocalize any sound(s), such*
              that the sounds are audible outside the room where she has been sleeping,
              on 8 of 12 consecutive opportunities.

Contexts/occasions for intervention:	Infant/child response:	Consequences for correct response:
When you notice that Fia is awake, in the morning, after a nap at home or at preschool	*Fia will vocalize any sounds, such that they are audible outside the room where she has been sleeping*	*Pick Fia up immediately and say, "Oh, you are ready to get up now!" and carry her out of the room.*

Physical positioning and/or materials:

On her right side, with a pillow between her knees and under her head, with her left knee and hip flexed

Intervention techniques:	Task analysis (if applicable):	Consequences for incorrect response:
1. *Approach Fia and talk to her until she vocalizes (do for 5 days).*	*n/a*	*Approach Fia and say, "Are you ready to get up?" Wait 6 seconds. If she vocalizes, respond as you would for a correct response. If she doesn't, leave the room for 6 seconds. If she vocalizes within the 6 seconds, pick her up immediately, If she doesn't, pick her up and try again next time.*
2. *Enter the room so Fia can see you, wait 6 seconds before talking to her. After 6 anticipated correct responses (within 6 sec. delay), move to step 3.*		
3. *Wait outside the room for 10 sec.*		

Figure 5-2 Instructional plan

is initially learning it. Teaching the child to share in three different situations concurrently, rather than waiting for learning to occur in one situation before moving on to the next, is training to generalize.

It is also necessary to develop data collection systems to monitor the effectiveness of instruction. The type of data collected must correspond to the criterion level specified in the goal. For example, if the child must share materials at least three times during three consecutive play sessions, then the number of times (or frequency) the child gives materials to a peer must be recorded. Data are graphed so that progress may be monitored. If progress does not occur, or occurs too slowly, the instructional plan should be modified. Chapter 6 provides a complete discussion of measurement, data collection, evaluation methods.

Step 6: Instructional Schedule

Identify Functional/Natural Times for Implementing Instructional Plans. Once instructional goals and plans have been developed, instructional opportunities must be identified and scheduled. A scheduling matrix (see Figure 5-3) is useful for creating an individualized schedule. The first step in filling out the matrix is to complete the left column by listing a daily schedule of activities. If the child is enrolled in a center-based or home-based infant program that meets one or two hours per week, two matrices may be developed—one for the infant program, and one for home on days when the infant does not receive services from the infant program. If the child attends childcare or preschool, the daily program schedule is listed as it occurs during the child's daily schedule.

The second step is to review the infant/young child's instructional plans. Activity goals also listed on the daily schedule are starred (*). In keeping with the naturalistic curriculum model, the times when activities naturally occur are the most appropriate times for instruction. Look for times when the other activity objectives that are not listed on the daily schedule could easily fit into the schedule.

Most of the instructional plans will indicate settings and situations for program implementation that provide ideas for fitting the activities into the routines of the early intervention programs, early childhood programs, or home/family routines. For example, if a toddler has a goal to share during playtime with neighborhood peers, but the child does not currently play with peers in the neighborhood, the family might indicate that it would be feasible to invite neighborhood children into their home after morning nap at least twice each week. The family's schedule is then altered to indicate playtime with neighborhood peers.

Next, list the remaining activity and basic skill goals across the top of the matrix. In the column below each goal, place a checkmark across from each activity in the daily schedule where the goal might naturally occur. The matrix is now complete and indicates naturally occurring opportunities for instruction, based on individual goals and individual daily schedules.

If most of the instruction is to occur in the home, the family must decide when they are best able to implement the instructional plans. A family may feel too pressed for time to work on a self-feeding plan in the morning while preparing for work and school, but may feel comfortable in implementing the instruction at the evening meal and at lunchtime on weekends. If the infant/young child attends childcare or a preschool program, the instructional needs (and individual matrices) of the other children, as well as staffing ratios, must be considered in finalizing the schedule for the entire group of children.

Daily schedule	Sitting	Reaching	Self-feeding	Dressing	Toy play	Take turns	Vocalize	Recept. label	Point to choice or request	
Infant/child: Fia Corrado									Date: 1/25/92	
Additional objectives										
6:30–6:45 A.M.										
Wash up										
Diaper change										
*Dressing										
6:45–7:15 A.M.										
Breakfast										
7:15–7:45 A.M.										
TV with brother										
7:45–9:00 A.M.										
Playpen										
(mom's chores)										
Diaper change										
9:00–9:30 A.M.										
Play with mom										
9:30–11:00 A.M.										
Nap										
Diaper change										
11:00–11:30 A.M.										
Lunch										
*Self-feeding										
11:30–noon										
In kitchen										
with mom										
noon–1:30 P.M.										
With mom										
Errands or										
park or										
walk										
1:30–2:00 P.M.										
Diaper change										
Clean up &										
relax										
2:00–3:00 P.M.										
Nap										
3:00–5:30 P.M.										
With sibling										
*Take turns										
Etc.										

Figure 5-3 Scheduling matrix

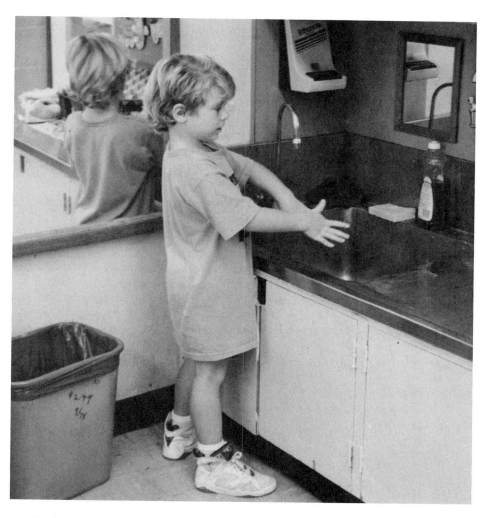

In the naturalistic curriculum model, instruction is implemented at functional times.

    The final step in establishing an individual instructional schedule is to decide which goals will be implemented during which activities. On the matrix, the checkmarks that correspond to the goals to be implemented in each activity may be circled. If it is not possible to implement all instructional plans as frequently as desired, the team (including the family) should establish priorities and decide which goals will receive the most attention. If there are not enough natural opportunities for implementing some of the instructional plans, then it may be necessary to create naturalistic occasions. For example, a preschool-age child may change her shirt after nap time if more instructional opportunities to work on a dressing goal are created.

Step 7: Instruction

Implement Instructional Plans. After the instructional plans have been developed and scheduled, instruction begins. Instructional plans are implemented as accurately as possible, so that their effectiveness can be determined. Program staff and family members who implement the same instructional plans observe each other periodically to be certain that they are implementing the plans in the same manner.

Step 8: Evaluation

Monitor Progress, Probe for Generalization, and Modify Instructional Plans as Necessary.   As noted above, progress on instructional plans should be monitored on an ongoing basis. How frequently data are collected will vary. For some instructional plans, very precise data will be collected by the infant specialist when the baby attends the infant program once each week. The family may keep general data (a checklist) indicating which days they were able to implement the instructional plan. If the young child attends a preschool program, data may be collected daily on high-priority instructional plans; lower priority goals may be monitored less frequently.

The more frequently data are collected, the more accurately progress can be monitored. When enough data have been collected and graphed to create a fairly clear picture of performance (usually five or six data points), the data are reviewed and a decision is made whether to continue the plan as is, or to change it. If progress is not as expected, only one part of the instructional plan is modified so that the effectiveness of the change can be evaluated (again, after five or six data points are collected). Frequent progress monitoring will result in a dynamic instructional plan that is responsive to individual differences and changing needs.

Given that most instructional objectives will be formulated as general case objectives, it is also necessary to assess if generalization has occurred. Generalization is assessed by observing the infant or young child in situations where the skill has not been taught, but where its use would be expected. For example, the skill of sharing was taught at preschool, with a sibling, and with neighborhood peers. Generalization is assessed by observing the child at a family picnic with cousins or with peers at a babysitter's home. Generalized objectives are mastered only when generalization to new (noninstructional) situations is demonstrated.

Eight steps have been described in the implementation of a naturalistic curriculum model:

1. Ecological assessment,
2. Establishment of priorities,

3. Present levels of performance,
4. Instructional objectives,
5. Instructional plans,
6. Instructional schedule,
7. Instruction, and
8. Evaluation.

These steps yield an individualized curriculum that is based on the unique ecology of an infant or young child and family beginning with the assessment process and continuing through the development, implementation, and ongoing evaluation of instructional plans. As noted previously, Chapter 6 describes the development and monitoring of instructional plans in detail.

Summary

The naturalistic curriculum model's focus on increased participation and interaction in natural environments is an important contribution to early intervention because it addresses empirical and social validity (Voeltz & Evans, 1983). Participation and interaction in natural environments are likely to be highly valued by the infants and young children and beneficial to their overall growth, development, and progress toward independence (empirical validity) for at least two reasons. First, goals involving environmental participation and interaction address developmental needs (for example, the fine motor goal of reach and touch), and do so by immediately applying the skills to natural, functional situations. For example, a naturalistic goal of pointing to an object to indicate preference is needed throughout an infant/young child's day (choosing a T-shirt, toy, activity, or food), and it requires the acquisition of developmental skills in fine motor and communication. Thus, environmental participation and interaction goals *include* developmental goals and address them in meaningful contexts. The value of the newly acquired skills is further enhanced because skills performed in natural, meaningful contexts are likely to be maintained over time by naturally occurring contingencies (Stokes & Baer, 1977).

Second, goals of environmental participation and interaction are empirically valid because they emphasize skills that increase the young child's ability to control the physical and social environment. Environmental control is a significant aspect of independence and personal freedom, and thus promotes human worth and dignity. Teaching young children to satisfy their desires and needs through communication, physical, social, or adaptive skills is teaching them new skills that have a high probability of increasing their quality of life.

Naturalistic goals address social validity because they are referenced to the infant/young child's typical routines within the home and community and are selected based on family priorities. Furthermore, naturalistic goals often involve enhancing social interaction with parents, siblings, and other significant individuals. Improving the quantity and quality of family interactions is likely to be reinforcing to the family and valued by them.

Activities

1. Use a developmental assessment and identify the skills that are "next" (potential objectives) for an infant or young child with a disability. Then ask the child's family to describe the child's daily routines. Through discussion with the family, identify potential goals related to improving or increasing the child's participation in daily routines. Bring the two lists of potential goals to class and be prepared to discuss the similarities and differences in the approaches to goal identification.

2. Review three or more published curricula for early intervention or early childhood special education. Identify the model (developmental, developmental-cognitive, behavioral, ecological) and the approach (content, content and instructional techniques, process) of each curriculum.

3. Observe the interaction of an infant (between 3 and 10 months) and parent. Note patterns of interaction that may serve as naturalistic teaching procedures. Explain why you think the patterns of interaction are instructional.

4. Interview infant specialists or preschool special education teachers. Ask them to describe the *process* they follow in identifying goals and objectives for the infants or young children they teach. Compare the process reported by the teachers to the process presented in the naturalistic curriculum model.

Review Questions

1. Describe the three traditional curriculum models in early intervention.
2. Discuss the difference between curriculum models characterized by (a) content, (b) content and instructional techniques, and (c) process.
3. Describe two examples of naturalistic trends in traditional curriculum models in early intervention.
4. State the goal of the naturalistic curriculum model.
5. Describe the general characteristics of the naturalistic curriculum model components:
   Content of instruction
   Instructional methods
   Evaluation methods
6. Describe and contrast appropriate content in the naturalistic curriculum model for 6-month-olds, 12-month-olds, 2-year-olds, and 4-year-olds. Discuss how the emphasis in instructional content changes relative to the infant or child's age.

7. Define *general case objective.* Explain why the naturalistic curriculum model emphasizes general case objectives.
8. Identify the six components of an instructional plan.
9. List and describe the eight steps of the naturalistic curriculum model.

Basic Instructional Principles

Objectives

1. Define systematic instruction.

2. Discuss a rationale for using systematic instruction in the naturalistic curriculum model in early intervention.

3. Describe the systematic instructional process.

4. State guidelines for providing effective prompts and encouragement.

5. Define general case instruction and five additional methods for promoting generalization.

6. Describe data-based methods for monitoring the effectiveness of systematic instruction.

*T*he purpose of an instructional strategy is to assist infants and young children with disabilities to acquire skills needed for participation in natural settings, now and in the future. This chapter will describe systematic instructional procedures for the naturalistic curriculum model. *Naturalistic* and *systematic* are not incompatible constructs. While systematic emphasizes consistent instruction, it does not require unnatural and mechanistic instruction. Furthermore, it does not require instructional plans be so rigid that the teacher or infant specialist responds without regard for the interests or spontaneity expressed by the infant/young child. Consistency *is* important to instructional effectiveness, but it must be balanced with sensitivity and responsiveness to the infant/young child.

A systematic instructional approach provides for program integrity and accountability. Strategies are precisely and clearly formulated and instruction is always conducted in a similar manner. Furthermore, when a teacher or infant specialist shares the plan with other members of the intervention team, the plan on paper is a true representation of what is being implemented. The extent to which a systematic instructional plan is teacher-directed and structured corresponds to the needs of the infants/young children. When new skills pose difficult challenges, a great deal of teacher direction may be needed; whereas, when skills are nearly accomplished, less structure and teacher direction are required. Finally, consistent instruction allows for objective evaluation of program effectiveness. Evaluation of the plan is important so that the plan can be modified if progress is not as expected. It is also important to the field of early intervention that effective procedures can be identified.

Systematic instruction is consistent instruction conducted according to an individualized plan. The purpose is to assist and encourage the infant/young child to learn a new skill. Assistance and encouragement is individualized to match the learning/developmental characteristics of the infant/young child. The type of assistance varies from arranging materials, to providing a reminder, to giving physical guidance. All types of assistance, however, have the effect of helping the infant/young child demonstrate a response. Encouragement refers to motivation. Encouragement procedures are included in instruction to arouse interest and reinforce desired responses. Although assistance and encouragement procedures will be defined and described separately, note that they often overlap in their function. For example, moving an infant's toy closer will make it easier for her to reach (assistance), and the movement attracts her attention and interest (motivation).

The purpose of this chapter is to describe the basic components of systematic instruction in natural environments. Later chapters expand on the application of these strategies.

Providing Assistance

The assistance component of systematic instruction is implemented *before* the infant/young child is expected to demonstrate a response. Asking an infant/young child to respond without teaching is using a trial-and-error method. When learning new responses, trial-and-error learning results in repeated errors (Bereiter & Englemann, 1966) and confusion. This is why assistance is provided. Assistance strategies include prompting, cuing, shaping, and fading.

Assistance procedures can also be provided *after* the infant/young child attempts a target response. If the infant/young child does not respond, or does not respond as desired, the assistance is a *correction procedure.* Correction procedures are different from the type of assistance initially provided because an ineffective procedure should not be repeated. They should also have a high probability of resulting in the desired response so that a second error does not occur. Assistance can also be provided after the infant/young child demonstrates a correct response to highlight the desired response. For example, a child says "Doll," and a parent says, "Doll—yes, that's your baby doll."

Prompts

Anything that assists an infant/young child to make a desired response is a *prompt* (Snell, 1987). There are natural and instructional prompts. Natural prompts are environmental stimuli that "occasion a response" (Holland & Skinner, 1961). Natural prompts do not cause or elicit a response; instead, they signal a response. This happens because of reinforcement when an appropriate response occurs. A toddler, for example, quickly learns that when Dad says "Let's watch cartoons!" (prompt), if she turns on the TV (response), Dad will watch cartoons and play with her (outcome). The predictability of the prompt-response-outcome relationship increases the likelihood that an appropriate response occurs when a natural prompt is present.

Instructional prompts are provided when natural prompts are inadequate or ineffective to teach a skill. An instructional prompt can be as subtle as a glance, or as intrusive as physical guidance. The amount of assistance provided by a prompt depends not only on its intensity but also on the infant/young child's ability to use it (Wilcox & Bellamy, 1982). If an infant does not understand speech, a verbal direction will not provide assistance. Likewise, if a child does not imitate, a model cannot serve as a prompt. For some infants and children, however, verbal directions and models are effective. Good prompts are ones that help a child make a response, rarely result in errors (LeBlanc & Ruggles, 1982), and are as least intrusive as possible while still being effective (Dunst et al., 1987).

Prompts can be identified by the type of assistance they provide. Common prompts include:

> *Indirect verbal:* Asking a question or making a statement that implies what is needed. For example, "What do we need to do now that we're home from our walk?" (meaning "Go to your room for a nap"), or "It's time for breakfast" (meaning "Raise your arms and I'll pick you up and take you into the kitchen").

Direct verbal: Making a specific statement to inform an infant/young child what needs to be done. "Say 'good morning'" or "Put your arm through the sleeve" are direct verbal prompts.

Gestural: Moving a hand or body part as a nonverbal prompt. It may be a conventional gesture that people are acquainted with, such as pointing, or an unconventional gesture known only to the child and/or her family, such as a sibling stomping his feet to prompt his sister to run to him.

Model: Demonstrating a desired response. The demonstration can be verbal or gestural. Verbal models might encourage a child to name things. Gestural models often prompt a child to engage in a variety of actions with objects (for example, demonstrating how to roll, bounce, or shake a small ball).

Tactile: Touching the child. The tactile prompt is used to get the infant/young child's attention, or as a reminder that a certain body part must be moved to make a response. Touching an infant's chin, for instance, prompts the infant to open her mouth to eat.

Partial physical assistance: Guiding an infant/young child by touching or manipulating a body part. The prompt is partial because complete guidance is not provided; the child must do some of the response. Guiding a child's elbow, or supporting the weight of an object as an infant picks it up, are examples of partial physical assistance.

Full physical assistance: Providing complete guidance by touching or manipulating a body part. Guiding an infant's hand and helping her push a button with her finger is a full physical assistance prompt.

Spatial: Placing a stimulus in a location that increases the likelihood of a correct response. Placing a preschooler's toothbrush in front of others on the counter is a spatial prompt.

Movement: Altering the location of a stimulus to attract attention. A parent may hold up two shirts and ask her child if she'd like to wear the blue one or the red one, shaking each shirt as she mentions it. The movement prompt assists the child to look at both shirts before choosing.

Visual/pictorial: Providing assistance through pictures (drawings or photographs), colors, or graphics. Placing a red mark on the back of an inside neckline, waistband, or clothing tag is an example of a visual/pictorial prompt.

Auditory: Using sound (other than speech) to assist a child to make a desired response. Tapping an object is an auditory prompt.

When formulating systematic instruction, prompts are operationally defined, not simply identified by type. For example, in a plan to teach a toddler to point and choose a toy, a partial physical assistance prompt is defined as "grasping her shoulders to maintain a forward and relaxed position." Clear definitions are necessary for consistent implementation.

Prompts can be used individually, in combination, or sequentially (Snell, 1987). When an *individual prompt* is used, the prompt is given once. When a *combination of prompts* is used, two or more prompts are *paired* and presented at the same time. Pairing increases the intensity of the prompt (Skinner, 1938) and may thereby increase effectiveness. In assisting a young child to pull up to stand, for example, a combination of three prompts is used: A sibling may (a) hold the child's hands and nudge her up, while a parent (b) provide trunk support, and (c) says "Up, up, up."

Natural prompts may be paired with artificial ones as a strategy to teach the infant/young child to recognize natural ones. For instance, in teaching a preschooler to say "Please," the natural prompt of "Would you like some _____?" is paired with the instructional prompt of saying "Pl." Pairing natural and instructional prompts is a particularly valuable strategy for teaching in natural situations.

A *prompt sequence* is a series of two or more prompts. For example, a three-step sequence consisting of a verbal direction, model, and physical guidance may be used to teach a toddler the initial step of putting his T-shirt on. The sequence begins with the teacher saying "Hold your T-shirt at the bottom." A second prompt is provided by modeling how to hold the T-shirt. If the child does not imitate the model (demonstrating the desired response), a third prompt is given as a correction by guiding the child's hands to grasp the shirt. The verbal direction and model provided prior to the response are a two-step prompt sequence; the physical guidance in the correction procedure creates a three-step prompt sequence. The prompt sequence is always implemented in the same manner.

Prompt Hierarchies

A *prompt hierarchy* is prompt sequence ordered according to the amount of assistance provided by each. The hierarchy can range from least to most assistance ("increasing assistance"), or from most to least ("decreasing assistance"). An example of a four-step hierarchy is:

1. Verbal,
2. Gestural,
3. Partial physical assistance,
4. Full physical assistance.

If the above hierarchy begins with the verbal prompt, it is a least-to-most hierarchy; if it begins with full physical assistance, it is a most-to-least hierarchy.

In implementing a *least-to-most assistance hierarchy,* the first prompt or "level of assistance" is provided. If the infant/young child does not respond as desired within a specified time period (for example, 5 seconds), the teacher or infant specialist proceeds through the prompt hierarchy, providing the next prompt and waiting the specified length of time. When the desired response is demonstrated, the infant/young child is reinforced. The least-to-most hierarchy provides only as much assistance as the infant/young child needs. More-intrusive prompts are automatically faded as the child responds to the less-intrusive prompts. Thus, the least-to-most assistance hierarchy is minimally intrusive.

Some infants/young children, however, become "prompt dependent" when a least-to-most hierarchy is used. They wait for prompts that provide more assistance because they learn that eventually they will be given help (Glendenning, Adams & Sternberg, 1983). Another problem with least-to-most hierarchies is that prompts that provide minimal assistance allow for errors (Csapo, 1981; Day, 1987).

A *most-to-least assistance hierarchy* may eliminate the problems of prompt dependency and high error rates associated with the least-to-most hierarchy. In a most-to-least hierarchy, the prompt that provides the most assistance is used first.

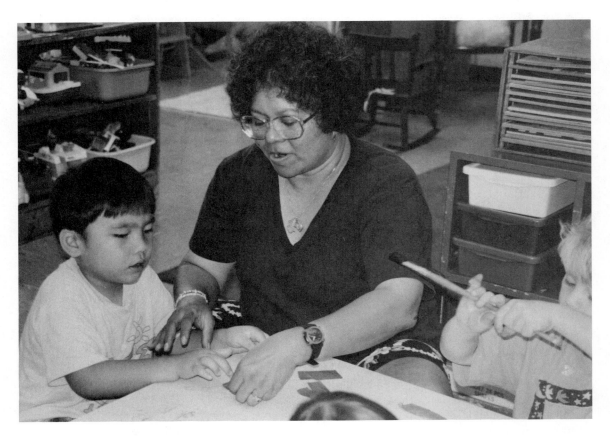

Physical prompts are one type of instructional assistance.

When the infant/young child demonstrates the response at a criterion level (for example, a specified number of times), instruction proceeds to the next level. Each subsequent level of the hierarchy is implemented when criterion is met at the current level. When an error occurs, the previous prompt level is implemented as a correction. If the criterion for progressing through each level is more conservative than necessary, instruction is not efficient. Errors, however, are kept to a minimum.

As noted earlier, not all prompts are equally effective for all infants and young children; some infants/young children will not use particular prompts. Prompt hierarchies, therefore, are formulated on an individualized basis. For example, a young child who is irritated by touch does not respond well to physical guidance. Such prompts are not included in prompt hierarchies for her. Or, for some children, a verbal prompt provides a great deal of assistance, and a slight gestural prompt is less assistance (Wilcox & Bellamy, 1982, pp. 108–109).

Graduated Guidance

A less structured prompting strategy, but one that is responsive to day-to-day performance, is *graduated guidance.* In graduated guidance, the teacher or infant specialist watches as the infant/young child attempts to determine how much assistance is needed. Initially, a great deal of assistance is provided. As the infant/young child acquires the skill, less assistance is given. This procedure is similar to the most-to-least hierarchy, because the amount of assistance is gradually reduced. The actual amount and kind of assistance, however, differs from the most-to-least hierarchy because the amount is sometimes increased. Furthermore, the amount and type of assistance is determined *while* the infant/young child is attempting the response, rather than being predetermined (Snell, 1987). In using graduated guidance to assist an infant to place toys in a container, the infant specialist sits close and watches. The infant's hand is guided to the container when it appears that he will miss it. More assistance is provided when it appears that he might drop the toy. When graduated guidance is properly implemented, errors rarely occur and only the least amount of assistance necessary is provided.

Cues

A *cue* is a prompt that directs attention to a particular dimension of a stimulus or task. For example, pointing and saying "Pick up your spoon" is a cue because it directs the child to a specific object. The most effective cues are ones that direct attention to the most important features of a stimulus. Pointing to the handle rather than at the the bowl of the spoon is a more precise cue, and potentially more effective, because it directs attention to where the child must place his hand.

Skilled teachers are keen observers of infants/young children, noting when cues are needed to direct attention to important stimulus features. Like prompts, cues can be of various forms: verbal, tactile, physical, movement, or spatial, for instance.

Errorless Procedures

As previously mentioned, the most desirable assistance procedures minimize errors. Some instructional procedures are virtually error free. *Time delay* is an errorless procedure in which an instructional prompt is paired with a natural one. Over successive trials, the time interval between the natural prompt and the instructional prompt is gradually increased, until the child responds to the natural prompt alone (Snell & Gast, 1981; Touchette, 1971). A mother may use time delay, for example, to teach her child to raise his arms when he wants to be picked up. When he is fussing and appears to want her to pick him up, she says "Do you want me to hold you?" (the natural prompt) and guides him to raise his arms (the instructional prompt). She repeats this 0-second delay procedure several times over the next 2 days whenever her son appears to want her to pick him up. On the fourth day, when he fusses, she asks if he wants to be held, and then pauses for 2 seconds. This pause gives her son a chance to raise his arms without assistance. If he does, she immediately lifts him up. If not, she guides him to raise his arms and lifts him up. She uses this 2-second-delay procedure for 2 days. Every 2 days, the interval increases by 2 seconds. Eventually, her son raises his arms before the prompt, responding independently to the natural cue "Do you want to be held?"

Several types of delay schedules have been shown to be effective (Snell, 1987). *Progressive schedules* begin with a 0-second delay (the natural and instructional prompts are paired), and the delay increases a fixed amount each trial (0 sec, 1 sec, 2 sec, 3 sec, etc.; or 0 sec, 2 sec, 4 sec, etc.). In *blocked schedules,* the initial trial(s) is at 0 seconds, and all subsequent trials are at a fixed interval (0 sec, 0 sec, 0 sec, 0 sec, 4 sec, 4 sec, 4 sec, 4 sec, 4 sec, etc.). This schedule is easier to implement accurately than the progressive schedule. A *blocked and progressive schedule,* the third alternative, begins with several trials at 0 seconds, and then progresses through a schedule of increasingly longer delays, with several trials at each level (0 sec, 0 sec, 0 sec, 2 sec, 2 sec, 2 sec, 4 sec, 4 sec, 4 sec, etc.). The progressive delay schedule moves through the delay intervals very quickly and may result in errors for infants/young children who have severe disabilities and do not "catch on" to the strategy. The blocked, or blocked and progressive, schedules provide a longer opportunity to learn to wait for prompts when the correct response is not known and thus minimizes errors.

In time delay, correct responses following the instructional prompt are *waited corrects,* and correct responses following the natural prompt are *anticipated corrects.* Both types of correct responses are reinforced. This decreases the likelihood of the child responding incorrectly during the delay. If the child doesn't know the correct response, she waits for the instructional prompt and responds correctly to receive reinforcement.

If an error occurs, a correction procedure is implemented. A typical correction procedure for time delay is to guide the correct response and return to the previous delay for a few trials. If several errors occur, the instructional plan is evaluated and modified. If the errors are occurring before the instructional prompt *(non-waited errors),* the reinforcer may not be effective and a different, more powerful one is needed. Sometimes non-waited errors occur because the child doesn't realize that if she waits, a prompt will be provided to help. Waited errors suggest that the instructional prompt is not effective and a different prompt is needed.

Stimulus shaping and fading procedures are prompting strategies in which an easily recognized prompt is gradually altered (stimulus shaping) or reduced (stimulus fading) until its appearance matches that of the natural prompt. A series of instructional prompts are prepared prior to implementing this procedure, with slight modifications to each successive stimulus. Modifications from one stimulus to the next are subtle so that the infant/young child responds correctly as the prompts gradually approximate the natural one. Figure 6-1 illustrates materials for stimulus shaping and fading.

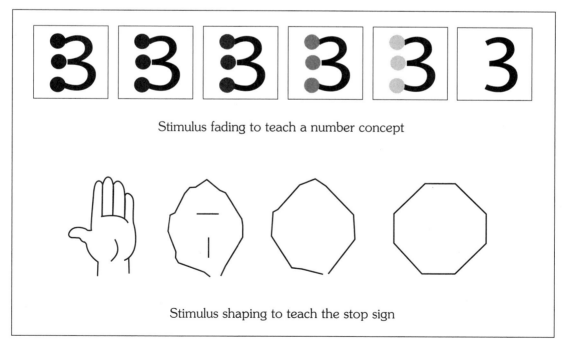

Stimulus fading to teach a number concept

Stimulus shaping to teach the stop sign

Figure 6-1   Sample materials for stimulus shaping and stimulus fading

Guidelines for Effective Prompting

As noted above, systematic instruction must be implemented accurately and consistently, regardless of which prompting procedures are used. Too often prompts are repeated even though an instructional plan specifies that the prompt be given once. If the infant/young child does not respond or responds incorrectly, the correction procedure specified in the instructional plan is implemented—the prompt is *not* repeated (unless that is the correction procedure). Repeating prompts leads to prompt dependency, the situation in which the infant/young child learns not to attend or respond because more help will be given. Adhere to the following guidelines for prompting:

1. Implement the prompting procedure as specified in the instructional plan. Do not repeat prompts unless indicated in the plan.
2. Be certain that the infant/young child is attending to you or to the relevant stimuli (for example, task materials) *before* implementing the prompt (Snell, 1987).
3. Deliver prompts so that they are clear and easily recognized (Snell, 1987).
4. Select prompts that are least intrusive, yet effective enough to minimize errors.
5. Change the prompt if the prompt is ineffective (the infant/young child makes several errors).
6. Use prompts and cues that help the infant/young child notice the naturally occurring ones. Natural and instructional prompts can be paired.
7. Use cues that focus attention on the most relevant characteristics of the stimuli.

Fading Prompts and Cues

Instructional prompts must be eliminated for the infant/young child to respond under natural conditions. A good instructional plan is one that provides assistance necessary for correct responses and gradually eliminates assistance while maintaining correct responding. A plan for fading prompts is a part of systematic instruction.

Prompt fading procedures all have one thing in common: they result in the instructional prompt becoming less noticeable. One method of fading is to decrease intensity. The intensity of a verbal prompt can be faded by speaking more and more softly (as in "Take another bite"). Physical assistance is faded by gradually moving the assistance away (for example, assisting a child to hold a crayon with hand-over-hand assistance can be faded by moving guidance from the hand to the wrist, the wrist to the forearm, to the elbow, and so on). Physical guidance is also faded by decreasing pressure (the touch associated with hand-over-hand assistance gets increasingly lighter until eliminated), or time (hand-over-hand assistance is first provided the entire time the child is coloring, then 90% of the time, 80% of the time, and so on).

Prompt fading strategies are related to the type of prompt: auditory prompts become quieter; spatial and movement prompts become smaller; visual prompts become lighter. The key is to make the prompt less noticeable in a subtle manner so that the infant/young child responds correctly as he did to the original prompt. Note that the most-to-least and least-to-most prompt hierarchies are complete prompt-fading strategies when the least intrusive prompt of the hierarchy is a natural one.

Errorless prompting techniques (time delay, stimulus shaping, and stimulus fading) incorporate prompt fading as a part of the strategy. In time delay, the instructional prompt is faded temporally; in stimulus shaping and fading, characteristics of the task materials/stimuli are gradually altered or reduced until only the natural ones remain.

Providing Encouragement

Encouragement, the motivational component of systematic instruction, is provided through reinforcement procedures *after* the infant/young child demonstrates the desired response. Motivation is addressed *before* the response is expected using interesting or enticing materials, settings, or situational arrangements. Selecting short-term objectives or skill steps that are challenging also provides motivation prior to response. *Well-formulated systematic instruction includes procedures that provide assistance and encouragement before and after the infant/young child's response.*

When encouragement is provided after the opportunity for demonstrating the response, it is usually *positive reinforcement.* Desired responses may also be encouraged by selectively reinforcing approximations of the response with *shaping strategies* or *changing criterion designs.* Motivational procedures implemented before a response are usually *environmental arrangements* that make the task more interesting or challenging, such as selecting attractive materials, teaching a basic skill in a play situation, or using the *interrupted chain procedure.*

Positive Reinforcement

Positive reinforcement is a consequence that increases the likelihood of a response being repeated. It is defined by its *effect.* Something that is reinforcing for one child or in one situation may not be reinforcing for another child or in another situation. Most infants/young children live in "reinforcement-rich" environments. Parents reinforce them with smiles, praise, frequent physical contact, and attention for *every* little thing they attempt or accomplish. Such naturally occurring encouragement, however, is not adequate for infants and young children with disabilities. They may not notice the encouragement, or the encouragement may not be powerful enough relative to the skill difficulty. When encouragement is not effective, the infant/young child is not receiving positive reinforcement. (Remember, positive reinforcement is defined by its effect.)

Infants/young children with special needs who have difficulty acquiring new skills or do not recognize naturally occurring encouragement should be provided with *instructional positive reinforcement*. Instructional positive reinforcement is "artificial" reinforcement that is not typical of a situation. It is provided as part of systematic instruction to address a specific skill need. Instructional positive reinforcement may include verbal praise ("Good, you got your toy!") or social praise such as hugs, smiles, pats on the back, or highly desired objects or actions (favorite toy or food, clapping). Ideally, instructional positive reinforcement is paired with naturally occurring reinforcement to help the infant/young child recognize naturally occurring reinforcement. For example, when an infant is learning to grasp objects, the natural reinforcement is obtaining the object and having the object available for play. Instructional positive reinforcement might include verbal praise ("Good, you touched it!") and smiles, plus assistance to shake and play with the toy.

When an infant/young child is first learning a skill, instructional positive reinforcement should be provided every time the response occurs. This is a continuous schedule of reinforcement *(CRF)*. As the child progresses in skill acquisition, instructional positive reinforcement is provided less often—such as every second response or every third response (a *fixed ratio schedule*), or perhaps every 30 seconds, or every minute (a *fixed interval schedule*). As the infant/young child approaches mastery of the skill, the instructional positive reinforcement is faded so that it is less recognizable. It is provided on a *variable ratio schedule* (for example, approximately every fifth occurrence), or on a *variable interval schedule* (approximately every 2 minutes).

Effective instructional positive reinforcement in the motivational component of systematic instruction highlights naturally occurring reinforcement and is gradually faded. When instructional reinforcement is eliminated, natural reinforcers maintain the behavior. Reinforcement is gradually faded by changing the reinforcement schedule. Reinforcement may also be made less noticeable by decreasing its intensity or quantity, or by delaying when it is delivered.

Shaping and Selective Reinforcement

Positive reinforcement provided contingent on an approximation of a desired response is called shaping. For example, any vocalization beginning with "b" is reinforced as an approximation to "bottle." As the toddler achieves success, an approximation of "buh" is required for reinforcement. In this way, verbalizing "bottle" is gradually shaped. This encouragement strategy is *reinforcing successive approximations* or *selective reinforcement*.

Shaping, or reinforcing successive approximations, can be implemented systematically by using a *changing criterion design*. In a changing criterion design, a response is reinforced when it meets a particular standard (criterion). The standard gradually changes (increases or decreases) until the desired standard is achieved. For example, a preschooler is reinforced for playing independently for 30 seconds. When the preschooler demonstrates 30 seconds of independent play on three occasions, the criterion is raised to 45 seconds. Each time the preschooler meets the criterion three times, it is increased by 15 seconds, until the objective of 5 minutes of independent play is achieved. The changing criterion design is effective because the reinforcement schedule remains predictable, even though it is thinned. Furthermore, natural reinforcers assume a more powerful role as the child learns a functional behavior and instructional reinforcers are delayed (for example, as the preschooler learns to play, the natural enjoyment of play is reinforcing).

When reinforcement is withheld from a previously reinforced behavior, the behavior is eventually eliminated. This is called *extinction*. If the criterion in the changing criterion design is altered too drastically or too quickly, extinction may inadvertently occur because the child does not anticipate reinforcement. Returning to the example of the preschooler learning to play, if the initial criterion of 30 seconds of play was doubled and raised to 1 minute (instead of 45 seconds), the child gives up after about 45 seconds not realizing that there is still an opportunity for reinforcement. After several occasions of playing alone for brief periods of time and not being reinforced, the child's independent play is extinguished.

Environmental Arrangements

As previously noted, environmental arrangements can provide encouragement. Environmental arrangements that can be modified to encourage learning include the (a) instructional situation, (b) materials, and (c) style of presentation. The *instructional situation* is the context of instruction—the where, when, why, and with-whom. The place and time is the where and when of instruction. Natural places and times ensure a real need for the skill, and natural reinforcers are available. For example, teaching a preschooler dressing skills weekly at the public swimming pool is a very motivating time and place. The why of instruction refers to the activity used for teaching. A meaningful activity teaches the purpose of a skill and thus provides motivation. Functional skills, such as dressing, are taught when activities that require the skills normally occur. Referring to the dressing example, there is no need to contrive opportunities to teach dressing. Morning and evening routines, and activities such as swimming, provide natural and motivating times for instruction. Basic skills, such as vocalizing, sitting, and reaching, should also be taught within meaningful activities. The with-whom of instruction involves the teacher or infant specialist, as well as other individuals. Including preferred people, such as parents, grandparents, siblings, or peers in an instructional situation increases motivation. A toddler, for example, is highly motivated to "be like his big brother," and makes more of an effort to work on his sitting skills while playing with his brother.

Materials provide another opportunity for enhancing motivation. Attractive, age-appropriate, and interesting materials are more appealing than drab materials. New or different materials increase motivation because they are novel (Dunst, 1981). And materials that correspond to the physical and intellectual capabilities of the infant/young child hold the child's attention because they contribute to the "do-ability" of a task or activity.

Style of presentation involves the affective characteristics of instruction. Most of what infants and young children do should be fun, and that requires that the instructional style be enthusiastic and appropriate to the activities in which they occur. If instruction is to be enjoyable, the *level* of task difficulty must be appropriate to the infant/young child's current levels of performance. An appropriate level of task difficulty is one in which the task is slightly beyond the child's present ability so that it is challenging. The task is not too easy or is it boring, nor so difficult that it seems insurmountable.

When a task is too difficult, it is broken down into component steps through *task analysis*. A task analysis is constructed by thinking through the steps of a task, doing the task yourself, observing a competent adult/child doing the task, or copying the steps from normal developmental sequences (Bailey & Wolery, 1984). Table 6-1 illustrates a task analysis that was constructed by observing a competent 2-year-old demonstrate the task. Task analyses should be individualized to the infant/young child: more and smaller steps for difficult tasks or difficult portions of tasks; and fewer and larger steps for easy tasks or easy portions of tasks (Gold, 1980).

Instruction for a skill that has been task analyzed is implemented one step at a time until each step is mastered, or it occurs for all steps concurrently *(total task)*. The total-task approach is more efficient than teaching one step at a time (Snell, 1987). If the skill is too difficult or complex for the total-task approach, the skill is taught one step at a time. There is the option to forward chain or backward chain the steps. In *forward chaining,* the first step is taught until it is mastered, then the first step plus the second step is taught until mastered, until the entire sequence is taught. In *backward chaining,* the last step of the task analysis is the first step taught. When it is mastered, the last step plus the second last step is taught, until the task analysis is completed. When forward or backward chaining is used, the infant/young child may be assisted to complete all of the steps in addition to the step(s) currently being taught, or someone else may complete the steps.

The decision to use forward or backward chaining is based on the infant/young child's present level of performance: begin in the task analysis where the infant/young child demonstrates partial acquisition (where the steps may be easier

TABLE 6-1

Example of a Task Analysis for Putting on Shorts Constructed by Observing a Competent 2-Year-Old Perform the Task

1. Grasp shorts at the waistband with hands on either side
2. Look for label on inside waistband; if necessary, turn shorts so that label faces the back
3. Squat and hold shorts close to floor
4. Insert left foot into left leg of shorts
5. Insert right foot into right leg of shorts
6. Pull up shorts to knees; first the left side, then the right side
7. Pull up shorts to hips, pulling up one side at a time until reaching the hips
8. Grasp shorts at back of waistband and pull shorts up over buttocks
9. Grasp front of shorts and pull shorts up to waist

and thus more motivating). If the level of task difficulty is similar throughout the task, backward chaining is the procedure of choice because of its motivational value: the last step of a task yields a functional outcome and immediate reinforcement. Figure 6-2 illustrates these approaches to chaining with a skill that has been task analyzed.

Goetz, Schuler, and Sailor (1983) hypothesized that performing skills in a sequence is motivating. They developed and demonstrated the *interrupted chain procedure.* In this procedure, children are interrupted as they perform a behavior chain. A relevant skill is taught at the point of interruption. For example, a child's hand is blocked as she attempts to push down a toaster lever, and she is taught to respond to the question "What do you want?" Children are allowed to complete the task if they respond correctly during the interruption. The interrupted chain strategy was demonstrated to be more efficient than teaching skills in isolation. This procedure is described in more detail in Chapter 8.

The idea that sequences of behavior are more motivating than behaviors performed in isolation is not new. Guess and his colleagues formulated the individualized curriculum sequencing (ICS) model, with motivation as a key part of the rationale (Guess et al., 1978; Sailor & Guess, 1983). In *curriculum sequences,* two to five instructional objectives are arranged in a logical order and instruction is implemented for each skill consecutively. Teaching skills in a logical sequence enhances motivation by providing an opportunity for the infant/young child to see the purpose of a skill and its relationship to other meaningful skills.

TOTAL TASK
Grasp spoon
Scoop food
Lift spoon to mouth
Open mouth
Insert spoon in mouth

FORWARD CHAINING
1. Grasp spoon
2. Grasp spoon
   Scoop food
3. Grasp spoon
   Scoop food
   Lift spoon to mouth
4. Grasp spoon
   Scoop food
   Lift spoon to mouth
   Open mouth
5. Grasp spoon
   Scoop food
   Lift spoon to mouth
   Open mouth
   Insert spoon in mouth

BACKWARD CHAINING
1. Insert spoon in mouth
2. Open mouth
   Insert spoon in mouth
3. Lift spoon to mouth
   Open mouth
   Insert spoon in mouth
4. Scoop food
   Lift spoon to mouth
   Open mouth
   Insert spoon in mouth
5. Grasp spoon
   Scoop food
   Lift spoon to mouth
   Open mouth
   Place spoon in mouth

Figure 6-2   Example of total task, forward chaining, and backward chaining

Guidelines for Providing Effective Encouragement

Infants and young children with special needs can be encouraged to learn by including motivational strategies within systematic instruction. Encouragement procedures are provided in two parts of instruction: first, in response to the infant/young child's attempt to demonstrate the desired response (reinforcement procedures), and second, prior to the infant/young child's attempt at the response (environmental arrangements). The following are guidelines for using encouragement procedures:

1. Provide instructional reinforcement on a continuous schedule for new skills.
2. Monitor the infant/young child's affective reaction to reinforcement and progress in the skill acquisition to be certain that the "reinforcer" is effective.
3. Pair instructional reinforcers with natural ones. Whenever possible, use the instructional reinforcer to highlight or accentuate the natural one.

4. As the infant/young child learns a new skill, fade the reinforcer by shifting to less frequent schedules of reinforcement or by decreasing the intensity or quantity of reinforcement.
5. Use selective reinforcement to encourage increasingly closer approximations to the desired skills (shaping, reinforcing successive approximations, and changing criterion designs).
6. Carefully select the setting, time, activity, and participants to make instruction as functional, interesting, and challenging as possible.
7. Use materials to aid in maintaining the infant/young child's attention. Remember that novel materials are effective in maintaining/increasing attention.
8. Be certain that task difficulty corresponds to the infant/young child's present level of performance: not too easy, not too difficult, but just difficult enough to be challenging.
9. When a task is too difficult, use task analysis to identify steps of the task. Teach the task-analyzed skill one step at a time or use a total-task approach. Select a forward or backward chaining technique to teach the infant/young child to perform the steps of the task successively.
10. Teach skills in sequences with other functional skills to enhance the meaningfulness.
11. Consider interrupting behavior chains to enhance motivation. Interrupt the chain at a point that arouses the infant/young child's attention but does not cause undue distress.

Promoting Generalization

The goal of the naturalistic curriculum model is to improve or increase participation and interaction in natural environments. The opportunities and needs for participation and interaction in natural environments are innumerable. There is not enough time to teach the endless number of skills required to address all the opportunities and needs. Rather than teaching a few discrete responses that are useful, the naturalistic curriculum model emphasizes instruction that promotes skill generalization. *Generalization occurs when an infant/young child demonstrates a response in an appropriate situation where instruction did not occur, and does not demonstrate the response in inappropriate situations.* When infants/young children acquire generalized skills, they are equipped to participate and interact in new and unforseen situations beyond the conditions of instruction. Thus they are provided with functional skills for complex and diverse environments.

There are two types of generalization, stimulus generalization and response generalization. *Stimulus generalization* occurs when a response is demonstrated across one or more untrained situations. For example, the child says "please" to his preschool teacher, his mother, and his father. Generalization across persons, settings, activities, conditions, or time are all considered stimulus generalization. The group of stimuli that yields a particular response is referred to as a *stimulus class*.

Response generalization occurs when a child demonstrates a response that is slightly different from the trained one. For example, if the child is taught to grasp her cup by the handle, and grasps it with one hand around the base of the cup, or with both hands around the cup, she demonstrates a generalized response. Slight variations in form among responses that serve the same function constitute a *response class*. Frequently stimulus generalization and response generalization occur together. A child may learn to unscrew container lids and demonstrate variations of grasping and turning when given a tube of toothpaste, peanut butter jar, and thermos.

The usefulness of a skill is often dependent on whether it is generalized or not. If an infant only lifts her head when receiving physical therapy, her ability to lift her head is not very useful. Likewise, the preschooler who says "mama," "ball," and "cup" when shown photographs, but does not use the words to make his desires known, lacks functional use of the words. Early intervention goals and objectives in the naturalistic curriculum model, therefore, are ones that target generalized skills and specify the parameters of the respective stimulus and response classes. They are referred to as *general case objectives* (Horner, Sprague & Wilcox, 1982).

Formulating General Case Objectives

As mentioned in Chapter 5, writing an instructional objective that addresses generalization relies on a procedure called *train sufficient exemplars* (Stokes & Baer, 1977). In using the sufficient exemplars procedure, the target skill is taught across several examples of stimuli that typically occasion the target skill. For example, in teaching a young child to identify "cup," a small plastic cup, a coffee mug, and a toddler "tippy cup" may be used as exemplars. The exemplars are trained concurrently rather than one at a time. The term *sufficient* suggests that an adequate, yet efficient, number of stimuli are selected (Anderson & Spradlin, 1980). Too few stimuli would not be likely to yield generalization; too many stimuli are unnecessary, inefficient, and fail to take advantage of the strategy. Horner and colleagues (1982) suggest that enough exemplars be selected to represent the common and diverse characteristics of the stimulus or response class targeted for generalization.

The response or stimulus class targeted for generalization is the *instructional universe* (Becker, Englemann & Thomas, 1975). Returning to the example of teaching a child to generalize a skill of identifying "cup," the instructional universe (the stimulus class of cups) and its features are identified. Note the variety of cups the child encounters at home, in childcare, and in the community. For example, the instructional universe might include a mug, a child's small cup, a "tippy cup," a styrofoam cup, and a softdrink cup. The features of this instructional universe are:

Material: ceramic, glass, plastic, styrofoam, paper
Breakability: breakable, nonbreakable
Handle(s): no handle, one handle, two handles
Size: small, medium, large
Weight: heavy, moderate, light
Color: white, yellow, blue, etc.; solid, multicolored

In selecting exemplars from the instructional universe, a few cups that best represent the range of features are chosen. Choosing the mug (large, one handle, heavy, solid color, breakable), plastic cup (small, no handles, lightweight, solid color, nonbreakable), and "tippy cup" (medium size, two handles, medium weight, multicolored, nonbreakable) samples most of the features of the stimulus class. If the child learns to recognize the three exemplars as cups, she is also likely to generalize and identify a styrofoam cup as a cup, an example that was not included in the training. Sufficient exemplar training is not limited to stimuli that are objects. It can be applied to people, places, times, situations, words, or activities. It may be used to promote response generalization by applying the same strategy of identifying the instructional universe (a response class, in this instance) and the range of features to which one wishes to generalize.

To formulate a general case objective, define the instructional universe: identify the extent to which the skill will be generalized, and whether the skill involves stimulus generalization, response generalization, or both. The scope and size of the instructional universe is a judgment based on the exemplars likely to be encountered by the infant/young child, and the extent to which the child is likely to generalize (appropriate level of task difficulty). Then write the behavioral objective (conditions, behavior, and criterion) with selected exemplars in parentheses. Examples of general case objectives are as follows:

STIMULUS GENERALIZATION:

Conditions: When a familiar person* (infant specialist Tina, Grandma, and Daddy) asks him if he'd like to be picked up,
Behavior: Lonnie will vocalize
Criteria: within 10 seconds for three consecutive opportunities.

   *(*Instructional universe of familiar persons:* Mom, Daddy, Grandma, Grandpa, cousin Tom, Uncle Kimo, Auntie Sue, neighbors Tom and Julie, infant specialist Tina)

RESPONSE GENERALIZATION:

Conditions: When she crawls to her toy box,
Behavior: Athline will request* a toy (by pointing to a toy in the toy box, by saying "toy," or by saying "please"),

Criteria: on four consecutive opportunities.

*(Instructional universe of requesting responses: reaching, pointing, vocalizing, naming request, saying "please," saying "more")

STIMULUS AND RESPONSE GENERALIZATION:
Conditions: When given finger foods* (crackers, raisins, and sandwich pieces),
Behavior: Darryl will grasp* the food, pick it up, and feed himself,
Criteria: at least five times per meal, four of five lunchtimes.

*(Instructional universe of finger foods: cookies, crackers, cereal, banana slices, orange slices, raisins, sandwich pieces; *Instructional universe of grasping:* light grasp, firm grasp, fine pincer, gross pincer, rake)

When general case objectives need to be further simplified to correspond to the infant/young child's current level of performance, two or more short-term, general case objectives can be formulated. It is important to include the multiple exemplars in each short-term objective; otherwise the general case nature of the objective is eliminated. An example of three short-term, general case objectives for the self-feeding objective is:

SHORT-TERM GENERAL CASE OBJECTIVE 1:
Conditions: When given finger foods (crackers, raisins, and sandwich pieces),
Behavior: Darryl will grasp the food,
Criteria: at least three times per meal, three consecutive lunchtimes.

SHORT-TERM GENERAL CASE OBJECTIVE 2:
Conditions: When given finger foods (crackers, raisins, and sandwich pieces),
Behavior: Darryl will pick up the food and raise it to his mouth,
Criteria: at least three times per meal, four of five lunchtimes.

SHORT-TERM GENERAL CASE OBJECTIVE 3:
Conditions: When given finger foods (crackers, raisins, and sandwich pieces),
Behavior: Darryl will pick up the food and feed himself,
Criteria: at least five times per meal, four of five lunchtimes.

Note that the last short-term objective is identical to the long-term objective.

General Case Instruction

General case instruction adheres to the guidelines specified earlier in this chapter for systematic instruction. Assistance and encouragement procedures are stated in an instructional plan and implemented exactly as stated in the plan. When an instructional plan is developed for a general case objective, the stimulus and/or response exemplars are specified. The plan is designed so that exemplars are taught concurrently, rather than separately. For example, for the short-term objective in which Darryl grasps raisins, crackers, and pieces of sandwich, the instructional plan includes daily opportunities for instruction with the three types of finger foods and the three types of grasp (this is in contrast to teaching Darryl to grasp raisins first, then to grasp crackers after grasping raisins has been mastered, and so on). Figure 6-3 is a general case instructional plan for this objective.

Other Generalization Procedures

A number of other methods have been demonstrated to facilitate generalization (Stokes & Baer, 1977). These methods can be incorporated into general case instructional plans to increase the likelihood of a generalization. There are five generalization procedures in addition to the sufficient exemplar strategy:

1. Program common stimuli,
2. Introduce to natural maintaining contingencies,
3. Use indiscriminable contingencies,
4. Mediate generalization, and
5. Train loosely.

Test Quest

Program Common Stimuli. In this technique, materials or stimuli from the generalization situations are used in the instructional situation. For example, if a preschooler must learn to drink with a straw from a milk carton for school, the family may assist their child to learn the skill at home. They implement the program common stimuli technique by using the same type of milk cartons and straws at home that are used at the preschool. When the child learns to drink from the milk carton at home, the child is likely to generalize and demonstrate the skill at school where the same stimuli are present. Program common stimuli is also a good generalization technique when instructional objectives address skills needed in subsequent environments (for example, teach cutting in preschool with the same types of scissors that will be used in kindergarten).

Introduce to Natural Maintaining Contingencies. Natural maintaining contingencies refer to the reinforcers and schedules of reinforcement that occur in settings where skills are needed. In this strategy, generalization is promoted by gradually shifting from instructional reinforcers and reinforcement schedules to natural ones. Natural and instructional reinforcers are initially paired, and then the instructional ones are faded. When assisting a toddler to pull her panties and shorts up, for example, a parent's verbal praise and hug is immediately followed by allowing the child to leave the bathroom and return to playing. Verbal praise and the hug are gradually eliminated, and returning to play (the natural reinforcer) continues to reinforce pulling her pants up. This natural contingency is in effect at childcare, and at grandma's house, and thus generalization is likely.

Date begun: ___4/1/92___

Infant/Child: ___Darryl___   Date completed: _____

Objective: ___Finger feeding (grasping finger food)___   Interventionist: ___Anna and Mom___

Conditions: ___When given finger foods (crackers, raisins, and sandwich pieces)___

Response: ___Darryl will grasp the food___

Criterion: ___At least 3 times per meal, 3 consecutive lunchtimes___

Intervention Context	*Prompting/Facilitation Techniques*	*Consequences*
Setting(s): ◆ Mondays: infant center ◆ Other days: home	*Positioning and Handling; Special Equipment/Materials:* ◆ Seated in adaptive high chair *with tray* ◆ Crackers, raisins, sandwich pieces	*Reinforcement:* ◆ Verbally praise Darryl for picking up food ◆ Provide physical assistance to help Darryl get food to his mouth
Routine(s)/Activity(ies): ◆ Lunch	*Environmental Modifications:* ◆ Place finger foods on plate with high lip	
Skill Sequence(s): ◆ Makes choice ◆ Grasps food ◆ Asks for "more"	*Prompting/Facilitation:* ◆ Guide Darryl's hand as needed toward food; wait 6 seconds *Additional Generalization Procedures:* ◆ Use same plate at home and infant center (program common stimuli)	*Corrections:* ◆ Place Darryl's hand on top of the food piece; wait 6 seconds. If he grasps the food, provide full physical assistance to help Darryl get food to his mouth ◆ If he still does not grasp the food, provide full physical assistance
Occasions for Incidental Intervention: n/a		

Figure 6-3   Instructional plan

Use Indiscriminable Contingencies. The term, *indiscriminable* means "difficult to notice" or "not too obvious." Reinforcers that are instructional are often obvious and contrived. Noticeable instructional reinforcers may be necessary in the early phases of learning, but interferes with generalization to other settings where the skill is needed and similar reinforcers are not available. Gradually decreasing the obtrusiveness of an instructional reinforcer enhances the likelihood of generalization. As noted earlier in this chapter, reinforcement is faded by decreasing its intensity (making verbal reinforcement quieter) or frequency (shifting to leaner and less predictable schedules of reinforcement, such as a variable interval schedule). For example, in assisting a preschooler to learn turn-taking in a game with a peer, the teacher initially sits close and briefly rubs the child's back as reinforcement. This is minimally intrusive because it does not interrupt play. As the child learns to take turns, the teacher rubs her back more briefly, and only every other time the child takes a turn. Eventually she simply touches the child's back a couple of times during a play session when the child is taking turns. Finally, the teacher moves away and withdraws the instructional reinforcement completely, as playing operates as the natural reinforcement for turn-taking.

Mediate Generalization. In this technique, a strategy is taught. Examples include naming the letters of the alphabet by singing a song, or saying a poem to remember which months of the year have 30 days and which have 31. These are cognitive strategies, and thus are applicable to toddlers and preschoolers. Other types of strategies could be included as mediational techniques. For example, teaching a child to put his shirt on by first laying it out on a flat surface such as the bed is a strategy that he can use across environments. Or, teaching a child with cerebral palsy to hold a peg on her wheelchair tray to stabilize movements is a mediational strategy that she can use across tasks requiring controlled fine motor movements (for example, self-feeding, art activities, communication board use).

Train Loosely. In the train loosely technique, generalization is facilitated by relaxing a systematic instruction that is typically implemented in a highly consistent manner. Instead of providing precisely the same prompt, reinforcement, and correction procedure each time instruction is conducted, the components of the instructional plan vary slightly from time to time. What constitutes an acceptable response may also vary, but the variation must not extend outside the response class. Minor variations in prompting, reinforcement, corrections, and acceptable responses increases the likelihood that when a similar, untrained situation is encountered, generalization will occur. There is a caution, however, that if the instructional plan is implemented *too* loosely, the infant/young child will fail to acquire the skill because the benefits of the systematic instructional plan are eliminated (that is, a predictable prompt-response-consequence relationship is no longer apparent).

When incorporating the train loosely strategy in systematic instruction, the plan should specify which components may be loosened, and acceptable examples of the components should be provided. For instance, if the prompt is trained loosely, then the plan might state: provide a simple verbal direction, such as "Please come with me," "Let's get into the car," or "Please sit in your carseat." In implementing the plan, any of the sample prompts may be used, or prompts that are similar to the examples may be used. Each component of the instructional plan that is trained loosely should be written in this manner.

Although train loosely appears to be similar to train sufficient exemplars, the technique differs in two important ways. First, in train sufficient exemplars the exemplars (the variations of the prompt or response) are selected to represent a stimulus or response class, and only those exemplars are used. In train loosely, specific exemplars are not preselected (although examples are provided), and instruction varies from the samples written in the plan. The second difference is that, in train sufficient exemplars, only the prompt and/or response portions of the plan include variations. In train loosely, any and all components of the plan may include variations.

One or more of the five generalization strategies described in this section (program common stimuli, introduce natural maintaining contingencies, use indiscriminable contingencies, mediate generalization, and train loosely) may be included in a systematic general case instructional plan to supplement the train sufficient-exemplar strategy that is the heart of general case instruction. Figures 6-4 and 6-5 demonstrate instructional plans incorporating these procedures.

 ## Implementation Considerations

There are three key variables associated with the successful implementation of systematic instruction. The first variable is the *amount of engaged time.* Engaged time refers to time in which the child is actively participating in instruction. The more time spent actively engaged in instruction, the greater the amount of learning (Anderson, 1976; McWilliam, 1991; Walker & Hops, 1976). Instruction is more likely to be effective if it is implemented frequently *and* requires active responding on the part of the infant (rather than the infant being a passive recipient of instruction).

The second implementation consideration is the *contingent arrangement of reinforcement.* This means that interesting stimuli are provided immediately and consistently when the infant/young child demonstrates an instructional target. It also means that we should only use stimulation contingently. In the past, noncontingent stimulation, such as auditory stimulation (ringing bells), was implemented in an effort to improve or heighten sensory functioning (auditory attending). Noncontingent sensory stimulation has been shown to be ineffective (Dunst, Cushing & Vance, 1985). Instead, specific responses should be taught. For example, rather than having a father hold his 1-year-old daughter on his lap and talk to her for 5 minutes to teach her to attend (noncontingent stimulation), he might bounce his daughter on his knee each time she attends to his rhyme about a bouncing baby (bouncing is arranged contingently).

Date begun: 3/6/92

Infant/Child: Maile

Date completed: ·

Objective: Signals to continue play   Interventionist: Karen, Mom, & Dad

Conditions: Given a pause during a repetitious song or rhyme game (e.g., pat-a-cake,
peek-a-book, row your boat, etc.)

Response: Maile will signal to continue play (e.g., eye contact, vocalizing, reaching out
for adult, attempting to begin song/game again, etc.)

Criterion: 3 times in 2 consecutive play periods

Intervention Context	Prompting/Facilitation Techniques	Consequences
Setting(s): ◆ After nap ◆ When Mom or Dad gets home from work	Positioning and Handling; Special Equipment/Materials: ◆ Sit Maile on your lap (legs apart) facing you; support her lower back	Reinforcement: ◆ Reinstate game more enthusiastically than before; smile and laugh enthusiastically
Routine(s)/Activity(ies): ◆ Repetitious song or rhyme games	Environmental Modifications: n/a	
Skill Sequence(s): n/a	Prompting/Facilitation: ◆ After several seconds of play, stop in the middle of a movement or phrase ◆ Look directly at Maile and wait 10 seconds Additional Generalization Procedures: ◆ Vary song and rhyme games ◆ Vary verbal corrections: "What?" "Whose turn is it?" "Do it again," etc. ◆ Accept *any* signal that seems to be a request to continue (train loosely)	Corrections: ◆ Provide a verbal prompt, such as "Do it again," or "What?" or "Whose turn is it?" Wait 5 more seconds. If she responds—reinforce ◆ If still incorrect, begin a different game and try again
Occasions for Incidental Intervention: n/a		

Figure 6-4   Instructional plan

Date begun: 6/15/92

Infant/Child: Hank

Date completed:

Objective: Toy play

Interventionist: Howard

Conditions: When playing with brother, cousin, or neighbor.

Response: Hank will shake or bang small toys (squeak ball, rattle, wooden spoon)

Criterion: For 3 or more seconds, 6 times

Intervention Context	Prompting/Facilitation Techniques	Consequences
Setting(s): ◆ Living room, brother's room, or lanai	*Positioning and Handling; Special Equipment/Materials:* ◆ Sidelying or prone over a pillow	*Reinforcement:* ◆ Praise both children for playing nicely; assist peer to help Hank bang or shake the toy 3 or 4 more times
Routine(s)/Activity(ies): ◆ While brother waits for school bus ◆ When Mom babysits neighbor and/or cousin	*Environmental Modifications:* ◆ Toys must be within easy reach	
Skill Sequence(s): n/a	*Prompting/Facilitation:* ◆ Shake or bang the toy 3 times within Hank's reach; wait 5 seconds *Additional Generalization Procedures:* ◆ After 2 consecutive correct, change to FR2 reinforcement schedule; after 2 more correct, change to VR3 (use indiscriminable contingencies)	*Corrections:* ◆ Tap Hank's arm and say "play with your toy"; if he does, reinforce as stated above ◆ If he still doesn't shake or bang the toy, physically assist him through a correct response; do not reinforce
Occasions for Incidental Intervention: ◆ Whenever Hank laughs at peer's play		

Figure 6-5 Instructional plan

A third implementation consideration is that instruction is more effective and efficient when *errors are kept to a minimum* (Bereiter & Englemann, 1966). Successful instructional techniques are those that help an infant/young child make a response and then provide reinforcement. If errors occur frequently and the infant/young child has few opportunities to experience the correct response and its resulting reinforcement, the instructional plan should be revised: more assistance, a different type of facilitation, or more powerful reinforcement may be necessary.

There are two concerns related to the exclusive use of errorless instruction. The first is the importance of allowing infants/young children to make errors and experience natural corrections. Children should have opportunities to experience naturally occurring corrections, particularly when the corrections include informative feedback. For example, if a toddler grabs a toy from her brother without asking, her brother may grab it back from her. The infant/young child's ability to use the natural corrections should also be monitored. If the infant/young child does not seem to understand them, it would be useful to pair instructional corrections with natural ones, and gradually fade the instructional corrections. In the example of the sister grabbing the toy from her brother, for instance, the sister might look confused when her brother grabs it back for himself. An instructional correction prompting the sister to ask her brother for a toy could be paired with the natural correction (the brother grabbing the toy back). This might help the sister understand why her brother grabbed the toy from her.

The second concern related to errorless instruction is the importance of providing opportunities for infants/young children to self-correct when errors occur (the preschooler whines, but no one comes to help him, so he self-corrects by raising his hand). Corrections should only be provided when no attempt is made to self-correct. There should also be consideration given to teaching infants/young children problem-solving skills that will enable them to generate possible solutions (that is, self-corrections) to minimize their dependence on adults and instructional corrections. Regardless of the specific type of instruction used, the three major variables associated with successful instruction—engaged time, contingent arrangement of reinforcement, and minimal errors—should be addressed.

Monitoring Systematic Instruction

A hallmark of systematic instruction is data-based decision making. A data-based decision is a judgment of whether to change or continue implementing an instructional program. Objective measurement of program effectiveness is determined by collecting data on skill acquisition, graphing the data, and interpreting the graphs. Traditionally, systematic instruction was characterized by extensive data collection (that is, data were collected continuously throughout all activities on a daily basis). In a naturalistic curriculum model, however, concerns for flexibility and unobtrusiveness must be balanced with the concern for objective measurement. Recommendations to achieve this balance are discussed following the descriptions of how to develop and implement data-collection procedures.

Measuring Instructional Progress

Chapter 4 described four common types of observational measurement systems for assessing social behavior: event (frequency), duration, interval, and time sampling. Although these measurement systems were described for assessing social behavior, they are applicable for monitoring skills across all domains. Recall that event recording is a count of each time a behavior occurs. If the opportunities for demonstrating a skill vary from day to day, the data may be reported as percent (9 correct responses out of 10 opportunities is 90%). Duration is the length of time a behavior occurs (one occurrence of a behavior or the total time of several occurrences of a behavior). Interval recording indicates if the behavior occurs or does not occur during a period of time (for example, 30-second intervals). In time sampling, the data indicate if the behavior occurs at the moment following a specified time interval (at 30 seconds, at 1 minute, at 1 minute 30 seconds, at 2 minutes).

Three other measurement systems are useful for data-based decision making: latency, rate, and permanent product. Latency is the time between a prompt (natural or instructional) and the response. For example, it is the time between a father taking a turn at pat-a-cake, and his child taking the next turn. Latency is a measurement concern when it affects the usefulness or functionality of a skill. If the child takes too long to respond to his father in the pat-a-cake game, the father assumes the child is not interested and quits the game. Latency is also a concern when a child's disability requires longer response times. A child with a developmental delay may respond slowly because it takes her several moments to recognize a prompt, and several moments more to determine how to respond. A child may also demonstrate long response latencies because of a physical impairment that interferes with movement. Families and others need to recognize a child's need for longer response latencies and adjust interaction patterns and expectations accordingly.

Rate is a measurement of how quickly or slowly responses occur (also known as fluency). For example, an infant may eat 23 spoonfuls of cereal in half an hour, that is, a rate of 0.76 spoonfuls per minute. Rate is calculated by dividing the number of responses by a unit of time: 23 spoonfuls divided by 30 minutes equals the number of spoonfuls per minute. Rate is typically reported as the number of responses per minute, per hour, per day, or per week. Similar to latency, rate is a concern when the quickness of a response influences whether it is functional or not. For example, a child feeds himself without adult assistance, but eats only 3 spoonfuls within 20 minutes. His family may not allow him to feed himself at home because it is impractical to spend so much time on meals. Increasing how quickly this child eats would be a meaningful objective, and rate would be the relevant measurement system.

Permanent product measures provide lasting evidence of responses and do not require direct observation. Through much of education, written tests provide permanent product measures of school achievement. In early intervention, a physical therapist asks a child reach as far as possible in different directions and mark on a paper with a magic marker. The marks remain as evidence of the child's range of motion. Videotapes and photographs also provide permanent product data. Permanent product measures are useful because the child's behavior (or the effect of the child's behavior) may be reviewed time and again. Skills measured by direct observation (that is, skills measured with systems such as frequency or duration) cannot be directly reviewed again.

Selecting a Measurement System.　The primary consideration in selecting a measurement system is choosing one that provides a clear indication of how well a child is performing a target skill relative to the criterion stated in the instructional objective. Matching the measurement system to the criterion is necessary to determine when a child has met an instructional objective. If the criterion states, for example, that the child will vocalize the initial sounds of familiar words beginning with "b," "p," and "m," on three consecutive opportunities, then each time the child says a word beginning with a designated consonant sound, the child's response is recorded as correct or incorrect (+ and −). This is event recording. When three consecutive plusses are recorded, the objective has been met.

Identifying Where and When to Collect Data.　The where and when of data collection is determined by three factors: (a) conditions stated in the instructional objective, (b) generalization concerns, and (c) practical and naturalistic considerations. The first factor, conditions stated in the objective, often indicates what times of day, or in what situations, the skill is to be performed. For example, an objective may state conditions such as "at breakfast, lunch, and dinner. . . ." Data must be collected during all three mealtimes, so that when the measurement system indicates that criterion is met, we are confident that the skill has been achieved as stated in the objective. We cannot assume that a skill demonstrated in one situation will also be demonstrated in other situations. The second factor that will influence where and when data are collected is generalization concerns. Sometimes generalization concerns are reflected in the conditions of the objective, as in the conditions of at "breakfast, lunch, and dinner. . . ." The criterion of an objective may also address generalization concerns. For example, the criterion of "three consecutive opportunities during free play and snack time" indicates that data must be collected at two times, free play and snack time.

Recall that a general case objective is considered mastered when generalization to one or more untrained exemplars from the instructional universe is demonstrated. The child's performance with untrained exemplars is measured with *generalization probes*. Generalization probes are conducted when skill acquisition has been demonstrated with the exemplars specified in the objective. To conduct a generalization probe, the infant/young child is presented with an untrained stimulus/situation from the instructional universe. The examples of general case instructional plans in Figures 6-3, 6-4, and 6-5 include generalization probe components. Note that generalization probes can also be conducted periodically (for example, weekly) prior to demonstrating complete skill mastery.

The third factor that influences where and when data are collected is practical and naturalistic considerations. Practical and naturalistic considerations go hand in hand. For example, it is impractical and unnaturalistic to expect a family to collect data on how quickly their child eats at every meal. In fact, for many families, it is impractical (and inconsiderate) to ask them to collect data. Instead, infant program personnel and early childhood teachers should assume primary responsibility for data collection. Practical and naturalistic considerations suggest that a teacher should not have a clipboard and stopwatch in hand through every activity. This would certainly interfere with a teacher's full participation in an activity, and more important, may interfere with a teacher's ability to provide instructional prompts and positioning and handling interventions.

The balance between the need to collect data and practical considerations is achieved by collecting data on a regular basis for the three to five objectives that are each family's highest priorities. When it is impractical to collect data every day on each instructional priority, data are collected every other day, or once a week. It should be noted, however, that the performance of infants and young children with disabilities varies considerably from day to day. Therefore, the more frequent the data collection, the more likely that the data will provide an accurate measure of child progress and program effectiveness. Data should be collected on lower-priority objectives every two to four weeks.

It may be impractical to collect data throughout an entire activity. When it is possible to address the criterion of an instructional objective with brief periods of measurement, it may be more practical to do so. For instance, data may be collected on a child's rate of self-feeding during the first 10 minutes of each meal rather than through an entire meal.

Figure 6-6 is a data sheet for the instructional program presented in Figure 6-5. Tally marks are used to record the frequency of toy play episodes that last 3 seconds or longer. Another option would have been to record the duration of toy play. Given that the duration criterion is brief (3 seconds), duration does not seem to be the most relevant feature to measure. Instead, the objective is concerned with building the frequency of brief play episodes.

Interpreting Instructional Data. To interpret child progress and program effectiveness from instructional data, it is necessary to chart the data on a graph. Because child performance data tend to be variable, it is difficult to judge whether the child is progressing by simply looking at numbers on a data sheet (Holvoet, O'Neil, Chazdon, Carr, & Warner, 1983). There are numerous graphing methods, but the most common is a line graph. On a line graph, the horizontal axis (abcissa) usually represents sessions or days, and the vertical axis (ordinate) is labeled as the variable being measured (for example, frequency, percent, latency). Figure 6-7 is a line graph depicting child progress as indicated on the data sheet in Figure 6-6.

Once the data are graphed, the next step is to judge whether progress is adequate or not. If the child is not progressing, or is not progressing as rapidly as desired, the instructional program is changed. The modified program is then implemented, and monitoring continues. Graphs should be reviewed every five or six data points. The following guidelines (based on the work of Browder, Demchak,

Frequency of Shaking or Banging a Toy for 3 Seconds or More

Week of	Monday	Tuesday	Wednesday	Thursday	Friday
2/10/92	I	II	II	I	I
2/17/92	I				

Figure 6-6 Sample data sheet for event recording

Heller & King, 1989; and Haring, Liberty & White, 1981) should be followed in making data-based instructional decisions:

1. If the graph suggests that the child is approaching criterion, no change should be made to the instructional program.
2. If the child's performance is highly variable and is not approaching criterion, change the instructional program to improve motivation.
3. If the child's performance is fairly steady and is not approaching criterion, change the instructional program to make it easier. For example, use a more detailed task analysis or use a different, more effective prompt.

In reviewing the data presented in Figure 6-7, Hank's toy play is not improving, and the data are fairly steady. Therefore, recommendation 3 applies: change the instructional program to make it easier. The prompting procedure in the

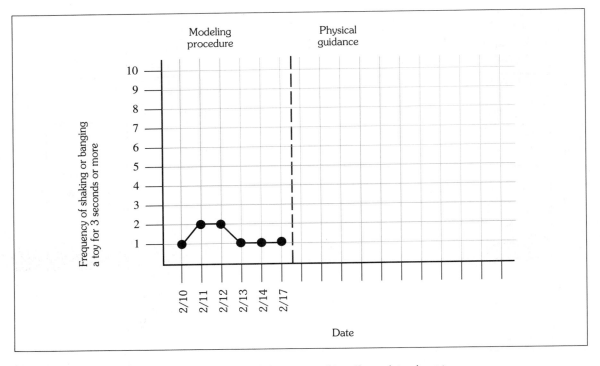

Figure 6-7   Sample graph for data-based decision making (from data sheet in
Figure 6-6)

instructional program is "Shake or bang the toy three times within Hank's reach and
wait 5 seconds" (see Figure 6-5). A prompt that provides more assistance is one way
to make the program easier. For example, a new prompting procedure is "Place the
toy in Hank's hand and shake it or bang it several times. Stop in the middle of a
banging or shaking motion." This prompt provides more direct practice prior to
expecting the response, and requires Hank to continue the response when it is
started for him.

 Summary

Systematic instruction is the consistent application of procedures designed to assist
and encourage an infant/young child with disabilities to acquire or improve skills
needed for participation in natural settings. Assistance procedures include a wide
variety of instructional prompting procedures, such as single prompts, multiple
prompts, prompt hierarchies, errorless procedures, and others. Encouragement
procedures are reinforcement techniques and environmental arrangement strate-

gies that help motivate an infant/young child to demonstrate a desired response. Systematic instruction can be designed to promote generalized skill acquisition by stating instructional goals as general case objectives, applying general case instruction, and/or incorporating additional generalization procedures (program common stimuli, introduce to natural maintaining contingencies, use indiscriminable contingencies, mediate generalization, and train loosely) into the instructional plan. When systematic instruction is implemented, the effectiveness of the instructional program is monitored through frequent data collection. Based on the data, program modifications are made when skill acquisition is not as expected.

Activities

1. Formulate general case objectives for the children and skills listed below. Begin by defining the instructional universe, and then selecting exemplars that best represent the various dimensions of the exemplars of the instructional universe. Be certain to specify naturalistic conditions and criteria in the objective.

Malia	1 year old	finger feeding
Joseph	2 years old	points to indicate request
Anna	3 years old	assists with dressing
Lonnie	4 years old	takes a turn in simple games

2. Select two of the skills listed in activity 1 and write a general case instructional plan for each. Be sure to provide assistance techniques that help the child make the correct response and minimize the need for corrections. Follow the instructional plan format presented in Figures 6-3, 6-4, and 6-5. Develop a data sheet and graph for each instructional plan. *(If you are working or in a practicum setting with infants or young children who have disabilities, do this assignment for a real child with real objectives.)*

3. Read two early intervention journal articles that describe or investigate an instructional procedure. Identify the (a) assistance techniques, (b) encouragement techniques, and (c) generalization techniques that characterize the instructional procedure. The following early intervention journals may be in your library:

Journal of Early Intervention
Topics in Early Childhood Special Education
Infant Toddler Intervention

1. Define the following terms:
   assistance procedure
   encouragement procedure
   prompt
   prompt hierarchy
   graduated guidance
   cue
   errorless teaching
   positive reinforcement
   shaping
   selective reinforcement
   generalization
   event recording
   duration
   interval recording
   time sampling
   percent
   latency
   rate
   permanent product
   data-based decision

2. Describe three examples of each of the following types of prompts: indirect verbal, direct verbal, gestural, model, tactile, partial physical assistance, full physical assistance, spatial, movement, visual/pictorial, auditory.

3. Discuss the similarities and differences among (a) least-to-most prompt hierarchies, (b) most-to-least prompt hierarchies, and (c) graduated guidance.

4. Describe a rationale for errorless instruction. Describe two errorless instructional procedures.

5. List seven guidelines for effective prompting.

6. Discuss two reasons why it is important to fade prompts and cues. Describe two methods for fading prompts and cues.

7. Discuss the use of selective reinforcement for shaping new skills.

8. Describe several ways that environmental arrangements can be used to provide encouragement as a part of an instructional plan.

9. Define general case instruction. How does it differ from the more traditional approach to instruction?

10. Define and provide an example of the following generalization procedures:
    a. program common stimuli
    b. introduce to natural maintaining contingencies

    c. use indiscriminable contingencies
    d. mediate generalization
    e. train loosely
11. Discuss the relationship between the criterion specified in an objective and the measurement system for an instructional program.
12. Identify and discuss three considerations in identifying where and when to collect instructional data.
13. Identify and describe three guidelines for making data-based instructional decisions.

7

Specialized Instructional Techniques

1. Describe specialized instructional techniques for communication, social, physical development, and self-help skills.

2. Discuss team and family involvement in selecting and implementing specialized instructional techniques.

*T*he assistance and encouragement procedures described in Chapter 6 apply across the instructional domains in early intervention (for example, home skills, community skills, and basic skills). This chapter describes the application of instructional techniques from Chapter 6 to the basic skill domains of communication, social, physical development, and self-help. It also describes specialized intervention techniques designed specifically for each basic skill domain. Some of the techniques derive from the study of "natural learning" opportunities in normal development (for example, communication strategies), and others derive from therapeutic approaches (for example, motor intervention techniques).

 # Communication Skills

Communication is using signals and symbols to effect changes in the environment and to fulfill one's needs and desires. Environmental control skills are the foundation of a communication repertoire. Recall from Chapter 5 that under the rubric of environmental control skills we include those social, cognitive, and communication behaviors that enable the infant/young child to reliably effect or cause certain events. For example, an infant who reaches toward his father controls his environment if his father consistently responds by picking him up. Once an initial communication repertoire of environmental control skills is established, the young child's repertoire expands: communication becomes more refined and efficient (Noonan & Siegel-Causey, 1990). For example, instead of crying out and vocalizing "ma ma" when hungry, the young child says "ba ba" to request her bottle.

Establishing Environmental Control Skills

The infants' earliest efforts to control the environment are simple, nonsymbolic behaviors such as eye contact, pointing, vocalizing, reaching, and touching. There are five phases in the development of environmental control skills:

1. *Attentional interactions:* Indicating awareness, recognizing, and/or anticipating persons, objects, or events (e.g., smiling in recognition of a familiar person);
2. *Contingency interactions:* Using simple behaviors to control reinforcing consequences (e.g., playing baby games, such as "so big," to maintain interaction with an adult);
3. *Differentiated interactions:* Controlling the behavior of others with responses that have socially recognized meanings (e.g., pointing, giving, or other nonverbal gestures);
4. *Encoded interactions:* Using behaviors that have precise meanings and are understood given the situation (e.g., using one or two word phrases or sign

language in response to environmental stimuli or events, such as saying, "Ball, Mommy" when a sibling comes into the room holding a ball);

5. *Symbolic interactions:* Using behaviors that have precise meanings (e.g., language or pretend play) to communicate, without reliance on the situation to be understood (e.g., saying "want drink"). (Dunst et al., 1987)

Instructional goals are based on the child's communication needs in daily, functional activities (derived from assessment strategies described in Chapters 3, 4, and 5). The goals build on what the infant/young child is currently doing and promote the child's development of skills in the next phase of environmental control. For example, in conducting a parent interview for Timmy, the parents indicate that they would like him to express his preferences at mealtimes and when playing with his sister. Presently, Timmy smiles and moves his arms excitedly when he sees his favorite foods and toys. One goal is for Timmy to look at a favorite food or toy for 5 seconds when given two choices. In requiring Timmy to look at a preferred food or toy, Timmy learns that looking controls getting what he wants. This goal moves Timmy from his present phase of awareness to the phase of contingent interactions.

There are three instructional approaches to assist infants and young children in progressing through the phases of environmental control skills: (a) enhance sensitivity, (b) create opportunities, and (c) establish routines (Noonan & Siegel-Causey, 1990; Siegel-Causey & Guess, 1989). All three approaches can be used concurrently.

Enhance Sensitivity.   Learn the ways in which an infant/young child tries to communicate nonsymbolically, and respond immediately when such behaviors are demonstrated. Also respond to behaviors that *might* be attempts to communicate nonverbally ("infer intent"). This strategy is particularly useful for enhancing parent-infant interactions when the infant's responses are difficult to detect, inconsistent, or infrequent. For example, Sally's mom notices that Sally stares at her when she is enjoying an interaction and fusses when she's tired. Mom responds immediately to Sally's staring and fussing, continuing to talk and play with her when she stares, and ending the interaction and comforting Sally when she fusses. Sally soon learns to use her attending and fussiness to control the length of interactions. As a result of mom's immediate responsiveness and Sally's ability to control the length of her interactions, interactions are more satisfying to Sally and her mom.

Create Opportunities.   Be careful not to eliminate an infant/young child's need to communicate by doing everything for him. Create communication opportunities by altering the environment, such as placing things out of reach or delaying expected events. For example, place only two pieces of finger food (slices of a sandwich, for example) on a toddler's highchair tray at a time. This will create the need to communicate a request for more food. *Interrupt behavior chains* to increase the infant/young child's motivation to communicate and complete the behavior chain. Interrupting Kayla as she selects a toy from the shelf is a motivating time to teach her to point to her communication card that says "please."

Establish Routines. Help an infant/young child develop expectations by establishing predictable routines, such as playing peek-a-boo during diapering. When the routine is well established, change it or insert a pause, to motivate a communication response. For example, hold the diaper above the infant, but don't begin peek-a-boo until the infant demonstrates some expectation of the game, such as giggling or reaching for the diaper.

Expanding Initial Environmental Control Skills

comm.
for attention
or pointing
↓
requesting, greeting
& protesting

Once a child is demonstrating environmental control skills with simple, nonsymbolic behaviors (such as vocalizing for attention, pointing to a desired toy), the next goal is to expand the child's skills to include communication responses serving more uses or functions. Examples of communicative functions include requesting, gaining attention, greeting, and protesting. These functions are typically demonstrated first through signals (for example, specific gestures such as waving "bye-bye," or as a grunt that communicates "I'm trying but I need help"). Later, these functions are demonstrated through symbols, such as words or sign language. A list of communicative functions (also known as pragmatics) expressed in one- and two-word utterances are in Table 7-1 (McCormick & Schiefelbusch, 1990).

When the child is using several communicative functions frequently and effectively, communication skills are expanded by increasing complexity. Complexity is increased in two ways. First, the content of what the child talks about can be

---

TABLE 7-1

Communicative Functions (Pragmatics) in Early Language Development

Pragmatic Function	*Example*
Attention	"look"
Request	"more play"
Protest	"no"
Commenting	"big ball"
Greeting	"bye-bye"
Answering	"mine (in response to question)

expanded. This is referred to as *semantics*. Children communicate about content such as people, places, events, and objects, and characteristics of people, places, events, and objects. Second, complexity is increased by expanding the structure of communication. This is *syntax.* Syntax is the form or grammar of language, described by terms such as nouns, verbs, and adjectives. Expanding what the child talks about, and the structures used to communicate, enables the child to communicate more precisely, and thus more effectively. Tables 7-2 and 7-3 list examples of semantic functions and syntax expressed in early language development (McCormick & Schiefelbusch, 1990). These sequences follow a simple to complex order.

Given the complexity of establishing goals that consider the pragmatic, semantic, and syntactic dimensions of communication, as well as needs related to home and community participation, a team approach is vital. As always, the family's role as decision maker is central to the team process. A speech-language pathologist (a professional with expertise in assessing communication needs and planning interventions) is an important team member.

The formulation of communication goals comes through a combined approach of ecological and developmentally based assessment. The broad goal is derived from ecological assessment, such as the parent interview described in Chapter 5 (Noonan & Siegel-Causey, 1990). For example, a goal to "initiate requests for desired activities with siblings" may be identified in analyzing the family routines in the parent inventory. Usually goals derived from ecological assessments will focus on communication use (the pragmatic dimension of communication). The

semantics
content

syntax
structure

TABLE 7-2

Semantic Functions Frequently Expressed in Two-Word Utterances

Semantic Function	Example
Existence	"this ball"
Negation	"no cookie"
Recurrence	"more juice"
Attribution	"big ball"
Possession	"mommy sock"
Locative	"sweater chair"
Agent-action	"mommy go"
Action-object	"drink juice"
Agent-object	"mommy baby"

TABLE 7-3
**Syntactic Forms Frequently Expressed
in Two-Word Utterances**

Syntactic Form	Example
Noun + noun	"sweater chair"
Verb + noun/pronoun	"hit it"
Noun/pronoun + verb	"mommy go"
Pronoun + noun	"my toy"
Relational word + object name	"it ball"
Adjective noun	"pretty baby"

ecological assessment is also the source for identifying needed vocabulary. In the play activity, for example, learning the names of games may be a vocabulary need.

The level or complexity of the goal is based on the child's present level of performance: syntax and semantics are expanded following developmental sequences (see Tables 7-2 and 7-3). Returning to the example of requesting an activity, the child is currently using one-word utterances: he's using a grammar that consists of nouns or verbs, and he's talking about actions and people performing actions. A syntactic goal is to use a "noun + verb" form; a semantic goal is to use an "agent + action" expression (for example, "Tommy + catch").

Alternative Communication Modes.   Another consideration in formulating communication goals is deciding on a communication mode. When speech is delayed, or when there is a reason to think that it may be delayed or not develop at all (for example, when the child has multiple disabilities, including a significant hearing loss), augmentative communication systems are considered. An augmentative communication system is an alternative means of communication to *supplement* speech. Examples of augmentative communication systems include sign language, gestures, pictures, line drawings, written words, and Blissymbols (an abstract symbol system). Figure 7-1 illustrates simple signs that are commonly used in augmentative communication systems for young children with disabilities. Figure 7-2 illustrates a communication board using line drawings arranged on the tray of a child's wheelchair. This type of communication board is a permanently displayed communication system. Electronic communication devices are also frequently used with augmentative systems.

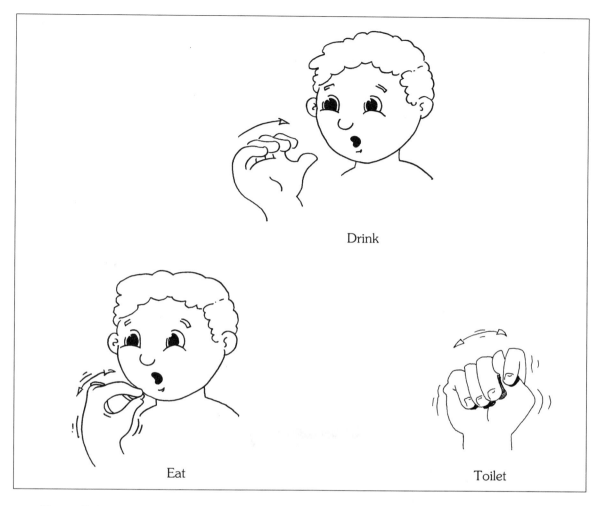

Drink

Eat

Toilet

Figure 7-1 Examples of signs commonly used with infants and young children with disabilities

The decision to use an augmentative system, and the selection of a system, is made by the early intervention team, including the family, speech/language pathologist, teacher or infant specialist, occupational therapist, and physical therapist. As noted throughout this text, parental preference should carry the most weight in decisions about their children. Decisions concerning the selection and use of an augmentative communication system are not one-time decisions. As the child

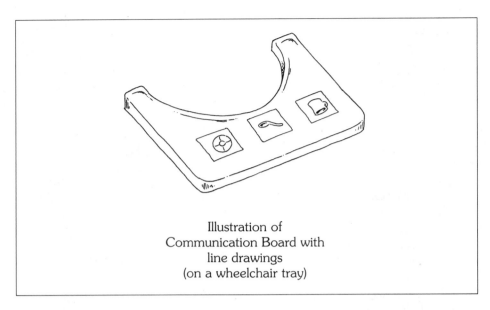

Illustration of
Communication Board with
line drawings
(on a wheelchair tray)

Figure 7-2   Illustration of communication board with line drawings (on a wheel-chair tray)

develops and circumstances change, needs and the appropriateness of the system are continually reevaluated.

In selecting an augmentative communication system, McCormick and Shane (1990) suggest that *modality sampling* be used. In modality sampling, a few skills in two or more systems are taught to determine if an infant/young child is ready to learn a system, and to determine which system may be easiest to learn. In selecting systems for modality sampling consider : (a) size of the audience (how many people will be able to communicate with the system); (b) size of the available vocabulary (gestures represent a limited vocabulary; American Sign Language has a large vocabulary); (c) cognitive abilities (is reading required?); (d) fine and gross motor abilities (for gesturing, signing, or pointing to a communication board); (e) portability (can the system be transported with the child or made available across settings?); and (f) visual discrimination skills (skills necessary to differentiate pictures, symbols, and so on). Given the ecological curriculum model's goal of increased participation and interaction in natural environments, augmentative systems easily understood by children and adults in the community (written words, pictures, and photographs) are preferred over gestural or sign language systems that are not likely to be understood by many other people.

In the field of education for children who are deaf, there is a long-standing concern by some professionals that the use of augmentative communication (primarily sign language) will impede the development of spoken language (Daniloff, Noll, Fristoe & Lloyd, 1982; Silverman, 1980). Empirical studies in the field of developmental disabilities, however, suggest that the use of augmentative communication systems does not delay the development of speech, and may even facilitate it. The position taken by these authors is that speech *and* augmentative communication goals should be considered whenever speech is significantly delayed.

Instructional Procedures. Naturalistic, or incidental, teaching procedures have been demonstrated to be particularly successful in assisting young children with disabilities to learn and use generalized communication skills (cf. Halle, Baer & Spradlin, 1981; Warren & Kaiser, 1986). As reviewed in Chapter 5, incidental teaching procedures are implemented contingent on a specific type of child behavior ("whenever Sue reaches for something"), rather than at a time or situation determined by the teacher or infant specialist. According to McCormick (1990c), there are four important characteristics of incidental teaching procedures:

1. Environmental arrangements are used to create a need for communication;
2. Instructional goals are based on the infant/young child's interests and skill levels, and opportunities occurring naturally;
3. Initiated responses by the infant/young child are responded to with requests for elaboration or expansion; and
4. Attempts to communicate, as well as specifically targeted communication forms, are reinforced.

Chapter 10 provides detailed descriptions of how to implement incidental teaching procedures.

Social Skills

Much of the social domain overlaps with the communication domain, particularly skills that develop during an infant's first year (for example, waving "bye-bye," taking turns). Social skills thought of as appropriate behaviors, such as "responding when called by name," or "playing cooperatively," are often overlooked in assessing social needs. Instead, social goals are most frequently targeted when inappropriate behaviors have been learned and need to be reduced or eliminated. This is despite the fact that from early childhood through adulthood, social skills needs are the single factor most accounting for failure in school, residential, recreational, and work settings (Rusch, 79; Schalock, Harper & Genung, 1981; Sutter, Mayeda, Call, Yanagi & Lee, 1985; Vincent et al., 1980). Social skills needs should be considered in formulating goals for *every* infant and young child with disabilities. Priority is placed on *teaching* appropriate social skills, rather than waiting until inappropriate social behaviors develop and require intervention.

Among the intervention procedures described in the behavior management literature for reducing inappropriate social behaviors are aversive techniques. Technically, aversive procedures are interventions that result in avoidance responses (Azrin & Holz, 1966; Bandura, 1969; Horner et al., 1990), cause pain, involve withholding basic human needs, or result in humiliation (Guess, 1988). From a more practical and broader perspective, any procedure that results in physical or psychological discomfort or harm to the infant/young child or the family is an aversive procedure. If the child reacts with noticeable discomfort, or if the family indicates discomfort with a procedure, the procedure should be discontinued and an alternative plan should be devised. In judging whether a procedure is appropriate or not, it is useful to ask if the procedure would be considered acceptable for nondisabled infants or young children. If the answer is no, the procedure is not acceptable. Involving the family in team-based intervention planning will help to avoid the selection of intervention procedures that are inappropriate or would make the family feel uncomfortable.

Teaching Appropriate Social Skills

The rationale for teaching skills in natural settings is more compelling when considering social skills than perhaps any other domain of behavior. The social demands of segregated settings, such as an early intervention program or special education preschool class, are unlike the social demands of integrated settings. The *only* situations in which naturalistic social situations occur are in natural environments. Naturalistic social environments, by their very nature, cannot be contrived.

There are at least three approaches to teaching social skills that have been demonstrated to be effective with infants and young children. The first is to provide frequent reinforcement for appropriate social behavior. Infants and young children should live and play in "reinforcement-rich" environments. If infants/young children receive an abundance of reinforcement for social behaviors, they are actively being taught which behaviors are acceptable or required. As Christophersen (1988) suggests, "Catch 'em being good" as often as possible. *"Every time you miss a chance to catch your child being good, you miss a chance to teach him how you would like him to behave"* (p. 13). Don't expect children to guess which behaviors are desirable, and don't provide attention only when they act out. Teach desirable behavior by actively and consistently reinforcing it. For most infants/young children, brief nonverbal physical contact is highly reinforcing and is easily provided frequently and unobtrusively.

Another rationale for providing infants/young children with reinforcement-rich environments is that high levels of reinforcement are associated with low levels of inappropriate behavior. Simply increasing the amount of reinforcement for appropriate behaviors is often effective in reducing inappropriate behavior.

The second approach to teaching social skills is to use direct instruction—the assistance and encouragement procedures described in Chapter 6. Identify and operationalize the social skill goal as any other instructional goal. Formulate a systematic plan with clearly defined assistance and encouragement procedures. It may be necessary to task analyze the social skill and teach the skill as a behavior chain. An example of direct instruction is to teach Michael "turn-taking" with his brother, James. Turn-taking for Michael is defined by the following task analysis:

1. Accepts toy from James
2. Plays with toy
3. Gives toy to James when he requests it

The assistance procedure is to provide physical guidance on each step as needed. James provides encouragement to Michael by talking to him as he plays appropriately, and saying thank you when Michael returns the toy to him upon request.

The third approach to teaching social skills to young children in integrated settings is to apply what has been learned about peer modeling (cf. Bricker, 1978). Young children tend to model peers with whom they identify—peers of the same age and same sex. They also tend to model peers whom they perceive as being more competent and of high status, and peers whom they observe being reinforced. For social skills instruction, this means that peer partners or groups selected for social skills instruction should be children with whom the target child identifies or whom the child seems to admire. The peers should be slightly more competent than the target child and should be reinforced for demonstrating the instructional goal in the presence of the target child. The child with disabilities is reinforced for imitating the social goal modeled by the peers. Prompts may also be used to assist the child with disabilities to watch and imitate his peers. This approach is discussed in detail in Chapter 10.

Reducing/Eliminating Inappropriate Behaviors

Intervention procedures for decreasing inappropriate behaviors have undergone significant changes during the last 15 to 20 years. The traditional perspective was that it was necessary to decrease inappropriate social behaviors prior to teaching appropriate behaviors. Eliminating inappropriate social behaviors was an essential component for a child to be "ready" to learn (Meyer & Evans, 1989). Our current perspective is quite different. Most behaviors of infants and young children with disabilities will not warrant reduction. Indeed, when infants or young children are said to have behavior problems, often the problem resides with the adult: the adult has inappropriate expectations (for example, expecting a 2-year-old to sit and wait quietly for 10 minutes); the adult is inconsistent (that is, the child can't possibly know what is expected because the adult's rules keep changing); or the adult is not sensitive to the child's needs or interests (for example, the adult persists in trying to get the child to play with a toy when the child is expressing interest in a different toy). When social development needs are present, they are most appropriately addressed by *teaching* new skills or arranging the environment to prevent behavior problems from occurring.

When a serious behavior problem is present, and teaching a new skill or modifying the environment is not an adequate or complete solution, a behavior reduction plan may be needed. The first step is to evaluate the seriousness of the problem by weighing what would happen if a formal intervention were not implemented, and what effect the behavior is having on the overall well-being of the child. If it is determined that the behavior is a serious problem (for example, it significantly interferes with the child's learning; it may lead to segregating the child; it is physically harmful), then a behavior reduction plan is needed. Two additional factors should be considered to determine if a behavior reduction plan is needed:

1. Consider the frequency, intensity, and durability of the behavior. If the behavior rarely occurs, is not too serious, or not likely to persist, a special intervention program may not be needed.
2. Is the behavior age appropriate? Some "inappropriate" behaviors are actually immature behaviors that are typical of young children at certain ages. If the behavior is developmentally age appropriate, a decision to implement a special intervention program may be delayed for a while.

If the behavior problem is serious enough to warrant a behavior reduction plan, the second step is to identify the purpose served by the inappropriate behavior. Formulate one or more hypotheses as to what purpose the inappropriate behavior serves (for example, Tina throws her spoon and dish *because she is full;* Tina throws her spoon and dish *because she wants Mom or Dad to feed her*). The third step is to test the most likely hypothesis by teaching a *socially acceptable behavior* that serves the same purpose (for example, teach Tina to say "ma ma" or "da da" instead of throwing her dish). The hoped-for result is that the undesirable behavior will cease because it is no longer needed (Meyer & Evans, 1989; O'Neill, Horner, Albin, Storey & Sprague, 1990).

Inappropriate behaviors that are of a less serious nature and seem to be maintained by adult attention or reinforcement (for example, occasionally slapping Mom and Dad, throwing toys when angry) may be reduced or eliminated using extinction or brief time out procedures. These procedures should only be considered if positive procedures (for example, increasing reinforcement) were implemented and found to be ineffective. *Extinction* (withholding reinforcement from a previously reinforced behavior) may be highly aversive to infants/young children in some situations. Typically, when a behavior is being extinguished, the behavior increases before it decreases and is eliminated. The infant or young child will try repeatedly to obtain the reinforcer with the same behavior that had previously been successful.

Furthermore, now and then the behavior is likely to recur (spontaneous recovery) before it is completely eliminated.

If the behavior to be eliminated is one that would be undesirable (or harmful) to increase for a brief period of time, then extinction should not be used. Likewise, if the infant/young child's reaction to the extinction procedure indicates that it is highly aversive (for example, the child cries and tantrums excessively), then another intervention procedure should be selected. Often, however, extinction can be used without causing undue anxiety to the infant/young child or anyone else. For example, if the objective is to assist the child in learning to sit attentively in a preschool group, the child's inappropriate requests for attention are ignored and attention is provided periodically (every 15 seconds) while the child sits attentively.

Undesirable behaviors can also be decreased or eliminated through a brief removal of the opportunity for reinforcement. This is the behavioral definition of *brief time out.* Having a preschooler sit on the sidelines for 30 seconds and watch his peers at play, or moving task materials out of reach for 10 seconds, are examples of brief time out. For time out to be effective, the environment must be rich with reinforcement opportunities; otherwise there will be no motivation to return. Note that both examples of time out are very brief (10 seconds; 30 seconds). Time out is most effective when the young child is returned quickly to an opportunity to obtain reinforcement. (It is common practice in early childhood settings to have children sit alone for a few moments to calm down when they have become upset. This should not be confused with the behavioral use of the term *time out.*)

In the past, many young children and individuals with developmental disabilities were subjected to abuse by the misapplication of time-out procedures. Children were placed in isolation (punished) in closets called time-out rooms for long periods of time, ranging from 30 minutes to several hours. Because time out has a history of being applied inappropriately, it should be used judiciously and with the family's full knowledge and consent. As a rule of thumb, Christophersen (1988, p. 51) advises that time out never exceed 5 seconds for infants (7- to 15-month-old), 3 minutes for toddlers (15- to 36-month-old), and 5 minutes for 3-year-olds (with 5 minutes being the maximum length of time out for a child of any age). In these authors' experiences, *very* brief periods of time out (for example, 10 seconds) are highly effective. Remember, *time out is most effective when the child is returned quickly to an opportunity to obtain reinforcement.*

Note that there is an ethical concern when a behavior is reduced or eliminated. Young children with disabilities have many skill needs in comparison to their peers who are not disabled. Further reducing their skills is difficult to justify. A "fair pair" rule should be followed: a functional skill must be taught or increased any time a behavior is reduced or eliminated (White & Haring, 1976).

Behavior Reduction Procedures to Be Avoided

Two behavior management procedures that are inappropriate in early intervention are punishment and negative reinforcement. They are defined here because sometimes they occur under natural circumstances. If recognized by a teacher or infant specialist, they can be eliminated—and more appropriate, positive motivational procedures can be implemented in their place.

Punishment is a stimulus (object, action, or event) applied contingent on a particular behavior that results in a decrease in the behavior. Like reinforcement, it is defined by its effect. Stimuli that function as punishment are perceived by the individual as aversive. Examples of stimuli that often function as punishers are verbal reprimands and spanking. Punishment *does* reduce behavior when applied consistently. There are, however, two serious ethical concerns. First, punishment is an aversive technique. Infants/young children should never be subjected to discomfort when it is avoidable. Second, punishment results in undesirable side effects including depression, generalized behavior reduction, emotional effects (such as crying and irritability), and aggression. Furthermore, the occurrence of aggression suggests that punishment *teaches* that aversive procedures are an effective way to control others. This is certainly not something we want to teach children.

Negative reinforcement is another aversive procedure to be avoided. Negative reinforcement occurs when the removal of an aversive stimulus results in an increase in a behavior. This procedure is inappropriate for infants/young children with special needs because it requires that the child be placed in a situation of discomfort. Letting a child get very thirsty as part of an intervention plan to teach a request for "drink" uses negative reinforcement (and is an inappropriate intervention). For some children, placing them prone (on their stomachs) over a wedge to encourage head control also functions as negative reinforcement. If the child expresses discomfort, this procedure should only be used for very brief periods of time, even though it may be recommended for therapeutic reasons.

Negative reinforcement is sometimes referred to as an "escape paradigm." Infants/young children may learn to escape difficult or disagreeable tasks by acting very upset, throwing tantrums, or even hitting themselves. This escape paradigm frequently accounts for how noncompliance is learned. When such behavior is observed, the adult usually attempts to calm the child by removing her from the situation. These behaviors may indicate that a task is too difficult or simply of no interest to the youngster (Meyer & Evans, 1989). These situations should be avoided by restructuring the activities or interventions to be more interesting and less demanding.

 ## Physical Development Skills

Many infants/young children with disabilities have physical development needs due to delayed development or neurological damage. As defined in Chapter 3, physical development refers to the acquisition of postural control and the necessary movement patterns to produce functional motor acts. Functional motor acts include gross motor and fine motor skills.

Gross motor skills are skills involving large muscle movements. The developmental sequence of gross motor includes the following important skills (important developmental skills are called *milestones*): head control, rolling, crawling, sitting, creeping, standing, and walking. Movements in and out of these positions are also important gross motor skills. Fine motor skills are smaller movements of the arms and hands. Important fine motor milestones include reaching, grasping, transferring objects from one hand to the other, and releasing objects. Coordination and refinement of fine motor skills requires control of the hips, trunk, and shoulders (the gross motor skills associated with postural stability). For this reason, gross motor development is the foundation of fine motor development.

Physical Development Difficulties

Gross and fine motor development is linked to the development of the central nervous system, a process that begins before birth and continues until about age 5. When motor development is delayed or abnormal, the lower brain centers persist in controlling movements. Movements controlled by the lower brain are primarily reflexive. Development of the higher brain centers is necessary for reflexes to be integrated and for more mature, voluntary movements to emerge (Molnar, 1979). An immature or maldeveloped central nervous system is characterized by delayed motor development and by one or more of the following problems: abnormal muscle tone, persistence of primitive reflexes, postural reaction deficits, and compensatory patterns. The extent to which these problems are manifested and interfere with normal motor development varies from slight to severe.

Abnormal Muscle Tone.　Muscle tone, the resting state of tenseness in a muscle (Copeland & Kimmel, 1989), may be too high ("hypertonia" or "spasticity"), too low ("hypotonia" or "flaccidity"), or fluctuating ("athetosis"). Abnormal tone interferes with the quantity and quality of movement: there is too little or too much movement, and movement is too fast, too slow, or jerky. Abnormal tone also interferes with the development of normal postures and movement patterns, and the ability to move from one position to another (for example, from creeping to sitting, or from lying down to sitting).

Persistence of Primitive Reflexes.　When the central nervous system is maldeveloped or immature, these reflexes tend to be abnormal in three ways:

1. They *persist* beyond the normal developmental time frame; in normal development these reflexes fade or become integrated with voluntary movement;

2. They are *exaggerated*, easily elicited, and usually fully demonstrated; they are not "fleeting" or "partial," as in normal development; and

3. They are *obligatory*; once elicited, posture and movement is restricted and bound by the pattern; they are never obligatory in normal development (Copeland & Kimmel, 1989).

Chapter 3 discussed the importance of reflexes in physical development.

Postural Reaction Deficits.   In infants/young children with motor delays or deficits, postural reactions (equilibrium and righting) do not develop or develop incompletely (Bobath, 1967). Without righting reactions, there is not a strong physiological urge to establish aligned and upright postures and movements. And without equilibrium reactions, normal postural and movement patterns are difficult to attain.

Compensatory Patterns.   The presence of abnormal muscle tone and primitive reflexes, and the lack of normal postural reactions, interfere with the infant/young child's opportunity to experience normal movement and postural sensations. This is true with mild motor disabilities as well as severe ones. Many of these infants/young children do achieve some postures and movements, but may do so through abnormal postures called *compensations*. Compensations are useful to the child (for example, accomplishing a head-in-midline posture), but they restrict movement and block subsequent motor development (Bly, 1983). Table 7-4 describes compensatory patterns that frequently occur among infants/young children with motor delays or disabilities.

Physical Development Intervention Procedures

Motor interventions should be conducted during functional activities. This is called *integrated therapy*. Integrated therapy teaches infants and young children the purpose of new motor skills and enhances generalization (Smith, 1989). Intervention for children with mild physical delays or disabilities will usually target the normal sequences of gross and fine motor. For children with severe physical delays or disabilities, the functional use of selected motor skills and adaptive skills will usually be targeted.

Mild Physical Disabilities.   Problems of abnormal muscle tone, persistent primitive reflexes, and compensatory patterns are not usually evident when physical development is only delayed, but may be present if the mild disabilities are due to central nervous system damage. When physical development is mildly delayed, it usually follows the sequences of normal development, only it proceeds more slowly. Delays in gross motor milestones are associated with delays in postural reactions. For example, delayed righting reactions will delay the development of sitting because the child does not have the urge to raise his trunk. Once the child finally

---

TABLE 7-4

**Compensatory Patterns that Interfere with Motor Development
in Infants/Young Children with Neuromotor Disabilities**

Pattern	Effect
Neck block: Neck hyperextension	Cannot bring head to midline in supine; lifts head with neck hyperextension; holds head erect by elevating shoulders; normal mobility of head, scapula, shoulders, and arms is blocked; jaw juts forward resulting in opening of the mouth
Neck block: Head and neck asymmetry	Posture dominated by ATNR; head is continually turned to one side; spine rotates in direction of head; child at risk for scoliosis and hip dislocation; reaches by swiping with one arm and has difficulty using both arms together
Shoulder block	Scapular stability does not develop; cannot bear weight on forearms, has limited upper extremity movement, poor protective extension, and poor fine motor skills
Pelvic hip block: Anterior pelvic tilt	Hyperextension of lumbar spine ("swayback") and hip flexion; cannot weight-shift from side to side; sits with "frog-legged' position; cannot creep, moves forward with "bunny hop" (moves both legs together); if able to stand, stands with feet far apart, and knees and thighs together (very unstable); at risk for contractures of hips, knees, and ankles
Pelvic hip block: Posterior pelvic tilt	Hyperextension of lumbar spine, hips, and lower extremities; limited movement in lower extremities; if placed in sitting, sits on sacrum with rounded back and flexed knees; child may learn to "W" sit for stability; may creep with bunny hop; not likely to stand

---

sits, it will take him a long time to learn balance and avoid falling because of delayed equilibrium reactions.

Delays in postural reactions result in postural instability (described earlier in Chapter 3). The problem of postural instability accentuates the problem of fine motor delays. For example, the preschooler with poor sitting balance will have difficulty feeding herself because her trunk and shoulders are unstable.

Intervention for gross motor skills when mild disabilities are present focuses on teaching the next skill in the developmental sequence and improving postural reactions, particularly the equilibrium (balance) reactions. Activities that encourage the child to practice a skill, and physical guidance, are common intervention procedures. For example, when a child is beginning to creep (move forward on hands and knees), encouragement is provided by enticing the child to creep toward

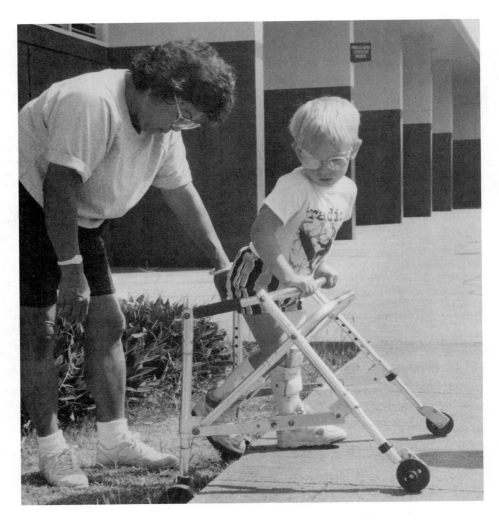

Adaptive equipment, such as a walker, can support the development of independent motor skills.

desired objects held a short distance away. Guided practice is provided by assisting the child to move her hips and legs back and forth in a creeping pattern. Balance reactions for creeping are encouraged by holding desired toys and objects off to the child's side, enticing the child to lift one arm and reach to the side for it. Reaching requires her to shift her weight to maintain the creeping position and avoid falling. If the child is unable to reach to the side, physical guidance to shift her weight is provided.

As noted above, children with mild physical disabilities will often have fine motor delays. Interventions that improve postural stability result in improved fine motor skills. These interventions can be provided through physical assistance or adaptations. For example, if a child is having difficulty controlling the movement of his toothbrush, he may be guided to spread his feet apart for a more solid base of support. He may also be assisted to hold the edge of the sink for balance. With a steadier base of support and assistance in balance, controlling the movement of his toothbrush is an easier task. An example of an adaptation to make the toothbrush easier to hold is to enlarge the handle by wrapping it with masking tape. Adaptations for gross and fine motor skills are discussed in more detail in Chapter 11.

Many fine motor tasks are performed while seated. Postural stability in a sitting position is critical to fine motor skills. Postural stability is enhanced when the child is seated in a chair of the proper size (its seat length is the distance from her buttocks to her knees) and she can place her feet flat on the floor or on a footrest. If the child has difficulty sitting upright with her hips at the back of the seat, a wide strap holding her hips in the back of the seat will improve stability. And finally, the table height may be modified to improve postural stability. The table height should be at least a few inches above the height of the child's elbows. For additional support, the table may be raised to a level slightly below the child's armpits.

Severe Physical Disabilities.   Usually severe physical disabilities are due to a developmental disorder rather than a delay, such as central nervous system damage or a neuromuscular disease. When a severe physical disability is present, the problems of abnormal muscle tone, persistent primitive reflexes, postural reaction deficits, and compensatory patterns are likely to characterize motor development. These problems affect the development of functional gross and fine motor skills.

The most common cause of severe physical disabilities in infants and young children is cerebral palsy. (Note that cerebral palsy can also cause mild physical delays.) Cerebral palsy is a nonprogressive disorder of movement and posture due to a lesion or damage in the immature brain. A common approach to intervention for severe physical disabilities is Neurodevelopmental Training (NDT) (Bobath, 1967). The goals of NDT are:

1. Facilitate normalized muscle tone,
2. Integrate primitive reflexes,
3. Facilitate postural reactions, and
4. Facilitate normalized posture and movement patterns.

It should be evident from the discussion of motor difficulties that goal 4, normalized posture and movement patterns, is dependent on the accomplishment of goals 1, 2, and 3. These goals are addressed during functional activities through positioning and carrying, and facilitation procedures.

Positioning and carrying procedures are therapeutic techniques that provide stable and aligned posture, normalize muscle tone, and inhibit abnormal reflexes (Clark & Allen, 1985; Copeland & Kimmel, 1989). Positions that appear to be opposite or counter to the abnormal patterns are usually effective. For example, when a child is placed in her highchair and demonstrates an asymmetrical tonic neck reflex (ATNR), her posture is characterized by too much muscle tone, asymmetry, and extension (her trunk, head, and neck rotate to one side, extremities are extended on her face side, and the opposite extremities flex). This abnormal pattern is broken up by using pillows, positioning inserts, or a special chair that aligns her body, limbs, and head; flexes her hips, knees, and ankles; and brings her head and shoulders slightly forward. Figure 7-3 illustrates this positioning example. Note that appropriate positioning and carrying procedures allow for normalized movement patterns. This implies that positioning must not be too confining: if an infant/young child is "over-positioned," movement will not be possible, and new motor skills will not be learned.

Using furniture, pillows, or specialized equipment *(adaptive equipment)* for positioning or carrying is called *static positioning*. The devices are fixed in place and cannot be readily adjusted in response to changes in muscle tone or movement, or situational demands. Static positioning and carrying procedures provide the infant/young child with independence from the adult, and free the adult for activities beyond the reach and confines of holding the child. An alternative to static

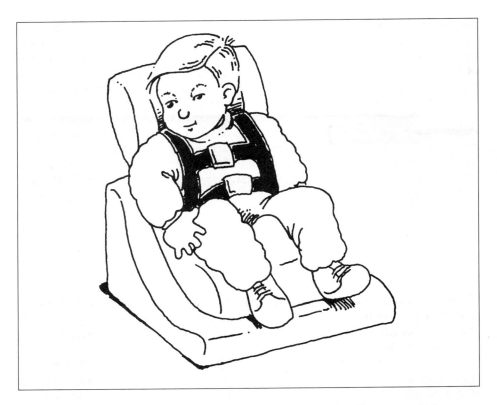

Figure 7-3 Example of positioning technique to "break up" asymmetrical extensor pattern

positioning and carrying is *dynamic positioning,* in which the adult's body (instead of equipment) is used to support the child in the desired position. The advantage of dynamic positioning and carrying is that the adult can respond immediately to child and situational needs. If the child's tone increases significantly, for example, the resistance from static positioning equipment might further increase tone because of discomfort. With dynamic positioning, the adult can relax positioning constraints and then reinstate support when the child's tone relaxes again.

Physical guidance and encouragement techniques that assist the infant/young child to accomplish normalized postures and movements (gross and fine motor skills and postural reactions) are called *facilitation* techniques. For example, while being assisted with dressing, a father holds his 2-year-old daughter on his lap, assisting her to prop herself with her hands on her knees. This position encourages and facilitates head and trunk control (holding her head and trunk upright) and discourages increased muscle tone. As her father helps her put on a T-shirt, he shifts her weight to one side, allowing her to lift her opposite arm into the T-shirt sleeve. As her weight is shifted to one side, she feels the weight bearing through her supporting arm. This facilitates an equilibrium reaction in sitting. It also facilitates a righting reaction associated with head and trunk control, encouraging her to realign and maintain her head and trunk upright. The procedure is repeated to the other side. Appropriate positioning and carrying procedures (including the use of adaptive equipment) ideally function as facilitation techniques, allowing and encouraging increasingly more independent postures and movement. Facilitation procedures are innumerable and must be responsive to the characteristics and needs of each child, as well as the postural and movement requirements of the situation.

Physical and occupational therapists typically have the responsibility of conducting the motor evaluation, developing an intervention plan, and teaching the other members of the transdisciplinary team to implement the plan, including the facilitation procedures. Although therapists have expertise in physical development, the team approach is critical to planning motor interventions that address infants' and children's movement needs associated with meaningful, functional activities.

Adaptive Development Skills

Adaptive development skills are personal care skills such as dressing, bathing, brushing teeth, toileting, and eating. Sequences of development and the ages at which adaptive development skills are acquired by normally developing infants and young children, is contained in most developmental assessment scales, such as the Early Intervention Developmental Profile (Schafer & Moersch, 1981). This information is useful in determining where to begin instruction and provides information on the age appropriateness of skills.

Adaptive development skills are usually taught using task analysis and the assistance and encouragement procedures described in Chapter 6. For example, in teaching a toddler to wash her hands, a task analysis assessment is first conducted. The steps of the task are delineated:

1. Turn on cold water faucet
2. Wet hands
3. Pick up soap
4. Lather palms
5. Replace soap
6. Lather back of hands
7. Rinse hands
8. Turn water off
9. Pick up towel
10. Dry hands
11. Replace towel

The toddler is assisted to wash her hands, and her performance on each step is assessed. When she is unable to perform a step, prompting and motivation procedures are provided to identify effective teaching strategies to be included in the instructional plan. The task analysis assessment also helps the teacher or infant specialist determine if the task has unnecessary steps that can be eliminated or combined with other steps, or if steps are too broad and additional steps are needed. Following the task analysis assessment, the instructional plan is formulated with the task analysis included (revised according to the assessment results). Prompting and motivation procedures are specified for each step. Figure 7-4 is a sample instructional plan for handwashing.

If an adaptive development goal is too difficult, or if it requires participation beyond the infant/young child's physical abilities, a *partial participation task analysis* may be developed (Snell, 1987). In a partial participation task analysis, steps within the child's physical capabilities that enable the child to participate *meaningfully* are delineated. For example, Snell (1987) described a partial participation task analysis for toothbrushing. The child's participation includes opening his mouth for the teacher to brush one quadrant of his teeth, and swallowing a drink of water after each quadrant has been brushed. Holding his mouth open and swallowing are important steps in assisted toothbrushing that make the task of the adult much easier. Figure 7-5 illustrates an instructional plan for handwashing that includes a partial participation task analysis.

Toileting and feeding are each a complex set of adaptive development skills that are critical to independence (Sailor & Guess, 1983). Therapeutic and specialized instructional procedures for facilitating these skills have been studied in depth and are described here.

Toileting

Toileting is comprised of several skills: recognizing the need, getting to the bathroom, lowering and raising clothing, getting on and off the toilet, sitting and

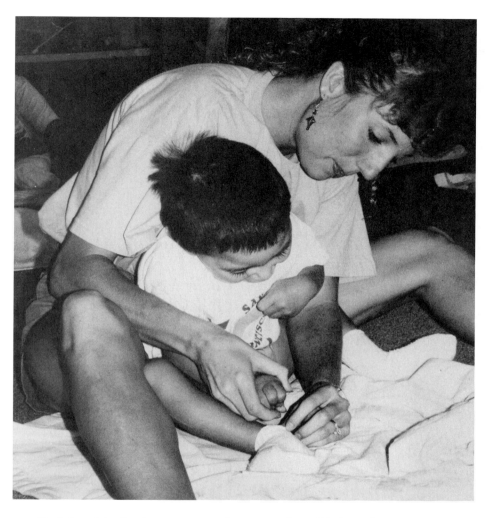

Partial participation is one way to adapt a complex self-help goal.

voiding, wiping, flushing, and washing and drying hands. Among normally developing children, toileting is typically achieved between 24 and 30 months of age. Toileting is not usually learned earlier than this because the following entry requirements seem to be essential (Snell, 1987):

1. The child's schedule of urination and bowel movements is fairly regular and does not include frequent dribbling.
2. The child remains dry for 1 to 2 hours on a fairly consistent schedule from day to day

		Date begun:	2/12/92

Infant/Child: Jillian

Date completed: _____

Objective: Handwashing

Interventionist: Molly and Dad

Conditions: Given a request to wash her hands

Response: Jillian will wash and dry her hands

Criterion: Independently, 3 of 4 consecutive times

Intervention Context	**Prompting/Facilitation Techniques**	**Consequences**
Setting(s): ♦At preschool, before lunch ♦At home, before dinner	*Positioning and Handling; Special Equipment/Materials; Environmental Modifications:* ♦ Stool at bathroom sink at home	*Reinforcement:* ♦ Verbally praise and state the desirable behavior (e.g., Good Jillian, you got the soap)
Routine(s)/Activity(ies): 1. Turn on cold water faucet 2. Wet hands 3. Pick up soap 4. Lather palms 5. Replace soap 6. Lather back of hands 7. Rinse hands 8. Turn water off 9. Pick up towel 10. Dry hands 11. Replace towel	*Prompting/Facilitation: (Wait 5 seconds after prompts)* 1. Point to faucet 2. Nudge hands toward water 3. Point to soap 4. Start motion of lathering hands 5. Point to soap dish 6. Place right hand on top of left hand 7. Nudge hands toward water 8. Point to faucet 9. Point to towel 10. Start motion of drying hands 11. Point to towel rack When all prompts are effective (no correctons needed), *delay* each prompt 4 seconds.	*Correction(s):* ♦ Physically guide Jillian through the steps

Figure 7-4   Intervention plan

Date begun: 6/6/92

Infant/Child: Todd

Date completed: _____

Objective: Assisted Handwashing

Interventionist: Selina and Mike

Conditions: Given a request to wash his hands

Response: Todd will assist in washing and drying his hands

Criterion: 5 consecutive times

Intervention Context	Prompting/Facilitation Techniques	Consequences
Setting(s): ◆At preschool, before lunch ◆At home, before dinner	Positioning and Handling; Special Equipment/Materials; Environmental Modifications: ◆ Position Todd in his feeder seat	Reinforcement: ◆ Smile and talk to Todd the entire time he is holding his hand(s) open
Routine(s)/Activity(ies): 1. Holds one hand up and keeps hand open with fingers apart (adult washes hand with wash rag) 2. Holds other hand up and keeps fingers apart (adults washes hand with wash rag) 3. Holds both hands out with fingers apart (adult dries both hands with towel)	Prompting/Facilitation: ◆ Tap hand(s) and say, "Let's wash (or dry) your hand(s)."	Correction(s): ◆ Shake arm(s) to relax tone ◆ Rub back of hand(s) and gently assist Todd to open his fingers

Figure 7-5 Intervention plan

3. The child is at least 18 months old if mild disabilities are present; and at least 2 ½ years old if more significant delays are present. This age consideration is included because studies suggest that sphincter control is delayed among young children with moderate and severe mental retardation.

Also note that in normal development, daytime toilet training is learned before nighttime toilet training.

While the child is learning the prerequisites, toileting needs are most easily managed through *timed toileting* (also known as "toilet regulation"). Timed toileting is placing the child on the toilet for a few minutes (not more than 10 minutes) at the times that she usually eliminates. If the child uses the toilet, reinforcement is provided. If the child does not eliminate, she is removed from the toilet without any consequences. Timed toileting helps the child learn why and when the toilet is used, and it eases caretaking responsibilities, although accidents may still occur. Timed toileting may also be an appropriate goal for a young child with physical disabilities affecting mobility or fine motor skills that interfere with independence.

For children with mild disabilities who are delayed in toileting but are learning in the prerequisite skills, task analysis and direct instruction procedures are used to assist them in learning dressing and handwashing. To teach them to recognize the need to use the toilet and to void in it, follow a procedure similar to the timed toileting. Keep a record of the times when the children are dry and wet by checking their diapers frequently (every half hour). Ask them if they need to use the toilet 5 to 10 minutes before they usually void. If the children say yes, place them on the toilet for about 5 minutes. Praise them if they eliminate in the toilet; comment that they should try later if they do not use the toilet. Most children with mild delays will learn toileting with this simple procedure.

For children with more severe disabilities, toileting is usually taught by increasing the intake of liquids so that they need to use the toilet more often. This increases the number of teaching opportunities. The toilet-training approach that popularized this procedure is the *rapid method* and is described in the paperback *Toilet Training in Less than a Day* (Azrin & Foxx, 1974).

Medical clearance should be obtained prior to implementing toilet-training procedures that involve increased in fluid intake. If hydration is to be used with a toilet-training procedure, care should be taken not to exceed normal daily water allowances: approximately 1 to 4 cups per day for children weighing between 4 and 22 lb, and approximately 4 to 7 cups per day for children between 22 and 88 lb (Thompson & Hanson, 1983). A substantial increase in fluids can cause overhydration (Snell, 1987). Overhydration symptoms include nausea, vomiting, muscle twitching, seizures, and coma. Some children have medical conditions for which increased fluid intake is contraindicated (hypertension, or abnormal functioning of the heart, liver, or kidneys, for example). Fluid intake procedures should *never* be used with children who have epilepsy, hydrocephaly, or a prior spinal injury.

Bedwetting (nocturnal enuresis) is a common problem among young children. Children are ready to begin nighttime toilet training when they are successful throughout 75% of the day with daytime toileting (Snell, 1987). There are three major types of intervention strategies for nighttime toilet training. The simplest procedure requires that the child's fluid intake be adjusted so that no fluids are provided 1 1/2 to 2 hours before bedtime. Awaken the child a few minutes before the times that he typically voids (most children will only need to use the toilet once during the night) and have him sit on the toilet for 5 minutes. Praise him for a dry bed and for eliminating in the toilet. If his bed is wet, change it without comment. Provide enthusiastic reinforcement in the morning if the child kept his bed dry. Gradually delay the wake-up (10-minute periods) to require that the child stay dry for increasingly longer periods of time.

The second procedure to eliminate nighttime bedwetting uses a *signaling device,* a pad that is placed under the bedsheet. This procedure is most appropriate for children who are at least 5 years of age. When the alarm sounds indicating a wet bed, awaken the child and assist him to practice toileting skills (going to the bathroom and using the toilet, changing pajamas and bedding). Provide praise when the child sleeps through the night without wetting the bed.

The third procedure is a rapid bedtime method (Azrin, Sneed, & Foxx, 1973; 1974), much like the daytime rapid training method. The procedure includes increased fluids, use of a signaling device on the bed, hourly checks, toileting practice, and praise for dry bed and eliminating in the toilet. It is not necessary to implement the procedure throughout the entire night; effectiveness has been demonstrated when the procedure was used from bedtime until 1 A.M. (Azrin & Besalel, 1979).

Feeding, Eating, and Drinking

Eating and drinking involve a complex set of motor and oral-motor skills. The normal sequence of these skills is described in Table 7-5. Table 7-5 can be used as a guide for determining developmentally appropriate mealtime goals. For infants and young children with mild disabilities, mealtime skills are taught using task analysis and direct instruction described in Chapter 6. For example, cup drinking may be task analyzed as follows:

1. Grasp cup
2. Lift cup to mouth
3. Drink a few swallows
4. Return cup to table
5. Release cup

Backwards chaining may be used to teach the task analysis. For instance, assist the child to perform the first four steps, and verbally prompt him to release the cup when it touches the table (the fifth step). When the child is successful with the fifth step, teach the fourth and fifth step together. As each new step is learned, add another step until the entire task analysis is acquired.

Hand-over-hand assistance is another direct instruction procedure frequently used with self-feeding skills. The adult lightly holds the child's hand and assists as necessary (for example, to hold a spoon, or to pick up a cracker). Figure 7-6 is an example of systematic instructional plan for a toddler who is delayed in using a spoon. Adaptive feeding equipment may also be included in the instructional plan to assist the child in acquiring independence (see Figure 7-7).

TABLE 7-5

Feeding development in normal children

Age	Skill
Birth	Sucking and swallowing Incomplete lip closure Unable to release nipple
4 weeks	Opens mouth, waiting for food Better lip closure Active lip movement when sucking Takes cereal from spoon
6 weeks	Pureed fruit from spoon
3 months	Anticipates feeding
4 months	Recognizes bottle, mouth ready for nipple Cup feeding may be introduced—very messy but enjoys process More control and movement of tongue is handled by child—not by reflexes Appetite is more erratic Will not consume three full feedings Tongue thrust seen more with cup feeding than spoon feeding
5 months	Mouth opens ready for spoon Uses hands to draw bottle to mouth but releases when nipple is inserted Tongue reversal after spoon removed, ejecting food involuntarily
5½ months	Good lip closure Overhand grasp with both hands to feed self with cup
6 months	Good control with lips and tongue Beginning definite chewing motion by gumming food
7 months	Spoon fed chunky foods Feeds self soft foods (banana, vegetables, etc.) Drooling noticed with mouth activity Reaches for food with head
8 months	Uses two hands on cup—messy Holds own bottle Picks up food with thumb and forefinger Finger feeds most of food Chokes easily when drinking from cup
9 months	Grows impatient when watching meal preparation Enjoys chewing Likes to finger feed self—messy Appetite finicky
10 months	Lateral movement of jaw Grasps and brings bottle to mouth Food is to be felt, tasted, smeared and dropped on floor Cup feeding still messy—may want to play with it

TABLE 7-5—*(continued)*

Age	Skill
11 months	Objects if mother tries to help complete feeding Can use cup by self
12 months	More choosy about food Independent about finishing meal—may dump remaining food on floor Lunch is least motivating meal
15 months	Holds cup with fingers—many spills Grasps spoon—poor manipulation Spoon inverted before insertion Shows definite preference for certain foods
18 months	Drinks from cup well Hands empty cup or dish to mother—if she doesn't see—child will drop item Chews meat well Better control with spoon
21 months	Handles cup well Very regimented in eating—wants everything on a routine schedule and presented same way each time
2 years	Can handle small glass with one hand, partially filled Moderate spillage from spoon Refuses previous favorite food Inserts food into mouth without turning over spoon Food preference may stem from taste, form, consistency, or just color
3 years	Minimum spilling from spoon Dawdles at mealtime Likes to spear food with fork
4 years	Sets table well Likes to serve self Washes and dries own face and hands
5 years	Appetite may increase, prefers simple food Beginning to use knife to spread Talkative during meals Doesn't always finish meal by self—may need assistance; often asks for help
6 years	Very active; cannot sit still Asks for more food than can consume Enjoys snacks more than mealtime Spills with milk—common at this age Breakfast may be most difficult meal Not interested in dessert May return to finger feeding
7 years	Appetite is less for girls; boys may have tremendous appetite May eat formerly disliked dishes Interested in desserts Use of napkin is spotty

TABLE 7-5—(continued)

Age	Skill
8 years	Girls hold fork in adult fashion; boys hold fork pronated Starting to cut with knife Shovels food into mouth Asks for seconds, even thirds
9 years	Appetite under better control Likes to help prepare meals Still has difficulty controlling and knowing what to do with napkin Difficulty in cutting food to appropriate size, tends to be too big
11 years	Has a satisfied feeling after meals
12 years	Bottomless pit—eating constantly
13 years	Appetite more stable
14 years	More like adult balance

SOURCE: From *Occupational Therapy for Mentally Retarded Children*, by M. Copeland, L. Ford, and N. Solon. Copyright © 1976 by University Park Press, Baltimore, MD. Data from Gesell and Amatruda (1947), Gesell and Ilg (1946), Ilg and Ames (1955), Rutherford (1971), Smart and Smart (1967), and Spock (1972). Reprinted by permission of the author.

For infants and young children with severe disabilities, special feeding techniques may be necessary. This is particularly true when a neuromotor disability, such as cerebral palsy, is present. The early intervention team works together to address mealtime problems; occupational, physical, and sometimes speech, therapists are the professionals on the early intervention team with expertise in feeding techniques. As always, family involvement and input is critical in planning interventions, particularly given that mealtimes are so much a part of family life.

Mealtime intervention plans for infants and young children with severe disabilities may include therapeutic positioning, adaptive equipment, pre-feeding techniques, therapeutic feeding techniques, and systematic instruction. As with the general principles of motor intervention, the purpose of therapeutic positioning for feeding, eating, and drinking is to normalize muscle tone, inhibit abnormal reflexes, and facilitate normal patterns of movement (including oral-motor patterns). There are several general positioning goals that are particularly critical when positioning an infant/young child for mealtimes. First, the infant/young child's body should be symmetrical and aligned. Usually, symmetry and alignment will inhibit abnormal postural and tonal patterns. An exception to this may be positioning the infant/young child with trunk rotation to facilitate relaxation and decrease hypertonicity. Second, unless an infant is still being bottle- or breast-fed, the young child should be positioned as upright as possible. The head should be in a slightly

	Date begun:	5/5/92

Infant/Child: _Francie_   Date completed: _____

Objective: _Scooping_   Interventionist: _Mom_

Conditions: _At lunch, when given a plate of ground and sticky food_

Response: _Francie will scoop and eat her lunch_

Criterion: _Without assistance for 10 minutes, 2 consecutive lunches_

Intervention Context	*Prompting/Facilitation Techniques*	*Consequences*
Setting(s): ♦ Lunchtime	*Positioning and Handling; Special Equipment/Materials; Environmental Modifications:* ♦ Use plate with high rim and small plastic coated spoon	*Reinforcement:* ♦ Provide a sip of juice
Routine(s)/Activity(ies): 1. Grasp spoon handle 2. Scoop food onto spoon 3. Raise spoon to mouth 4. Place spoon in mouth and remove food 5. Return spoon to bowl or table	*Prompting/Facilitation:* 1. Point to spoon handle 2. (Wait 6 seconds) 3. Model opening your mouth 4. Model opening your mouth 5. (Wait 6 seconds) *Backwards chain:* Assist through steps not being taught, prompt and correct current step as noted in this plan *Criterion is 2 consecutive corrects for adding previous step to intervention chain	*Correction(s):* 1. Physically assist Francie to grasp and lift spoon 2. Assist Francie to *start* scooping 3. Physically assist Francie to make correct response

Figure 7-6 Intervention plan

forward position with a slight downward tilt for swallowing. Alignment, symmetry, and an upright posture are critical to normal swallowing, the coordination of breathing and swallowing, and preventing food or liquids passing into the trachea or lungs (aspiration) or choking. Third, the infant/young child's feet should be flat on the floor or on a support to provide postural stability. Fourth, the shoulders and

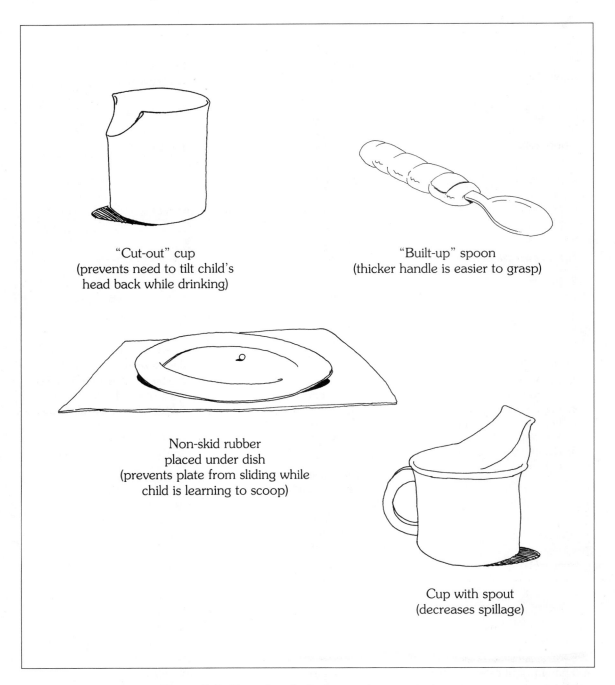

"Cut-out" cup
(prevents need to tilt child's
head back while drinking)

"Built-up" spoon
(thicker handle is easier to grasp)

Non-skid rubber
placed under dish
(prevents plate from sliding while
child is learning to scoop)

Cup with spout
(decreases spillage)

Figure 7-7 Examples of adaptive mealtime equipment

TABLE 7-6
Pre-Feeding Techniques for Infants/Young Children Who Have Oral-Motor Problems Due to Neuromotor Disabilities

Problem	Pre-Feeding Technique
Hypertonus throughout the body	Relax child prior to mealtime by gentle rocking and trunk rotation. Proper positioning for mealtime should help maintain normalized tone.
Tactile hypersensitivity in and around mouth	Provide tactile stimulation outside mouth by patting the cheeks and firm rubbing (terry cloth may be used). Stroke firmly and downward above the upper lip and upward toward the lower lip; apply quick stretching to corners of mouth (outward). Massage outside area of upper and lower gums with horizontal strokes (keeping fingers away from teeth). Avoid wiping mouth area during mealtime with spoon or rag. If necessary to wipe mouth area, pat area with terry cloth.
Lack of jaw closure	Apply quick stretching to jaw muscles, stroking downward just below cheekbones.
Lack of lip closure	Apply quick stretching to upper lip (upward), lower lip (downward), and corners of mouth (outward).
Hypersensitive gag reflex	Hold jaw open (grasping jaw just below ears) and firmly tap the tongue with a swizzle stick or tongue depressor, slowly "walking" the stick from the tip of the tongue to the middle of the tongue. Stop when the tongue "humps" in the middle or if gagging begins to occur.

arms should be relaxed and free to move, so that the young child can accomplish hand-to-mouth movements and participate in self-feeding. Occupational and physical therapists on the early intervention team are involved in identifying optimal mealtime position(s) for an infant/young child with neuromotor disabilities.

Pre-feeding techniques include rubbing and stroking to decrease hypersensitivity around and inside the mouth, and stretching techniques to facilitate normalized tone and movement of the facial muscles. Table 7-6 lists eating and drinking problems and describes pre-feeding techniques that address the problems (Copeland & Kimmel, 1989).

Therapeutic feeding techniques are strategies to inhibit abnormal oral-motor patterns and facilitate normalized oral-motor patterns. The positioning and pre-feeding techniques described above are important components of therapeutic feeding techniques. There are also techniques to assist a child with eating and drinking skills such as jaw control, lip closure, tongue control, chewing, and swallowing. Table 7-7 describes common eating and drinking problems and interventions to facilitate normalized oral-motor patterns (Copeland & Kimmel, 1989).

TABLE 7-7

Feeding Techniques for Infants/Young Children Who Have Oral-Motor Problems Due to Neuromotor Disabilities

Problem	*Feeding Technique*
Lack of jaw control; inability to grade jaw movements	Assist with jaw closure/grading by holding child's chin in cupped hand. Be careful not to extend child's neck while providing jaw control.
Lack of lip closure	Assist lip closure by placing index and second fingers above and below the child's lips and using a "scissors" motion to close the lips. If assistance for jaw closure is also needed, support jaw with baby finger.
	Place spoon on front third of tongue and apply firm downward pressure. Remove spoon at 45° angle and avoid scraping food off spoon with teeth (food should be removed with lips).
Tongue thrust	Provide jaw control and lip closure.
Hypersensitive bite reflex	Use small rubber-coated spoon for feeding. Place spoon on front third of tongue and apply firm downward pressure. Remove spoon at 45° angle and avoid scraping food off spoon with teeth (food should be removed with lips).
Lack of rotary chewing and/or tongue lateralization (side-to-side movements)	Place scoop of food or soft finger foods on back molars (alternating sides from bite to bite). Use lip and jaw control as necessary to assist in keeping mouth closed. Massage jaws (below cheekbones) in forward circular motion. Apply pressure to center of chin.
	When placing food on molars is effective, occasionally place spoon on front third of tongue and apply firm downward pressure. Remove spoon at 45° angle and avoid scraping food off spoon with teeth (food should be removed with lips).
Lack of normal swallowing; swallowing is delayed or associated with suck-swallow reflex	With mouth closed (assist with jaw and/or lip closure support if necessary), stroke downward under chin.
Cannot drink from cup	Provide least amount of assistance as necessary; lower lip closure, upper and lower lip closure, and lip closure with jaw control.

Infants and young children with severe eating and drinking problems are at risk for choking. Choking occurs when food or some other object or material obstructs the infant/young child's airway. If the infant/young child is coughing, the airway is not totally obstructed. Allow the child to cough, and assist the child to lean forward. An infant may be turned upside down. In both situations, gravity can assist in clearing the airway. If the infant/young child appears unable to breathe and is unable to cough, the airway may be completely obstructed. Emergency action is required. If it is an infant or small child who is choking, turn the infant/small child upside down with her face and head lower than her chest. Hit her back four times rapidly between her shoulder blades (Hafen & Karren, 1984). This maneuver requires holding the child with one hand, so that the other hand is free to administer the back blows. The blows should be sharp and firm, but not too hard, or the child may be injured. If the child is too large to invert completely and quickly, the Heimlich maneuver should be administered immediately (Hafen & Karren, 1984). Early interventionists should receive first aid and emergency care training annually so they can respond competently and quickly to choking and other emergencies that may arise.

For infants and young children who are unable to obtain adequate nutrition and hydration orally, feeding tubes (*gavage* feedings) may be used. A feeding tube is inserted through the abdomen wall *(gastrostomy)*, nose *(nasogastric tube)*, or mouth *(oralgastric tube)*. Food is administered through a gravity method or pump method (kangaroo bag). In the gravity method, food is placed in a large syringe attached to the feeding tube. The syringe is elevated 4 to 5 inches above the child's abdomen if a gastrostomy tube is used, or 4 to 5 inches above the child's head if a nasogastric or oralgastric tube is used. The food passes slowly through the tube and into the abdomen. Water may be given through the tube after feeding. The pump method is identical to the gravity method, except an electric pump is used to move the food from the bag through the feeding tube. Nasogastric and gastrostomy tubes may be left in place and taped to the skin when not in use. Oralgastric tubes are usually inserted for each feeding and removed afterward.

The insertion of feeding tubes requires special training. Although parents are frequently trained by a nurse or physician to insert the tube, school districts usually require that a licensed health care worker (physician or nurse) insert the tube (California State Department of Education, 1980; Pathfinder & School Nurse Organization of Minnesota, 1986). *Teachers and infant specialists should be aware that there are health concerns associated with feeding tubes:* there is a risk of infection, particularly at the site of a gastrostomy, and there is a risk of aspiration when nasogastric or oralgastric feeding tubes are used.

Summary

The systematic instructional procedures described in Chapter 6 can be applied to most skill needs demonstrated by infants/young children with disabilities. There are specific procedures, however, that have been proven to be particularly effective with certain skill domains. Some of these techniques are behavioral (for example, toilet-training procedures), some derive from studies of "natural learning" (such as environmental control skills), and others are therapeutic techniques (for example, feeding or eating). The specialized procedures should always be applied in meaningful contexts, even though they may have been developed in clinical situations. Furthermore, integrating the specialized procedures with systematic instructional procedures may enhance the effectiveness of the intervention by clarifying steps and including additional assistance or motivational procedures in instruction.

Activities

1. Interview an early childhood special education teacher and ask the teacher to describe an augmentative communication system currently being used with one of the students. Ask the teacher to describe the factors considered in selecting the augmentative system and determining the initial vocabulary.

2. Read and write a summary of two recent journal articles investigating the use of nonaversive behavior management procedures for reducing or eliminating serious behavior problems. Comment on the appropriateness and applicability of the procedures for young children with severe behavior problems. Articles on nonaversive behavior management techniques can be found in the following journals.

Journal of the Association for Persons with Severe Handicaps
Journal of Applied Behavior Analysis
Mental Retardation

3. Meet with a physical therapist at an early intervention or preschool special education program. Ask the physical therapist to demonstrate appropriate positioning and handling techniques for an infant or young child with severe physical disabilities. Be sure to find out the rationale for each procedure demonstrated.

4. Observe a nondisabled 4- or 5-year-old perform the following self-help skills:

removing a T-shirt
handwashing

As you observe, develop a task analysis for each skill, listing what the child does, step by step. Bring the task analyses to class, and discuss similarities and differences in each student's task analyses.

Review Questions

1. Define *environmental control skills.* Explain why these skills are considered communication skills.
2. Describe three examples of environmental control skills typically demonstrated by nondisabled infants and young children.
3. Describe three strategies for teaching environmental control skills.
4. Define the following terms: *syntax, semantics,* and *pragmatics.*
5. Identify and provide an example of three pragmatic functions.
6. Describe a goal for expanding a child's environmental control skills.
7. Define *augmentative communication system.* When are augmentative communication systems used?
8. Discuss how "modality sampling" is used to select an augmentative communication system.
9. Discuss three approaches to teaching social skills to young children with disabilities.
10. Discuss a positive approach to eliminating a serious behavior problem.
11. Describe appropriate and inappropriate applications of the time-out procedure for young children with disabilities. Be sure to comment on appropriate time intervals for time out.
12. Describe the fair pair rule.
13. Describe two behavior reduction procedures to be avoided, and explain why the procedures are not appropriate procedures.
14. Define and describe gross and fine motor skills.
15. Discuss typical problems associated with physical development difficulties.
16. Discuss approaches to intervention for infants and young children with mild physical disabilities and severe physical disabilities.
17. Identify and describe the most frequently used instructional approach for teaching self-help skills to infants and young children with disabilities.
18. Describe two approaches to daytime toilet training.
19. Define pre-feeding and therapeutic feeding techniques.
20. Describe appropriate methods for dealing with choking.

Intervention in Natural Environments

Objectives

1. Describe naturalistic teaching approaches and techniques.

2. Discuss arranging the environment to enhance learning and participation of infants and young children with disabilities.

3. Discuss adapting curricula to accommodate children with special needs.

4. Discuss adapting instruction methods for children with disabilities.

5. Suggest data collection strategies for natural environments.

*T*here are many references to "natural environments," "natural contexts," "naturalistic teaching approaches," or "naturalistic training techniques" in the early intervention literature. There is also reference to natural environments in the recent reauthorization of Part H (IDEA Amendments of 1991). One of the important additions to this legislation is the requirement that the IFSP include a statement of the natural environments where early intervention services will be provided.

What are "natural environments"? At the broadest level, the term *natural environments* refers to all integrated community settings. This includes homes, schools, parks, shopping centers, stores, fast-food restaurants, and all other settings where the majority of participants are nondisabled persons. Activities that typically occur in a natural environment are natural activities.

Environments designed specifically for specialized services (a segregated preschool class, a clinic for children with cerebral palsy) are not natural environments. Though there are some activities in these specialized environments that seem like natural activities (such as snack time in the segregated preschool program, a parent diapering an infant in the clinic waiting room, a 4-year-old and a speech-language pathologist having a lively interaction at a computer), they are not natural activities. It is not possible to have natural activities in environments that are inherently restrictive. Because specialized environments share few of the rich and varied physical and social stimuli found in natural environments, generalization of skills learned in these settings is at best tenuous.

Natural environments are the ideal settings for instruction of natural activities. For example, the regular preschool classroom is the best setting for activities that typically take place in a preschool classroom setting. Similarly, natural activities are the ideal context for instruction of functional skills. For example, snack time is an ideal activity for instruction of social and language and communication skills.

Naturalistic Teaching Approaches and Techniques

Instruction in natural environments necessarily involves naturalistic teaching approaches. As discussed in Chapter 6, "natural" or "naturalistic" does not mean haphazard: it does not mean that there is no "tampering with Mother Nature." Instruction is carefully planned and intentional.

When naturalistic teaching approaches are being implemented, the environment is not natural in the strictest sense of the word. The environment may be altered (in an unobtrusive manner) to increase the probability that the desired behavior—or some approximation of the desired behavior—will occur. Naturalistic teaching approaches share these characteristics (Kaiser & Warren, 1988):

1. Teaching occurs in the natural environment.
2. Individual teaching interactions are typically very brief and distributed or spaced over a period of hours and days.

3. Instructional interactions are typically child-initiated.
4. Instruction uses natural consequences (objects and events are highly salient and desired by the child).

The last characteristic, natural consequences, is significant. In the broad class of external reinforcers, there are two categories of reinforcers: natural and instructional. Natural consequences are events that occur naturally as a result of a child's behavior. For example, when a child asks for a drink of water, the child is given a glass of water. The objective is to teach the child that certain behaviors function to obtain desired objects, activities, and services. Instructional reinforcers are motivators that are introduced strictly for the purpose of teaching or increasing the strength of a particular skill. There is always the possibility that a skill acquired using instructional reinforcers will not maintain when they are withdrawn.

Most naturalistic teaching approaches feature variations of a small subset of techniques. These techniques, sometimes called *milieu teaching,* were first described by Hart and Risley (1968) in the late sixties and early seventies. Probably the best-known milieu teaching approach is *incidental teaching,* which was expanded on by Hart and Rogers-Warren (1978), Rogers-Warren and Warren (1980a), and Warren, McQuarter, and Rogers-Warren (1984).

The incidental teaching language intervention approach involves (a) arranging the environment to increase the likelihood that the child will initiate a request or comment to an adult; (b) selecting language targets appropriate to the child's level, interest, and opportunities; (c) responding to the child's initiations with requests for elaborated language forms; and (d) reinforcing the child's communicative efforts by providing attention and access to the desired objects or events (Warren and Kaiser, 1986). The technique of incidental teaching is one element of the incidental teaching language intervention approach: the approach also incorporates three other procedures: (a) modeling; (b) the mand-model procedure ("Mand" is a term used by Skinner (1957) for a command, request, or demand); and (c) the time-delay procedure.

[handwritten marginalia: Key Elements of Incidental Language Teaching]

Other naturalistic approaches include conversational teaching (MacDonald, 1985); child-oriented teaching (Fey, 1986); unobtrusive training (Wutz, Meyers, Klein, Hill & Waldo, 1982); and coincidental teaching (Stowitschek et al., 1985). While much of the research considering naturalistic teaching approaches has dealt with language and communication objectives (Halle, 1982; Halle, Alpert & Anderson, 1984; Kaiser & Warren, 1988; Rogers-Warren & Warren, 1980a), there is evidence that naturalistic teaching approaches are effective in teaching other functional skills. Oliver and Halle (1982) found naturalistic training strategies effective in facilitating manual signing. Peck (1985) and Stowitschek and colleagues (1985) found naturalistic training strategies effective for teaching social skills. Kayser, Billingsly, and Neel (1986) used naturalistic teaching strategies to teach self-care behaviors such as zipping a coat and brushing teeth. Additionally, it is important to recognize that most instruction that parents andother caregivers provide for infants and young children is naturalistic teaching.

The rationale for naturalistic teaching applies across skill domains. Major reasons for using naturalistic training procedures for instruction of functional skill are: (a) to avoid (or at least reduce) problems related to generalization; (b) to increase daily interactions that will continue even after training has ended; and (c) to increase the likelihood that what is taught will be functional.

Naturalistic teaching approaches tend to employ one or another (or some combination) of these instructional techniques: (a) incidental teaching, (b) verbal prompts, (c) time-delay prompts, (d) interrupted routines, (e) interrupted behavior chains, (f) interesting materials, and (g) behavior trapping. Note the potential confusion related to the term *incidental teaching*. It is used three ways. It is used to refer to the specific naturalistic language training approach developed and expanded by Hart and colleagues (Hart & Risley, 1974; Hart & Rogers-Warren, 1978). It is also a specific naturalistic teaching technique. Finally, the term is sometimes used in the broadest sense as a synonym for naturalistic teaching.

Incidental Teaching Technique

The broadest definition for incidental teaching is taking advantage of naturally occurring child-adult interactions in order to teach specific functional skills. When the child demonstrates an interest in some object or event, either by looking at it, asking for it, or examining it, the expression of interest is viewed as a request for instruction and the occasion is used as a teaching opportunity.

Dunst and McWilliam (1988) describe application of the incidental teaching technique to facilitating cognitive skills with young children with severe and multiple impairments. These are the steps involved in using the incidental teaching strategy to encourage complex interactions with the environment.

Step 1: Arrange the environment to be interesting and fun for the child. Provide stimulus events that are known to elicit and maintain the child's attention.

Examples: Surround the child with interesting objects and materials.

Arrange for peers to interact with the child.

Take the child to a place where there are especially interesting activities.

Step 2: Watch the child carefully to determine what he finds interesting and fun. It is generally safe to assume that persons, objects, and particular features of objects that maintain the child's attention will be effective reinforcers.

Examples: Note what the child listens to.

Note what the child looks at.

Note what the child plays with.

Note who the child plays with.

Step 3: Get the child to interact with (or act upon) interesting objects or persons. Engage the child in interactions in which natural reinforcers are contingent on certain behaviors.

Examples: Encourage the child to pick up a toy or object.

Encourage the child to play with a toy or other object.

Encourage the child to talk to peers or to adults.

Step 4: Intervene (prompt, model, or rearrange the environment) to elicit ~~produce~~ more complex behaviors. Get the child to elaborate in a manner that successively approximates the desired behavior. To produce variations in the child's behavior, get the child to perform the behavior differently, complete the task, do it more smoothly, or take more time.

Examples: Prompt the child to do something different with the toy or object.

Prompt the child to name the toy or object or person.

Prompt the child to play cooperatively with peers.

Model appropriate labels or requests.

Step 5: Focus on development of conventional behavior. Most important is to make the behavior functional for the child. The behavior should be effective in helping the child achieve desired goals.

Examples: Help the child play independently with toys or other objects.

Prompt the child to initiate play with peers.

Encourage clear communication.

In summary, the idea is to follow the child's attentiveness to different features of the environment, and evoke successively more elaborate elaborations until the child's behavior approximates conventional behavior. Thus, in contrast to teaching procedures that emphasize bringing the learner under stimulus control, the incidental teaching technique parallels "developmentally appropriate practice" (Bredekamp, 1987), using procedures that are child-centered, child-directed, and teacher-guided.

Verbal Prompts

As discussed in Chapter 6, the goal of prompting is to help the child make a correct response with the least amount of assistance possible. Included under the heading of verbal prompts are (a) task directions, (b) questions, (c) requests, and (d) models of the correct response (for the child to imitate). Verbal prompts are somewhat more intrusive than time-delay prompts (discussed later). Another name for the verbal prompting strategy is the *mand-model procedure.* This is what it is called when used as part of the incidental teaching approach (Rogers-Warren & Warren, 1980a).

Verbal prompts vary according to the particular situation, the child's ability level, and what the child is learning. The verbal prompting strategy differs from the incidental teaching strategy in that the adult need not wait for the child to initiate an interaction. It is similar to the incidental teaching strategy, in that the environment is arranged to make a variety of interesting and desired objects available to the child. Here are the steps for implementing the verbal prompt strategy:

Step 1: Provide a direction, question, or request to perform the target behavior. When the child approaches a desired object or activity, provide a direction or instruction to perform the desired behavior. For example, if communication is the target skill, say "Tell me what you want." The direction, question, or request is always related to whatever is maintaining the child's attention at that moment.

Step 2: Give feedback and verbal expansion if the child responds correctly. The feedback will vary, depending on the situation. For example, if the child responds with the desired label, providing the desired object or material constitutes feedback. In most instances, verbal confirmation and expansion are also provided ("Here it is, your favorite puzzle," or "OK, I'll push you in the swing").

Step 3: Provide a model of the correct response if the child does not respond or responds incorrectly. Using the above example, the model might be "Say *puzzle*," or "Say *swing*."

One variation on the above procedures is called the *model-lead-test procedure*. The adult provides the model or the direction, instruction, or request on initial trials ("What do you want? Say *puzzle*.") On subsequent trials the child is expected to respond without a model or other prompt (Wolery and Brookfield-Norman, 1988). The latter trials are considered test trials. Corrective feedback is provided for errors, and correct responses are confirmed by providing the desired object or action.

Time-Delay Prompts

The time-delay prompting strategy is a systematic "wait procedure." When the child shows an interest in an object or activity or needs a particular object (food, materials, toys) or an action (assistance), the adult waits for the child to emit some behavior related to that object or activity (looking at the adult expectantly, saying "more"). The time-delay strategy teaches a child to initiate an interaction and is probably the least intrusive way to assist responding. It is similar to the incidental teaching strategy in that the child is expected to respond to physical or visual cues in the environment rather than adult verbalizations. Time-delay is widely used to teach language and other discrete responses to preschoolers and older students with moderate to severe handicaps (Halle, Alpert, & Anderson, 1984; Snell & Gast, 1981). Halle, Baer, and

Spradlin (1981) used the time-delay strategy to teach requesting to six young children with developmental delays.

The steps in the time-delay strategy are:

Step 1: Face the child with an expectant look and display a desired object. This may be a pitcher of orange juice, a favorite toy, or a crayon to finish a picture in progress.

Step 2: Wait a specified time (for example, 4 seconds) for the child to request or label the desired object. Wait silently while maintaining *eye* contact with the child.

Step 3: If the child responds correctly, provide the desired object. With this strategy, as with the other naturalistic teaching strategies, positive feedback generally takes two forms: provision of the desired object or action *and* verbal confirmation or expansion.

Step 4: Provide a verbal prompt or physical prompt if the child does not respond or responds incorrectly. Then reinforce the prompted response by providing the desired object or action and verbal confirmation.

Interrupted Routines

A routine is a sequence of actions or events that is repeated frequently and always in the same way. Frequent routines for toddlers and preschoolers include (a) social routines, (b) caregiving routines, (c) entertainment routines, and (d) activity routines. Examples of social routines are "Good morning" routines and other predictable interactions involving amenities and courtesies ("Please pass the cookies") and celebration routines such as birthday parties. There are a variety of caregiving routines centered around such tasks as washing, toileting, and brushing teeth. Entertainment routines typically involve music, dancing, toys, and games. Examples of activity routines are snack time and morning circle.

The defining characteristic of all routines is that they involve a predictable sequence of actions and events. Once children learn a routine, they anticipate the action or event that will happen next. Thus, routines provide a context in which to teach language and other functional skills. For example, a mother and child are involved in a daily dressing routine. The mother describes the dressing actions as she and the child perform them. She also labels pieces of clothing. The child is exposed to the same words and concepts several times a day, every day for weeks and months and in different settings (different rooms of the house). In time the child begins to produce parts of the descriptions and labels in the activity context. When the well-established routine is interrupted, there is a high probability that the child will "fill in the slot" (produce the behavior that is expected at the point of interruption). This is an enormously productive teaching strategy. For example, in the dressing routine the child learns (a) object labels, (b) rules for participation in a routine in different contexts, and (c) words to describe actions associated with the routine.

In addition to being an excellent context for teaching language and communication skills, routines are an ideal context for teaching social, cognitive, self-care, and motor skills (Halle, Alpert, & Anderson, 1984). There is no need to develop new routines, as numerous routines are already in place in natural environments.

Almost any routines can be used, but some are better than others. When considering the routines that are in place in the environment, look for these characteristics (Halle et al., 1984):

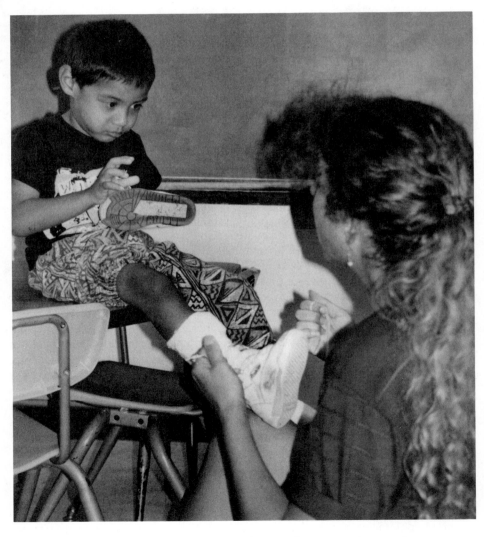

Routine activities such as dressing provide naturalistic antecedents and consequences for skill acquisition.

1. The routine should involve a variety of objects and materials that the child finds attractive, interesting, and desirable.
2. The whole routine or component subroutines should be completed quickly so that there are maximum opportunities for interactions.
3. The routine should require many repeated actions because each repeated action is potentially an opportunity for interaction.
4. The routine should be functional to ensure that skills learned within the context of the routine will generalize.

Once a routine is established and the child learns to anticipate the events in the routine, the decision becomes when and how to interrupt the routine to encourage interaction. There are three procedures for interrupting an established routine (Halle et al., 1984):

1. Withhold or delay provision of expected and desired objects or event. Withholding expected objects or actions creates opportunities for interactions (gaining attention, making requests, indicating desires). For example, assume that the typical sequence after the children are seated at snack time is to pass napkins, pour juice or milk, and then distribute pieces of fruit. When the teacher "forgets" a child's napkin or "forgets" to pour a child's juice or "forgets" to pass the plate of fruit to everyone, there is a high probability that the child who did not receive the expected object (or a peer) will protest the oversight or request a serving of fruit. This technique is especially useful in a group because peers typically prompt one another to request the expected action (a turn to stir the cookie batter) or object (a share of apple pieces): "Tell Miss Miller you didn't get a napkin," or "Tell Auntie you didn't get a turn."

2. Provide an incomplete set of materials. Many routines such as games, art activities, and cooking projects require a set of materials. Not providing all needed materials for a project will typically prompt an interaction (perhaps an attention-getting behavior and a request). The adult simply waits until the child says something about the "mistake." There are two requirements for this procedure to be effective: the routine must be inherently reinforcing and it must require a prescribed set of materials.

3. Make "silly" mistakes. Intentionally violating an object's function or what children know to be correct will almost invariably elicit protests or informational exchanges. Some examples are "mistakenly" offering another child's sweater or "mistakenly" holding a coat upside down. Other more obvious silly mistakes include taking a toothbrush from a purse and beginning to brush one's hair or holding a book upside down at story time. In addition to prompting spontaneous protest, this type of calculated "silliness" helps children develop a sense of humor.

Interrupted Behavior Chains

The interrupted behavior chain strategy (Goetz, Schuler & Sailor, 1983; Goetz, Gee & Sailor, 1985; Hunt, Goetz, Alwell & Sailor, 1986) is a variation of the interrupted routine technique. A behavior or response chain is a sequence of behaviors that is either performed spontaneously and independently (for example, playing with a toy) or is being taught through systematic instruction (such as brushing teeth). The criterion for selection of a sequence is a minimum of three steps in the behavior chain, with each step initiated by the child.

The interrupted behavior chain strategy is implemented by inserting an instructional trial into the middle of an ongoing response chain. For example, the behavior chain being interrupted might be getting food from the refrigerator; the target response might be a request for juice.

The first step in planning the interrupted chain procedure is to identify the specific response chains that will be used in the training. Goetz and colleagues (1985) suggest two considerations when selecting a chain that can be used effectively in the interrupted chain teaching strategy. A first consideration is whether the behavior sequence is one that the child will attempt to complete if performance of the chain is interrupted. A second consideration is the child's frustration level when performance of the chain is interrupted. Goetz and colleagues suggest evaluating the child's frustration level on a three-point scale (lowest rating would be a 1 for low or no frustration; 3 would be high frustration). Use response chains if the child attempts to complete at least two out of three trials and where the child's average level of frustration is judged to be moderate (1.5 to 2.5).

This example from a study by Hunt and colleagues (1986) illustrates how the interrupted chain strategy works. Nate is a 6-year-old nonverbal student with severe mental retardation. When Nate wants a hug, he walks up to the teacher or other familiar adult and reaches out to put his arms around her neck or he pushes his head against the adult's body. When he wants help with dressing or to go outside, he grabs and pulls the hand of the nearest adult. When he does not want to do something he indicates this by crying, pushing objects away, averting or closing his eyes, or physically leaving the situation.

The instructional goal for Nate is to teach him to use a picture communication book. His communication book has only two cards: a "want" card and a blank card (as a distractor). The book is attached by a key clip to the waistband of his pants. The first objective is for Nate to point to the "want" card. The initial step toward this objective is for Nate to pull the open communication book up to above waist level.

The four response chains selected for Nate are (a) playing catch in the classroom or at recess, (b) preparing to go out to recess, (c) approaching and hugging an adult, and (d) playing with a See'n Say during leisure time. The first three sequences are independent and spontaneous response chains; the fourth is an instructed response chain. In the first chain, an interruption is planned after Nate throws the ball to his partner in a six-step ball-play chain. In the second chain, an interruption is planned just after Nate's classmates and nondisabled peers are dismissed to go to recess in a four-step chain for recess preparation. In the third chain, an interruption is planned while Nate's arms are around an adult in a three-step hugging behavior chain. In the fourth chain, an interruption is planned while Nate is pulling on the cord of the See'n Say® in a toy-play chain with five steps.

The first instructional target for Nate—pulling his open communication book with the word "want" printed on it to above waist level—is inserted into the first chain at the predetermined point in the sequence. Instruction occurs twice daily at times when the sequence is normally performed. When Nate reaches criterion on the first instructional target, a second training phase is implemented. In this second phase there is instruction on a second target within the second behavior chain and so on until the desired target responses have all been acquired. Data provided by Hunt and colleagues (1986) indicate that all four target responses were acquired and maintained at a high level of consistent performance.

Interesting Materials

In order to learn, children must interact in developmentally and contextually appropriate ways with their environment. This is called *engagement.* Children's engagement with materials depends on the novelty and the appeal of the materials.

McGee, Daly, Izeman, Mann, and Risley (1991) describe a toy rotation plan used in an integrated program (the Walden project) in Massachusetts that serves children with autism and nondisabled preschoolers. These are the steps in implementing this toy rotation plan:

Step 1: Code all classroom toy and play materials according to the dimensions of size, complexity, developmental level, category, and sensory quality.

Step 2: Divide toys and materials into sets, each of which includes a mix of toys and materials representing each dimension. (In the Walden classroom, toys have been divided into 12 sets, each containing ten items.) It is important that each category of toys (manipulatives, building materials, dramatic play objects, and visual motor toys) be represented by at least one item in each set and that all sensory preferences are addressed. Also, each set should include at least one low-development toy (6 months to 24 months) and one high-development toy (4 years to 6 years), as well as several items that can be used in different ways by children at any level.

Step 3: Begin with two sets of toys and materials available in the classroom and then systematically rotate one set each week. Begin with sets 1 and 2. At the end of the week, remove set 1 and replace it with set 3. At the end of the second week, replace set 2 with set 4. Thus, each week half of the toys are "new" to the children.

The toy rotation plan does not include all toys and materials in the Walden classroom. Some items, such as dolls, dress-up clothes, books, and blocks, are not rotated. They are always available. Engagement with these permanent toys or items is increased with the toy rotation plan because there is the potential to use them in new ways as sets are rotated. There are at least three benefits from using some type of toy rotation: (a) increased engagement, (b) more varied play skills, and (c) increased sharing, cooperative play, and peer modeling of imaginative and creative play (McGee et al., 1991).

Behavior Trapping

In behavior trapping the goal is for the natural environment to take over subsequent teaching and maintenance of the new behavior. The notion of behavior trapping was first conceptualized by Baer and Wolf (1970). It is closely related to what is called the Relevance of Behavior Rule described by Ayllon and Azrin (1968). The Relevance of Behavior Rule states that when selecting intervention targets you should select those behaviors that receive reinforcement in the natural environment. This is because behaviors that are rewarded in the natural environment are more likely to be maintained once the arrangements contrived to change the behavior have been withdrawn.

The essence of behavior trapping is to arrange a situation that is powerfully attractive to the child, one requiring only a relatively simple response from the child in order to participate. Once the child becomes interested and engages in the activity, the natural reinforcers in the situation will take over to increase and maintain engagement. Social and play behaviors are examples of behaviors that lend themselves to this paradigm. If an isolate child can be provided sufficient social skills to gain acceptance in a peer play group, there is a good possibility that, once a member of the group, the child will continue to acquire appropriate social skills and that her social skills will be maintained.

In summary, this section has described seven instructional techniques that can be implemented in the context of everyday routines and activities in natural environments. These strategies are suitable for use in regular developmentally appropriate preschools as well as specialized classrooms. As Kostelnik (1992) notes, many curricular objectives in a developmentally appropriate preschool are addressed through pervasive classroom routines such as dressing to go outside, preparing for the snack, and cleaning up. In the developmentally appropriate classroom, teachers influence children's learning directly as well as indirectly. They provide certain activities in which the focus is on children's self-discovery and exploration. They also use a variety of instructional strategies: they pose questions, offer suggestions, suggest explorations, and provide information and challenges that help children move beyond their current concepts and skills.

 ## Adaptations for Natural Environments

Infants and young children with disabilities can and should learn in natural environments. Generally, only minimum adaptations are necessary. Because adaptations of the physical environment are often the easiest and the most natural, they should be considered before exploring adaptations of other aspects of the program.

Adapting the Physical Environment

The physical environment includes all nonsocial dimensions of the environment. The most important dimensions of the physical environment are environmental design, materials and equipment, and grouping and scheduling.

Environmental Design. Environmental design refers to the amount of space available and how it is arranged. Most states have regulations pertaining to the minimum amount of square footage necessary per child in a childcare program. Typically this is in the range of 35 square feet of usable indoor space and 75 square feet of outdoor play space for each child (National Academy of Early Childhood Programs, 1984). Somewhat more space may be necessary when a program integrates young children who require adaptive or supportive equipment. Otherwise, space adaptations for children with disabilities should be kept to a minimum.

There are two reasons for this. One is so as not to call undue attention to children's disabilities. The other reason to avoid all but the most essential adaptations of the physical environment is that children with disabilities need to learn to move around in and accommodate (to the extent possible) to the constraints of natural environments. Learning to negotiate the barriers of a physical environment without special adaptations is one of the important benefits of the mainstream setting.

Children with severe physical or visual disabilities provide an exception to the general rule to minimize adaptations. As noted above, children with wheelchairs and other mobility aids may require more space. Some adaptations are essential to ensure that children with severe physical and visual disabilities have the same safe and independent access to all aspects of the environment as their nondisabled peers.

The major considerations in planning the indoor space for an integrated program are the same as for any regular preschool or childcare program. First is how to organize the available space. There is evidence of a higher level of child engagement in activities when the indoor space is arranged into *well-defined activity areas* (Moore, 1986). Well-defined activity areas have these characteristics: a specific location, visible boundaries, surfaces for both work and sitting, adequate space for storage and materials display, and bright colors and soft materials (Olds, 1987).

Most preschools provide at least these activity centers:

1. Block play center (with blocks of different sizes, shapes, and materials)
2. Pretend play center (with housekeeping toys, dress-up clothes, dolls, puppets)

3. Messy activities center (with sandbox, water table, paint, and easels)
4. Sensory materials center (with child-sized tables and chairs and drawing, coloring, cutting materials)
5. Quiet center (with carpet and large pillows, books)
6. Manipulative play center (with puzzles, small toys, pegboards, popbeads)
7. Gross motor play center (with crawling tunnels, trampolines, small slides)

Generally the only activity center accommodations that are necessary for children with severe physical disabilities have to do with furniture height and space. Tables should be high enough for a wheelchair to fit underneath and entrances to activity centers must be wide enough, and unobstructed, so as not to block a wheelchair or walker.

It is a good idea to begin with a diagram when planning an indoor space arrangement that meets the needs of all children in the program. Sketch the room out on graph paper and assign locations to those activities that have particular space, materials, or equipment requirements. For example, the art center should be near water and have a washable floor surface. The block center should be large and carpeted to reduce noise. Place it away from main pathways to minimize the possibility that children will stumble on constructions or stray blocks. The location of electrical outlets is another consideration at this first stage of planning, as some classroom equipment will require outlets.

Next, plan for the visible barriers that will separate activity centers. They should be high enough to give children a feeling of privacy, but not so high that activities cannot be observed by adults in other parts of the room.

Materials and Equipment.   Equipment refers to furniture and other large items such as easels and climbing structures. Materials are the smaller items in a program such as puzzles, games, books, and toys. The first consideration when purchasing materials and equipment is safety. Then consider design and attractiveness. Well-designed equipment and materials can help children develop large and small muscle coordination, concepts about the physical world, creativity, social skills, and self-awareness. Equipment and materials should have sensory appeal (color, texture, sound) and they should be physically responsive so that children can experience the effects of their behavior.

In addition to basic child-size furnishings (tables, chairs, storage cubbyholes, bookshelves) the typical preschool setting includes natural materials such as sand, clay, and water, active play materials such as tires, seesaws, and tricycles, construction toys such as blocks, Legos®, Lincoln Logs®, and Tinker Toys®, and manipulative toys such as puzzles, beads, pegboards, and games. There will be media materials such as paint, crayons, glue, and clay, and shelves with a supply of good-quality children's books. Dramatic play materials in most classrooms include dolls, dress-up clothes, child-size kitchen furnishings and kitchenware, and furnishings and materials for other themes such as store, bus, or restaurant. Additionally, most early childhood settings have tape players and tapes, record players and records, a VCR, and ideally, one or more computers with appropriate peripherals and software.

Grouping and Scheduling. Early childhood programs typically have routines associated with arrival, self-care, mealtimes and snacks, rest time, and departure. There are several fairly large blocks of time (indoors and outdoors) when children choose their own activities and other blocks of time designated for large group activities guided by the teacher. These activity blocks are linked by a sequence of transition routines. Separate scheduling for children with disabilities should be avoided. To the extent possible they should follow the same consistent schedule and daily routines as other children in the program.

Transitions occur when children are finishing one activity or routine and preparing to start another. There is a high probability for disruptive behavior before, during, and after a transition (with nondisabled children as well as children with disabilities). Three sets of circumstances increase the probability for disruptive behavior during transitions: (a) if children have to be told or are confused as to what to do next, (b) if children do not have adequate time to end one activity and clean up before preparing for the next, and (c) if the direction to change activities is announced by a bell or buzzer without ample warning.

The key to smooth transition routines (and other routines) is preparation. Figure 8-1 provides some suggestions to increase the likelihood of smooth transitions.

Planning Goals and Objectives

Successful integration requires thoughtful planning and decision making prior to placement and then careful monitoring once the child is enrolled in the mainstream program. Because all children do not flourish equally well in the same curriculum model, preplacement decisions should be influenced by the program's curricular approach and the extent to which staff are willing to individualize for children's special needs.

---

1. **Provide a 5-minute warning that an activity will end shortly**
2. **Provide self-directed activities for children who finish early, and allow children to move independently to these activities when they finish**
3. **Use the time productively when waiting for children to assemble for a large group activity** (for example, sit with already assembled children and look at pictures in the book that will be read when all have assembled)
4. **Specifically instruct transition behaviors** (where and how to line up, where and how to put away materials, acceptable quiet activities to engage in while waiting for other to finish, and so on).

Figure 8-1 Suggestions for smooth transitions

There are several ways to adapt a curriculum to accommodate children with special needs: (a) develop different (but related) goals for group activities; (b) add new goals and objectives; and (c) modify input and response options (for example, Braille for the child with severe visual impairment, pointing for the child with severe language disorders).

Individualizing.   Many early childhood curricula are organized by unit plans with class goals for the various activities in the unit. For example, in a Montessori preschool program, there may be a goal for children to sequence objects by size. The children have activity choices involving a variety of materials that can be arranged and ordered by size, such as pets to be lined up according to increasing height, or a circle puzzle with circles to be arranged by increasing diameter. In this context, individualizing can mean developing one or more different but related goals for the child with disabilities. For example, one of the child's goals might be to identify the largest object in each group of objects (rather than arrange and order the objects by size). Another goal might be for the child to indicate a choice of activities. Although both of these goals are different from the sequencing goal that the other children are achieving, they are related. The child is participating in the same activity as the other children and, at the same time, his special needs are being met.

Adding New Goals and Objectives.   Early childhood programs may choose to add new goals and objectives to the curriculum. While these goals and objectives are added to accommodate the needs of children with disabilities, they also have value for nondisabled children. Among the goals that may be added for children with disabilities are:

1. Learning to interact with peers
2. Learning to participate in typical routines
3. Learning functional skills
4. Learning survival skills

Many children with disabilities need specific instruction in peer-related social skills (to be discussed in Chapter 10). These are the skills required for peer-related social interactions and participation in typical classroom routines (initiating interactions, taking turns, waiting in line, communicating wants and needs, and terminating an interaction). They also need to learn the functional skills that will enable them to participate in integrated home environments (setting the table, using a microwave, washing dishes, hanging clothes on hangers). Finally, young children with disabilities need systematic instruction in skills that will help them be successful in future educational environments—especially kindergarten and first grade.

Modifying Input and Response Options.   Children with physical or sensory impairments may require modified input and response options to participate fully in integrated settings. For example, a child with a physical disability may need Velcro® attachments on her hands and some materials to enable her to pick up the materials and use them. It may be necessary to give instructions with pictures as well as orally for a child with hearing impairment.

Creative adaptations in the way instructions are presented (for example, using concrete examples) and required response modes (for example, accepting pointing to a picture rather than labeling) will often benefit and increase the participation of nondisabled children, as well as those with disabilities. Possibly one of the greatest benefits of creative adaptions is that they demonstrate in a very concrete manner for nondisabled children that adults accept and accommodate individual differences. (Specific adaptations are presented in the next section.)

Adapting Instructional Methods

There is no single instructional method that is likely to be effective with all children in a setting or with all skill/content areas. For example, some children learn to put materials away by following verbal directions. Others need more prompts, such as the teacher pointing to where the materials belong. Most important is to arrange the environment to maximize the potential for learning *and* to provide children with disabilities with specific instruction. You must do both. Do not assume that learning will occur without specific instruction just because the environment is arranged in a particular way.

Figure 8-2 provides general suggestions for arranging the environment and adapting instruction. What follows are some specific instructional adaptations for children with hearing or visual impairments, health impairments, or a physical disability.

Children with Hearing Impairment.   Many children with significant hearing impairment participate in both a specialized program and an integrated program. The reasons for integrating children with hearing impairment are the same as for other children with disabilities: to provide age-appropriate language models and opportunities for normal social and play activities.

The following suggestions for children with hearing impairment are equally appropriate and desirable for nondisabled children:

1. **Speak naturally in a normal teaching voice.** There is no need to over-enunciate or speak loudly. Use natural gestures to supplement oral presentations.
2. **Call the child's name when addressing her.** Wait until you have the child's attention before speaking.
3. **Give the child a full view of your face when speaking.** The child needs all the visual cues that a speaker provides, so be careful not to talk while facing away from the child.
4. **Indicate the referent for any person- or object-specific comment.** When referring to someone or something in the room, touch, point, or nod in the direction of the referent.

To Help Children Learn to Pay Attention:

Seat children in a location where there are no extraneous noise sources (air conditioner or traffic).

Position children in a circle for group activities (so they can see each other).

Teach children always to face the speaker when being spoken to.

To Help Children Learn to Follow Directions:

Use concrete examples, pictures, and gestures as well as words when giving directions.

Show children that following directions is a desirable behavior by praising those who follow directions.

Be sure that instructions are relevant and specific and provided in a vocabulary that the children understand.

To Teach Children to Succeed:

Let children know that you think they can master the task and that you will help if needed.

Provide structure and support to help children recognize cause/effect relationships and feel confident that they can succeed.

Provide specific and concrete verbal feedback so that children do not have to guess whether they are doing what is being requested.

Be sure that your verbal and nonverbal behaviors are consistent (that praise is delivered in an enthusiastic tone and accompanied by smiles).

Be sensitive to fatigue and recognize the exceptional effort that even a seemingly simple task may require of a child with disabilities.

Provide ample opportunity for practice of new skills.

Provide concrete examples and demonstrations, allowing children to attempt new tasks with maximum teacher support.

"Talk the child through" new materials and experiences.

Figure 8-2   Instructional adaptations for young children with disabilities

5. **Be careful not to stand in front of a strong light source.** This makes speech reading difficult because your face is in the dark.
6. **Consider amplification as an option for enhancing speech input.** Consider wearing a small lavalier® microphone for voice amplification.

Children with Severe Visual Impairment.   Children with severe visual impairment are placed in mainstream programs at an early age. Special services are provided by a consultant, itinerant teacher, resource teacher, or other teacher with specialization in visual impairment. Special services may include:

- ◆ Recommendations related to special materials, such as Braille, large print, recorded materials, magnifiers, and special equipment (for example, tape recorder)
- ◆ Demonstrations of the proper use of the above materials and equipment
- ◆ Advice and counselling for parents and teachers
- ◆ Assistance in teaching orientation, mobility, and the use of residual vision

The major difficulties of children whose visual impairment is not complicated by secondary conditions (for example, motor or hearing impairment) center around concept development, mobility, and social competence. Reduced vision restricts access to the environmental experiences necessary for concept development, limits mobility, and prevents imitation (the process through which many personal and social skills are acquired).

The following are some suggestions to assist children with vision impairments:

1. Seat the child to minimize the interference of glare and shadows and maximize desirable natural light. Allow the child to move or adjust her seating as needed for different activities and light conditions.

2. Check frequently to be sure that the floor is free of objects and doors are not left ajar. Never change the room arrangement without informing the child. Familiarize her with any new additions to materials and equipment.

3. Prompt the child to "use words to make things happen." It is critical for the child to become aware of the association between words and events and the potential of language to control the environment.

4. Be careful not to overestimate the child's understanding. The child's language skills may suggest greater understanding than the child actually possesses. This "mismatch" between expressive language and cognitive skills sometimes occurs because the child misses important details or components of an experience.

Children with Physical and Health Impairments.   Children with physical and health impairments are an extremely heterogeneous group. Children with health impairments such as asthma, allergies, diabetes, rheumatic fever, or leukemia may require medical consultation and dietary supervision. Be aware that allergies and many medications can affect classroom behavior. For example, the most commonly prescribed asthma medication is correlated with inattentiveness, hyperactivity, drowsiness, and withdrawn behavior (McLoughlin et al., 1983).

There are a number of ways that physical disabilities affect overall developmental progress and ability to participate in daily routines. First, there may be many interruptions of home, school, and peer group experiences because of the child's need for intensive medical intervention, such as surgeries and repeated or prolonged hospitalizations. Second, if a child has cerebral palsy and abnormal reflex patterns, there may be interference with normal movement and development of motor skills. Third, abnormal muscle tone may affect physical growth. Finally, restricted movement can interfere with cognitive development because the child

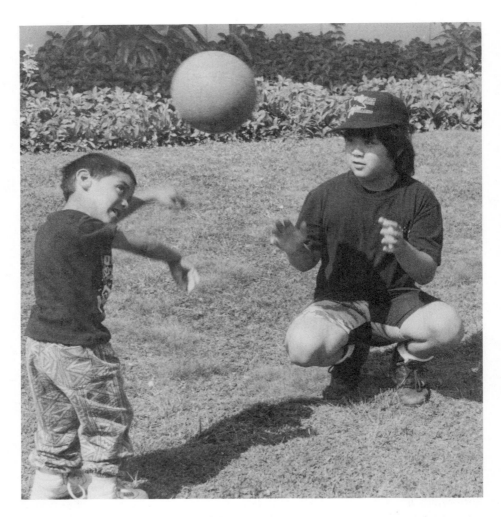

Cerebral palsy interferes with normal movement and the development of motor skills.

does not have opportunities for the range of experiences necessary to learn about and from the environment.

Speech, language, and communication skills and mobility are major problems for young children with physical disabilities. Some children cannot produce intelligible speech because their disabilities affect the processes necessary for speech production: respiration, phonation, resonation, and articulation. Those children who develop functional speech may demonstrate language disturbances such as echolalia (repeating what others say) or saying words or phrases out of context. The mobility of children with a physical disability requiring the use of crutches, a walker, or a wheelchair is restricted compared to nondisabled peers.

The following are some suggestions for assisting children with physical or health impairments:

1. Be sure to have written authorization from a parent *and* the physician on file if medication is administered at school. Teachers may administer medication, but it is preferable for the parents to administer it at home or for it to be administered by a nurse. Store medication in a locked compartment and be sure to keep careful records that include specific directions for administration.

2. Establish a means of regular communication with the parents or caregivers and therapist(s). If time constraints prevent regular team meetings, try to establish some other vehicle for exchange of information. The parents or caregivers may act as liaisons between teachers and therapists to assure that information and reports are shared.

3. Learn how to position, carry, lift, and transfer the child. The parents or caregivers and the physical or occupational therapist(s) can teach these skills. Practice with supervision until they are performed with comfort and confidence.

4. Become familiar with the child's orthotic or prosthetic devices. These devices can restrict range of motion, cause discomfort and abrasions, or interfere with circulation if they do not fit properly. The physical or occupational therapist(s) will provide the necessary information and remain available to answer questions.

5. Ask for help to adjust standard equipment. The therapists and/or parents or caregivers will help with equipment adjustments. For example, for most children, all that is necessary to adjust a tricycle is to move the handlebars to an upright position (so that the child does not need to lean forward) and secure the child's feet on the pedals with Velcro® straps. Chairs can be used for mobility if the floor is carpeted. The child moves around the room by pushing a chair in front for support.

6. Use special adaptive equipment for sitting, standing, and floor activities. If the child cannot use a standard chair, ask parents or caregivers and therapists to provide a special adaptive chair. Additionally, a supported stander, adaptive boards, wedges, and other supports should be made available if the child needs this equipment.

7. Ask parents and therapists to assist adapting equipment for independent printing, drawing, painting, coloring, cutting, and eating. If the child cannot use the same materials as peers, consider adapted scissors and adaptations to other hand-held implements to help the child write, draw, paint, and color. In most cases it is a good idea to tape the child's paper to the table when there is a printing or art activity. This keeps the paper in place. The child may need adaptive spoons with a built-up handle or a swivel and scoop dishes and cups in order to eat independently.

8. Teach all children safety precautions associated with the use of a walker, crutches, or a wheelchair. The most critical safety precautions are (a) wiping up spills immediately, (b) keeping the floor clear, and (c) not pushing or running in the classroom or the halls.

This section has not dealt with adaptations for children with speech, language, communication, cognitive, or socialization difficulties, as these disabilities are addressed in other chapters. The key to planning effective intervention in natural environments is to focus on children's strengths and the similarities among children. The suggestions provided in this section are good teaching practices.

Once whatever adaptations are necessary have been made for children with special needs, the next step is planning *when* facilitation and instruction of desired skills will be embedded into the daily routine. It may be throughout the day, or over some part of the day. One method to facilitate planning is to use a matrix. The planning matrix is versatile, in that it can be used for any setting and it can be used in different ways. Here are some suggestions:

1. For a child with several skill objectives: List daily activities (the classroom or home schedule) in the left column and briefly note skill objectives for the child across the top. Decide which activities provide a context for facilitation and instruction of the skills and place a check in the appropriate cells. See Figure 8-5 for suggestions to help make decisions about activities that lend themselves to embedding objectives. (Chapter 5 shows an example of this type of matrix.)

2. For several children who need help with a single skill (the same skill or different skills): List daily activities in the left column and the names of the children across the top. Decide which activities provide a context for facilitation and instruction of the skills and place a check in the appropriate cells.

3. For several children who need help with specific skills in a particular activity: List the steps and subskills required for the activity in the left column and the names of the children across the top. Place some notation in the appropriate cells to indicate subskills each child needs help with or has acquired. (Figure 8-3 shows an example of this type of activity matrix.)

4. Make multiple copies of a child's matrix and use the matrix as a data collection form to monitor daily performance on targeted skills. (Figure 8-4 shows an example of a matrix used as a data collection form.)

Bricker, Cripe, and Norstad (1990) provide some suggestions for selecting activities that will provide a context for facilitation and instruction of specific skills (see Figure 8-5). The vast majority of activities in childcare programs (center-based or home-based) and preschool programs that use developmentally appropriate practice (Bredekamp, 1987) would easily meet these criteria.

After deciding *when* new skills will be taught, decide *how* to facilitate the skills in the context of natural activities using naturally occurring antecedents and consequences. Bricker and Cripe (1992) call this *activity-based intervention (ABI)*.

Activity: **Washing hands**

	Todd	Emily	Adam	Jason	Julie
Turns on water	*	*	ok	*	*
Wets hands	*	ok	*	*	*
Locates soap	*	ok	ok	ok	*
Lathers hands	*	*	ok	ok	ok
Rinses soap off	*	ok	ok	ok	ok
Puts soap in dish	ok	ok	*	*	*
Turns off water	*	ok	*	*	*
Locates towel	*	ok	ok	ok	ok
Dries hands	ok	ok	ok	*	ok
Hangs up towel	*	*	*	*	*

* - needs help
ok - acquired

Figure 8-3 Planning matrix for washing hands

Activity-based intervention is similar to the interrupted routines and interrupted behavior chain strategies except that there is no interruption in the activities. Activities are carefully planned and implemented to provide opportunities for teaching and practice of specific skill objectives.

Activity-based intervention is an ideal vehicle for demonstration of teaming skills. The team works together to enhance the activity for specific children and for all children who are potential participants. Bricker and Cripe (1992) give the example of planning for the needs of Jasmine, a multiply handicapped child in a

Name: __Mark Guerrero__   Date: __4-18-92__
Teacher/Recorder: __Wells__

	Prepositions "in" and "on"	Plurals	"Wh" questions	Requests	Increase vocabulary ✱	Standing/ stand-up table	Sitting with support
Arrival 8:00-8:15	+++ꜩ	θθ	+ θ	++	+		
Toileting 8:15-8:30	++	+	ꜩ	++			
Free Play 8:30-9:00	+				++		
Large Group 9:00-9:30	+ꜩꜩ+			+	+		+
Snack 9:30-9:50	+++	++	+++θθ+ꜩθ+	+			
Science 9:50-10:30				+++++	+++	+	+
Music/Art 10:30-11:00	++	θθθ			+++	+	+
Toileting 11:00-11:15	+	+	+++				
Lunch 11:15-12:00	++		++				+
Rest/Story 12:00-1:15			+				
Outside Play 1:15-1:30							
Bus Prep. 1:30-1:45	+++	++	+++	+θθ	+		

✱ mand - model new words

Opportunity   = —
Correct Response   = +
No Response   = θ
Incorrect Response = ꜩ

Figure 8-4 Matrix used for daily data collection

1. **Select activities that permit grouping of similar objectives for different children.** For example, telling stories with puppets is an activity for circle time that lends itself to facilitation and instruction of objectives related to the ability to identify objects by function.

2. **Select activities that allow grouping different goals for the same child.** Most activities meet this criterion. For example, at least three of Brendyn's objectives—his language objective (naming familiar objects), his cognitive objective (matching colors and shapes), and his fine motor/selfcare objectives (pouring and stirring)—can be facilitated in the context of the activity of snack preparation.

3. **Select activities that can be adapted for varying ages and skill levels.** For example, the activity "Yes you can," which teaches children to help with simple household tasks, easily lends itself to adaptation for varying ages and skills levels. Less competent children can be assigned the easier steps in dusting the bookshelves and setting the table.

4. **Select activities that require minimal adult direction and assistance.** For example, "Dress-up teatime" requires lots of props (clothing, play furniture, dishes, pots and pans) but minimal adult direction or assistance once play begins.

5. **Select activities that provide many opportunities for child initiations.** For example, an activity called "Up, up, and away," in which children say the name of a peer and then pass a balloon to that peer, provides myriad opportunities for children to initiate interactions with peers.

6. **Select activities that are motivating and interesting.** Activities that are fun are inherently reinforcing and there is a greater probability that children will become actively engaged and learn from them.

SOURCE: Adapted from *Activity-Based Intervention* by D. Bricker, J. Cripe, and S. Norstad. Paper presented at Post Conference Workshop, Council for Exceptional Children Conference, October, 1990, Albuquerque, New Mexico.

Figure 8-5   Considerations when selecting activities

sand-play activity: The occupational therapist suggests storing the toys for sand in large plastic jars with lids so that Jasmine will get functional practice of wrist rotation. The physical therapist suggests placing the sand in tubs on the floor rather than having a table-height sandtable so that Jasmine and the other two children in the class who have special positioning needs will have better access. The speech-language pathologist helps the teacher identify toys for the activity that contain Jasmine's articulation target which is use of /k/ at the beginning of words. They assemble an assortment of cups, cookie cutters, and cans.

Sometimes children do not demonstrate desired skills (or skill approximations) in planned activities as anticipated. When this happens, consider one or another of the techniques described earlier in the chapter: incidental teaching, verbal prompts, time-delay prompts, interrupted routines, interrupted chains, more interesting materials, or behavior trapping. Finally, once intervention procedures have been described, plan data collections procedures.

Data Collection Strategies

Data collection procedures for discrete trial teaching are straightforward because (a) training typically involves presentation of repeated trials with the same or similar responses, and (b) teaching generally takes place in a separate location, one which is set aside specifically for instruction. Data collection procedures for naturalistic teaching strategies in natural environments are not so straightforward. The most obvious measurement difficulty is related to the fact that strategies are implemented in the context of routines and activities where there are many distractors. Naturalistic teaching opportunities are dispersed throughout the day among numerous activities and settings, making it difficult to have a data sheet readily available and the time to record child responses. Other factors contributing to measurement difficulties are (a) the number of steps in the process (for both the intervener *and* the child), and (b) the rapid pace of instruction.

There are several possibilities for data collection with naturalistic teaching strategies. One suggestion is to scan among children, collecting data on only one or two different children each day. The planning matrix can be adapted for this purpose with opportunities with correct responses recorded in the appropriate cells. Many copies of the matrix will be needed if it is to be used in this way, because each data collection day will require a separate form. One method to avoid the need for duplicate data sheets is to copy the matrix on transparency film. Record daily data with a felt pen and erase (wipe off) the data each day after they have been transferred to a graph or other permanent record (Sherman, 1989).

Another possibility in the classroom is to place data sheets near the activity centers where different routines take place. For example, data sheets for the arrival routine are posted near the door. Data sheets for snack preparation are posted on the refrigerator where snacks are kept. Data sheets may be created from an enlarged script of the routine, or they may be as simple as a blank index card. Most important is to keep some record of (a) opportunities for demonstration of targeted skills, and (b) the nature of children's responses.

Helping Others Use Naturalistic Teaching Strategies

Naturalistic teaching strategies are based on observations of normal modes of adult-child interaction in natural environments (the type of unplanned teaching interactions that occur naturally between parent and child or teacher and child in natural environments). Because the strategies are familiar and generally "feel right" to adults, it is not difficult to help therapists, new staff, parents, volunteers, and paraprofessionals to learn to apply them in a systematic fashion (Cavallaro &

Poulson, 1985; Halle et al., 1981; Mudd & Wolery, 1987; Peck, 1985). Once learned and practiced, even for a limited time, staff view the procedures as useful and successful (an important social validity measure), so use of procedures is generalized across activities (Halle et al., 1981).

Use of modeling, role-playing, and other means of active participation in a didactic workshop format increases the likelihood that staff and parents will generalize the procedures beyond the training sessions. Mudd and Wolery (1987) suggest that inservice training should emphasize procedures for requesting elaborations, use of models, and use of confirmation.

Home intervention can maximize intervention outcomes, but whatever training is provided by parents and other family members at home must be compatible with the natural structure of the family's life—the family's routines, activities, and interactions. Parents are particularly good with naturalistic training strategies because they have substantial experience with adult-child interactions on which to draw (Culatta & Horn, 1981; Salzberg & Villani, 1983).

When training cannot be provided at home, there are other options for helping parents learn naturalistic teaching strategies. Innocenti, Rule, Killoran, and Stowitschek (1983) suggest a workshop format. They have developed a curriculum for parents to teach their children social skills. Parents learn to use prompting strategies to engage their children in appropriate behaviors and to deliver praise. The curriculum consists of three teaching strategies that parents can use with lessons that cover 26 different social skills.

Wutz and colleagues (1982) take a slightly different approach in their home-centered communication training program. They suggest an interview format to help parents learn to recognize potential naturalistic training opportunities. Together, the teacher and parent(s) list (a) the child's favorite activities; (b) the child's modes for communicating desired objects and events (for example, reaching, smiling); and (c) the situations in which the child emits these responses. The major goal of the interview is to sensitize parents to the form of their child's communicative behavior and the occasions when these behaviors are likely to occur. The interview also provides an opportunity to direct parents' attention to critical features involved in communicative interactions, including their own behavior in communicative situations, and teach them the specific strategies to use when the target responses do not occur spontaneously. They also learn how to provide reinforcement for appropriate behavior, how to model desired actions, and how to use the other naturalistic teaching strategies.

Summary

The approaches and techniques described in this chapter are enormously powerful procedures that can enhance and facilitate instruction of all skills in any natural environments. Most efforts to intervene in natural contexts will integrate two or more of the naturalistic teaching strategies. Probably the greatest advantage of these teaching strategies is not so much their ability to teach targeted responses (this can also be accomplished with direct instruction) as their ability to teach children to perform targeted behaviors spontaneously at the appropriate times, and thus the increased potential for generalization of new skills.

Activities

1. Construct a simple observation checklist and observe an integrated preschool or childcare program. Look for (a) demonstrations of the naturalistic procedures presented in this chapter, and (b) transition procedures. Observe the program for at least 2 hours and record which procedures are used and how often.

2. Draw a diagram of the floor plan for a preschool classroom with appropriate activity areas and equipment/furnishings. Show where modifications may be necessary for a child in a wheelchair. What about a child who uses a walker? Describe how each activity area would be defined.

3. Develop a planning matrix for Jesse Aloha. Use the daily schedule on the matrix shown in Figure 8-4 and formulate one objective for each goal on Jesse's IEP (Chapter 4).

4. Select a routine preschool activity such as an art activity using construction paper, scissors, crayons, and paste, and describe how the activity could be modified for a child with sensory or physical impairments.

Review Questions

1. List four characteristics common to naturalistic teaching approaches.
2. Define and give an example of how each of these procedures is implemented in a naturalistic environment: incidental teaching, verbal prompts, time-delay prompts, interrupted routines, interrupted behavior chains, interesting materials, behavioral trapping.
3. Describe space adaptations for children with physical or visual impairments.

4. Give two reasons why adaptations for children with disabilities should be kept to a minimum.

5. List the activity centers included in most preschools and describe how they can be defined.

6. Provide suggestions for smooth transitions between activities.

7. Describe and illustrate application of each of the three methods for adapting a curriculum to accommodate children with special needs.

8. Describe ways to adapt instructional methods for (a) children with hearing impairment, (b) children with severe visual impairment, and (c) children with physical and health impairments.

9. Describe how to use a matrix form to plan when targeted skills will be encouraged and facilitated and to collect data.

Group Instruction

1. Describe a rationale for using group instruction with infants and young children who have disabilities.

2. Describe the characteristics of instructional groups.

3. Discuss strategies and provide examples of planning group instruction.

4. Identify strategies for using groups to enhance the instructional process.

*I*nfants and young children are often among peers, particularly if they spend time in childcare, preschool, or kindergarten settings. Same-age peer groups may also be present at home (if there are two or more siblings who are close in age), at family gatherings, with neighborhood children, and in public recreational environments such as the beach or playground. These situations provide opportunities for infants and young children with disabilities to learn to play and socialize with their age-mates. The skills associated with group play and socialization are particularly important curriculum goals for infants and young children with disabilities. They have needs in this area that are far greater than would be expected, considering their intellectual functioning (Guralnick & Groom, 1985; 1987; Guralnick & Weinhouse, 1984).

Instruction with two or more infants/young children simultaneously is *group instruction*. Group instruction provides opportunities to prepare infants and young children to participate in mainstream educational (Fink & Sandall, 1978; Vincent et al., 1980) and social situations (Alberto, Jobes, Sizemore & Doran, 1980). Successful participation in educational and social groups requires a wide range of skills, such as following group directions, responding to group-directed teaching techniques, following rules and routines, working/playing independently in close proximity to others, working/playing cooperatively with peers, turn-taking, sharing, and waiting. These skills can *only* be taught in group situations.

In addition to preparing infants and young children for less restrictive environments, group instruction increases skill gains. One reason group instruction promotes skill gains is that it provides opportunities for observational learning when children of differing abilities are grouped together (Brown & Holvoet, 1982; Westling, Ferrell & Swenson, 1982). In a toddler group, for example, Tommy, who does not say words, learns to vocalize for adult attention when he observes Kimi gaining attention by speaking. Another benefit of group instruction is that it increases the total amount of time in which children are actively engaged in instruction. Rather than dividing 30 minutes into three 10-minute individual instructional sessions for three children, all three children receive group instruction for the entire 30 minutes. As noted in Chapter 6, the more time spent actively participating in instruction, the greater the gains (Anderson, 1976; McWilliam, 1991; Walker & Hops, 1976).

Group instruction also benefits families and interventionists. It creates opportunities for families to meet one another to form relationships and support networks. In early intervention programs serving infants and toddlers, families might otherwise meet only program staff. Group instruction is a more efficient use of teachers' and infant specialists' time (Brown, Holvoet, Guess & Mulligan, 1980; Collins, Gast, Ault & Wolery, 1991). The one-to-one staff-child instructional arrangement is extremely costly and time-intensive in terms of staff resources.

The Nature of Groups

Participation in group instruction should be considered for all infants/young children with disabilities. The task is to match the child with the group. Groups can be characterized by their composition, interaction, and content.

Group Composition

The number and types of infants/young children included in a group are group composition considerations. Instructional groups have a minimum of two infants/young children. The largest groups occur in childcare and preschool programs serving a majority of infants/young children who are nondisabled: group size in these settings may approach 25 to 30. For a particular child, the decision of group size is based on these questions:

1. In what size group could the infant/young child demonstrate the instructional objectives?
2. What size group is typical among the infant/young child's peers?
3. For what size group does the infant/young child possess group skills?
4. What is a group size that the teacher or infant specialist can *effectively* manage?

Most groups in early intervention settings are small, composed of three to five infants/young children. Expectations for group skills should consider each child's developmental level and developmental norms. A child's developmental level provides information for individualizing expectations. For example, a 3-year-old child who becomes upset in noisy situations initially participates in a group with only two other children. When the child becomes comfortable in the small group situation, participation in slightly larger groups is appropriate.

Developmental norms must also be considered. Normally developing young children from 6 to 24 months of age engage in simple social interactions (for example, smiling, or turn-taking in games such as peek-a-boo); from 24 to 30 months of age they tend to play alone with toys; from 30 to 42 months they continue playing alone but near other children; and from 42 months of age and on, children play with their peers cooperatively (Bailey & Wolery, 1984).

interesting

Group composition may be homogeneous or heterogeneous (Collins et al., 1991). *Homogeneous groups* include infants/young children who are at similar functioning levels or within an age span of 6 months for infants (birth through 12 to 16 months), or an age span of 1 year for toddlers through kindergartners (ages 12 to 16 months through 5 years). *Heterogeneous groups* include children with different functioning levels, an age span of more than 6 months for infants, or an age span of more than 1 year for older preschoolers.

Homogeneous groups are easier for instruction because tinfants/young children at similar performance levels and ages are likely to have similar goals. Likewise, an activity that is of interest to one child in a homogeneous group is likely to be of interest to the others. Homogeneous groups have a major disadvantage: they do not have children who can also be models for the others in the group. Additionally, if all children in the group have severe delays, significant physical handicaps, or are nonverbal, there is limited active participation. Planning and implementing instruction for heterogeneous groups is more challenging for the teacher or infant specialist, but the advantages outweigh the costs.

Group Interaction

A major rationale for group instruction is teaching social interaction skills. If social interaction skills are taught in the group (for example, Joseph is taught to turn toward named peer), or if an element of social interaction is included within the group activity (as when children pass materials to one another, or peers reinforce one another), the group is referred to as an *intersequential* group. When there is no interaction among group members, the group is *intrasequential* (Brown et al., 1980). Although *intersequential* groups are the more desirable group arrangement, groups that do not involve interaction also have benefits. *Intrasequential* groups provide opportunities for incidental learning, and they are an efficient use of the teacher's or infant specialist's time.

Group Content

Most groups have a theme or purpose. The content or theme should *always* be age appropriate. Organizing and planning around themes is a *unit curriculum approach*. A theme is selected for a specified period of time (for example, 1 week, 2 weeks, 1 month) and carried out in activities, materials, and songs. For example, Valentine's Day may be the theme in February. Valentine bulletin boards are designed, numbers for the calendar are written on hearts, Valentine songs are sung during morning circle, Valentine stories are are placed in the book corner, and art activities including valentines are conducted each day. In addition to holidays, common unit themes for early childhood settings include seasons, animals, birds, transportation, family, neighborhood, occupations, and so on. Many inexpensive books with ideas for implementing the unit approach are commercially available (cf. Bernstein, 1989; Dodge & Colker, 1992; Grayson, 1962; Kingore & Higbee, 1988; Spencer, 1976).

It is possible to organize children in groups even though each child is participating in a different activity. This occurs in childcare and preschools when children are allowed to select activities for independent "work" time.

Group instruction is conducted in the context of an activity. Some group members have similar goals and others have different goals. Goals are most likely to be different for each group member when the group is heterogeneous. The group activity serves as the *context* for instruction. Goals of each group member are addressed in the activity. In a toddler group, for example, an activity with apples and oranges involves naming, noting color, feeling texture, and tasting. One toddler practices *reaching and touching* when the apple and orange are presented; another toddler is encouraged to *imitate names of the fruit,* and *point to her peer when it is that peer's turn.*

[handwritten margin note: 2 goals / 2 diff. chn. / 1 activity]

Group Participation Skills/Objectives

Among the social and communication skills acquired during the early childhood years, there are a number of skills that are relevant to participation in groups. Children learn skills for at least three types of group situations: (a) social/play; (b) independent work/play; and (c) instructional/recreational. Examples of the types of skills required for each type of group situation are as follows:

a. *Social/play groups:*
   sharing
   turn-taking
   helping
   cooperating
   waiting
b. *Independent work/play groups:*
   attending to task
   working/playing without assistance
   not bothering peers
c. *Instructional/recreational groups:*
   following group directions
   following rules and routines
   asking questions in turn
   speaking in turn
   staying with the group
   waiting/walking in lines

Many of the group skills listed here are learned in the toddler years (Murphy & Vincent, 1989); the others are learned later, with learning continuing into the school years, and through adulthood. Table 9-1 lists the group skills identified by teachers as important for success in preschool (Noonan et al., 1992) and kindergarten (Vincent et al., 1980).

If a child does not demonstrate the group skills in Table 9-1, these skills are appropriate goals. Also, developmental assessment instruments, such as the *Brigance Inventory of Early Development* (Brigance, 1978) and the *Learning Accomplishment Profile* (LeMay et al., 1977), include some skills for group

---

TABLE 9-1
Group Skills Included on Survival Skills Lists

Preschool Group Skills[1]	*Kindergarten Group Skills*[2]
Makes transitions from one activity to another	Initiates interactions with adults and peers
Complies with directions	Interacts with adults and peers when not the initiator
Follows rules and routines	
Focuses on task	Listens and attends to speaker in large group
Focuses attention on speaker	Demonstrates turn-taking in a small group
Socializes with others	
Communicates with peers	Attends to task for minimum of 15 minutes
Communicates with adults	
Takes turns	Adapts to transitions between activities throughout the day
Shares materials/toys with peers	
Cooperates with/helps others	Communicates with peers and adults
Does not disturb others	Asks questions of others
Uses voice appropriate to activity	Can "line up" and stay in line
	Raises hand and/or gets teacher attention when necessary
	Waits to take turns and shares
	Controls voice in classroom
	Stays in "own space" for activity

[1]Noonan et al., 1992.
[2]Vincent et al., 1980.

participation. Note that the *preschool* group skills in Table 9-1 were validated as in the repertoire of nondisabled 3-year-olds (Noonan et al., 1992).

Planning Group Instruction

There are many considerations when planning group instruction. Decisions about when and how objectives will be included must be made, and instructional techniques that facilitate group participation and take advantage of learning opportunities must be selected. Each of these important elements of groups (teaching group skills, organizing groups, facilitating group participation, and using group situations to support the instructional process) will be discussed.

Teaching Group Skills

Children as young as age 2 can be taught group participation skills, such as sitting in a group for 5 to 15 minutes and taking turns. When group participation is a problem, as it often is for children with disabilities, begin by rewarding the child for interacting and participating with only one other child. When the child learns to participate in this smallest group arrangement, add other children one at a time (Koegel & Rincover, 1974). Systematically increasing the size of the group is called a *tandem group* arrangement (Collins et al., 1991; Koegel & Rincover, 1974).

If the infant/young child participates appropriately in a group situation but is not making progress with individual goals, it may be necessary to have individual teaching sessions. This is called a *1:1 supplement* (Collins et al., 1991; Faw, Reid, Schepis, Fitzgerald & Welty, 1981). The 1:1 supplement is an alternative to discontinuing the child's participation in the group when the child is not progressing. The extra assistance of the 1:1 supplement may provide enough extra help to allow the child to benefit from group instruction. The 1:1 supplement is discontinued when the child demonstrates adequate progress.

Organizing Group Instruction

Ideally, *all* infants/young children with disabilities receive instruction on *at least one* goal during a group activity. As noted above, children may have the same goals, or they may have different goals. There are two approaches to incorporating instruction of specific goals/objectives into groups: skill embedding and skill sequencing.

Skill Embedding. Skill embedding is much like the activity-based approach to instruction described in Chapter 8. The first step is to select an age-appropriate group activity. The activity may be a self-care or play activity (for example, brushing teeth, playing "house"), or a daily routine (such as circle time). The activity may also be a child's "activity objective" (derived from the parent interview, see Chapter 6).

After selecting an age-appropriate group activity, review the child's objectives and select one or more objectives that fit logically into the activity. If there is more than one infant/young child with a disability in the group, select only two to four objectives per child. Imagine, for example, how Kimi's objectives of "grasping," "asking for more," and "manipulating objects" could be embedded in the activity of "playing with the kitchen bowls and utensils." All three skills can be taught during the bowls-and-utensils activity: Kimi grasps the bowls and utensils when passing or receiving them from another child in the group, and she grasps the utensils while "stirring" in the bowls; Kimi asks for "more" when the bowl is moved out of her reach; and Kimi manipulates objects by examining the utensils and bowls when they are given to her.

After selecting the activity and each child's objective(s), the next task is to write out the group activity like a script and indicate when each child's instructional trials will be presented. Figure 9-1 is an example of a group instruction plan that includes Kimi and the kitchen play activity. (With experience, such detailed scripting may not be necessary.) For each skill in italics, systematic instruction is implemented.

Skill Sequencing. Skill sequencing (Guess et al., 1978) is similar to skill embedding. The difference is that objectives are chained rather than distributed throughout the activity. Group skill sequences are constructed by first listing the objectives of the infants/children who will be in the group. An age-appropriate activity or theme is then selected. Next, one to three objectives for each child are identified on the basis of their logical relationship to one another. The final step is to write the sequence as a script, indicating the order in which instruction will be conducted for each objective. (Figure 9-2 is a sample script for the skill sequence delineated.) If the kitchen play group in Figure 9-1 was reconstructed as a skill sequence, the plan might be as follows:

1. Kawiki: *Look* when his name is called
2. Kawiki: *Point* to named objects
3. Darron: *Visually track* the utensils and bowl (when given to Kawiki)
4. Darron: *Visually track* the utensils and bowl (when given to Darron)
5. Darron: *Visually track* the utensils and bowl (when given to Kimi)
6. Kimi: *Grasp* the spoon and *manipulate*
7. Kimi: *Ask for more* (e.g., "more play" when the bowl is removed)

Activity: Kitchen Play

Group: Kimi (12 months), Darron (14 months), & Kawiki (11 months)

Implementation time: Mondays, 9–9:30

Interventionist: Allen

Date Initiated: 5/20/92   Ending Date:

Pass out two metal mixing bowls and a wooden fork and spoon to each child. Name each child and talk about the bowls and utensils as they are distributed.

> Darron: *Visually track* the utensils and bowl when they are presented to him.
> Kawiki: *Look when his name is called* (when the bowls and utensils are given to him).

Encourage the children to look at and pick up the bowls and utensils, assisting as necessary.

Demonstrate different ways to play with the bowls and utensils: turning them over, banging them on the floor, banging a utensil on the outside of the bowl, banging a utensil on the inside of the bowl, "stirring" with a utensil, etc.

> Kimi: *Grasp* the spoon and *manipulate*.
> Kimi: As she repeatedly bangs on the bowl, move the bowl out of reach and look at Kimi expectantly. Kimi will *ask for more*.
> Darron: *Visually track* the bowl and spoon as the interventionist bangs them together and moves them slowly in an arc, from right to left, and then left to right.
> Kawiki: *Points to named objects* when the interventionist holds up the bowl and a spoon.

Continue to encourage the children to play with the bowls and utensils. Repeat the above sequence (Kimi grasping and manipulating, Kimi asking for "more," Darron tracking, and Kawiki pointing to named objects) at least two more times.

Figure 9-1   Sample group instructional plan with embedded objectives

In this skill sequence, after Kawiki looks when his name is called, he is asked to point to something. There is a logical progression from the skill of looking to a skill that requires participation in the group (point to something). Darron visually tracks the utensils and bowl as they are passed to Kawiki. It is meaningful for him to do this after Kawiki has pointed to the objects and is receiving them. The relationship between the skills enhances motivation to perform the skills. In skill sequencing, infants/young children have opportunities to learn the logical relationships between skills learning, relationships that are likely to be present under natural conditions.

Activity:	Kitchen Play	
Group:	Kimi (12 months), Darron (14 months), & Kawiki (11 months)	
Implementation time:	Mondays, 9–9:30	
Interventionist:	Allen	
Date Initiated:	5/20/92	Ending Date:

Kawiki	*Darron*	*Kimi*
1. Look when name is called 2. Point to named objects		
	3. Visually track items given to Kawiki 4. Visually track items given to Darron 5. Visually track items given to Kimi	
		6. Grasp 7. Manipulate 8. Ask for more

Figure 9-2   Sample group skill sequence plan

Note that the group activity is not likely to occur in lockstep as scripted in the instructional plan: The behavior of infants and young children is rarely that predictable. The script is a *guide*.

Facilitating Group Participation

Effective instruction requires frequent and appropriate participation by all children in the group. Participation is evidence that the children are actively engaged. Some techniques to enhance group participation include (a) quick pacing, (b) selective attention, (c) partial/adaptive participation, (d) group interaction, (e) group responding, and (f) group contingencies.

Quick Pacing. Pace refers to the speed with which the teacher or infant specialist moves from one child to the next in the group. Quick pacing has three advantages: (a) it results in frequent instruction for all children, (b) it helps children attend to the activity, and (c) it decreases the likelihood of boredom and behavior problems. Typically the teacher or infant specialist focuses attention on each infant or young child for several moments, one at a time, to instruct specific skills. With practice, a teacher or infant specialist can become skilled at quick pacing.

Periodic attention is a technique associated with pacing. Occasionally, the teacher or infant specialist calls different children by name or uses some other strategy (*eye* contact, pointing, smiling) to maintain or regain the children's attention. In addition to redirecting children to attend to the group activity, periodic attention rewards those children who are attending.

Selective Attention.   Selective attention is another way to enhance group participation. Praise those infants/young children who are attending and partici-

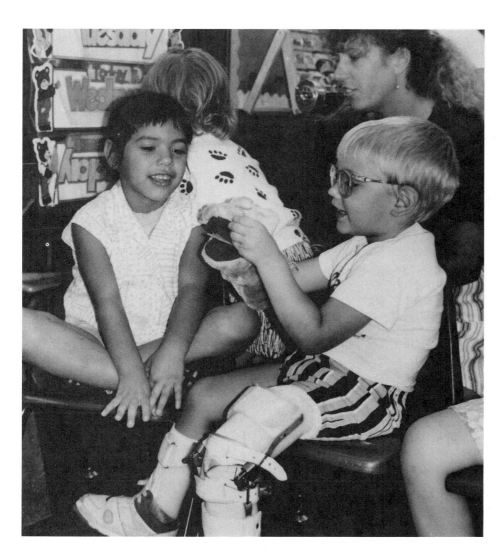

Group instruction may be conducted with as few as two children.

pating. Social reinforcement should be delivered quickly and individually. In addition to praise, visual attention, smiling, gentle touching, or other social reinforcers may be used.

Ideally, children who are not reinforced will notice that they have been bypassed when their peers receive reinforcement, and attempt to imitate those who were successful in obtaining reinforcement.

Partial/Adapted Participation. Some children are not able to participate in typical group activities. Thus, requirements for participation must be modified. This is *partial or adapted participation*. Partial participation and adapted participation are slightly different. When only a portion of the response is required, it is partial participation. When response requirements are changed and a response that serves the same purpose but is accomplished through an alternative means is substituted, it is called adapted participation. For example, if children are expected to reach and grasp materials, and one child is unable to maintain a grasp, partial participation suggests that child will reach for the materials and open her hand, and an adult or peer will assist her to grasp and bring the materials to her lap. Adaptive participation is another option for this child. She could wear a strap on her hand fitted with Velcro®. After reaching, the materials are secured to her hand, and she completes the response by bringing them to her lap. Partial participation and response adaptations are discussed in greater detail in Chapter 11.

Group Interaction. Much of early intervention involves didactic interactions between infants/young children and one or more adults. This is true even in group situations. To take full advantage of opportunities provided in group instruction, social interaction among the group members should be promoted. (As noted in the rationale for group instruction, group activities are the only context where it is possible to enhance peer-related social competence.) The most obvious way to promote interaction is to identify and target one or more social interaction objectives for children in the group. Socialization objectives may be embedded in the group activity or taught through skill sequencing.

Figure 9-3 shows an intersequential group activity in which preschoolers are passing materials one at a time. Passing materials is not an objective (objectives are designated with an asterisk in the figure); it is included to create the need for social interaction and to teach the children to take turns. Specific social interaction objectives are also included in the group sequence for three of the four preschoolers (indicated in bold print in the sequence). The fourth child, Daria, practices attending to the activity four times each time the sequence is conducted.

Group instruction can also teach *task interdependence* among group members. Task interdependence occurs when each child's participation in the activity can only occur if another group member fulfills a participation requirement. Each child has a clear and necessary role. Group members must attend to what their peers are doing in order to know when it is their turn. In the example in Figure 9-2, the requirement that children pass the materials for their peers to take their turns

Activity:	Sand or Water Play

Group: Tomiko (36 months), Sean (32 months), Matthew (40 months), and Daria (37 months)

Implementation time:	Tuesdays 10–10:20	Interventionist:	Francie

Date Initiated:	1/12/92	Ending Date:	

Tomiko	*Sean*	*Matthew*	*Daria*
*Pour from one container to another (*use both hands in fine motor activity*)*			***Attend to activity (watch peer)**
Pass containers to Sean— — — —			
	*Say "thank you"		***Attend to activity (watch peer)**
	*Imitate Tomiko		***Attend to activity (watch peer)**
	Pass containers to Matthew— — — —	*Pour from one container to another*	
		*Identify named peer	
		Pass containers to Daria— — — —	***Attend to activity (receive containers)**
			Pour from one container to another
			Pass containers to Tomiko

Repeat sequence four more times, using different actions requiring Tomiko to use both hands with objects in the sand or water play.

*Instructional objectives

Figure 9-3 Sample intersequential group skill sequence (with social skill objectives in bold print)

sets up an interdependent situation. Usually, however, task interdependence involves a complex goal. For example, if preschoolers have the task of setting the table, one may have the task of wiping the table clean, another may be required to count out the appropriate number of dishes, cups, and napkins, and the third may be required to set the table. The group is interdependent because the dishes, cups, and napkins cannot be placed on the table until the table has been cleaned by the first member of the group and the second member has given the materials to the third.

Group Responding.   In the examples of group instructional plans presented thus far, most participation has been one child at a time. Group members may respond together. Group responding increases each child's opportunities for active responding. Group responding can be verbal, with children answering questions, singing songs, or rote reciting (for example, counting), or nonverbal, with children performing a motor response. Making hand motions to a song, imitating the teacher or infant specialist demonstrating a task (such as folding a paper in four), or playing with the activity materials (for example, musical instruments) are examples of nonverbal group responding.

During group responding it is a good idea for the teacher to shift eye contact and attention quickly among the children, to let them know that their participation is appropriate. This requires that the group be in close proximity to one another. Whether the response is verbal, nonverbal, or both, group responding has two important advantages: (a) it assists group members to attend and participate in the activity, and (b) it minimizes the time that children must wait for a turn.

Group responding is more difficult when group composition is heterogeneous. Group responding may be included for only one or two components of group instruction. For example, all children may be asked to point at pictures as they are named in a story. Then there may be individual requirements. One child, for example, is required to vocalize and another to say a word during the group response. (Note that individualized response requirements may include partial participation or adaptive participation.)

Group Contingencies.   A group contingency is an instructional arrangement whereby reinforcement is provided when all group members demonstrate a required response. Most of us are familiar with group contingencies from elementary school expeiences in which we lost or gained privileges depending on the behavior of the entire class. If the entire class did their spelling homework, for example, the class could earn 10 minutes of free time after reading. If one or more members of the class did not do the homework, however, the class did not earn the free time or was penalized. Because group contingencies rely on peer pressure (anticipated peer acceptance or rejection) for their effectiveness, they are not likely to be effective for infants and very young children. They have been demonstrated to be as effective

not particularly effective

as individual contingencies, however, when teaching social skills to preschoolers with disabilities (cf. Kohler, Strain, Maretsky & DeCesare, 1990).

Using Groups to Support the Instructional Process

Group instruction provides unique teaching opportunities. In addition to providing opportunities to teach social interaction skills, group situations are well suited for assistance, encouragement, and generalization strategies.

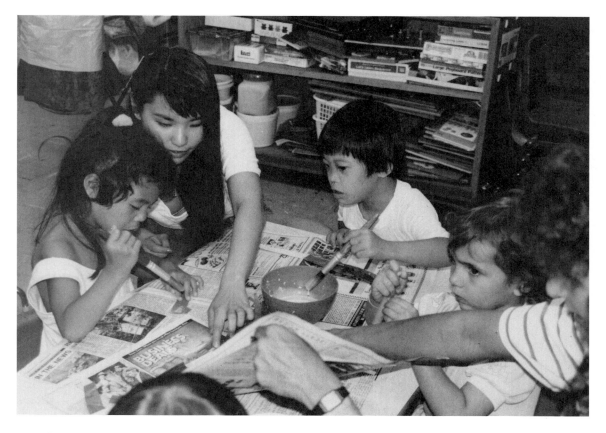

Group instruction provides opportunities for children to learn from one another.

Assistance Procedures. Possibly the most important advantage of group instruction is the opportunity for observational learning. Observational learning, however, should not be left to chance. Rather than just hoping children will imitate, praise attending and imitating peers ("I see you're doing it just like Carmen, that's good!"). Observational learning can also be facilitated by encouraging children to reinforce one another. Have children clap for one another, or have a child give stickers to peers when they make correct responses. Delivering reinforcement to peers enhances attention to peers, and facilitates observational learning (Brown & Holvoet, 1982).

Peer modeling can be used to prompt desired behavior. For example, Jason is asked to demonstrate how to spread paste with his finger. Brendyn observes Jason spreading the paste on the back of his Santa face *and* he also sees that Jason gets praised for the skill. So Brendyn spreads paste in the same way. Children imitate more competent peers and peers they observe receiving reinforcement. Peer modeling is a good technique to teach social or communicative interactions —skills that cannot be modeled by the teacher or infant specialist.

Group instruction also provides opportunities for peer tutoring/prompting. *Peer tutoring/prompting* uses other children in the group (usually more competent children) to provide assistance and encouragement for a particular child. (This is discussed at length in Chapter 10.) Research has demonstrated that socially competent preschoolers can deliver prompts effectively if they are directly taught to do so (Kohler et al., 1990). Prompting is maintained through group reinforcement contingencies (a reward is earned by the group rather than a single child). All children are reinforced if the children learning the new skills are successful. A kindergarten teacher might use peer tutoring and a group contingency to teach her students to walk to the cafeteria quietly and in a line. Peer tutors are assigned and told to remind their partners to "use a quiet voice" when they talk loudly, and to "walk slowly and stay in line" when they leave the group. All the children earn an extra story during story time if the entire class walks quietly in a line to the cafeteria.

In homogeneous groups where more than one infant/young child has the same objective, the effectiveness of instruction is enhanced by repetition of the same (or similar) instructional procedures. A child may observe instruction implemented one or more times before he is required to respond. This repetition has the effect of providing additional instruction. Similarly, repetition of the prompt highlights and thus increases the effectiveness of the prompt (Skinner, 1938). And if a peer is working on the same objective, but receiving a less intrusive prompt, the target child may learn to respond to the less intrusive prompt (Brown et al., 1980). For example, Jimmy, a toddler who needs hand-over-hand assistance to pull up his shorts, observes his peer pulling up his shorts after a demonstration. Jimmy attempts to imitate, thus responding to a less intrusive prompt assistance.

Encouragement Procedures. Attention is critical for effective instruction. Use selective attention to reward children's attention to prompts: if the child attends, give him a turn. Group instruction also provides opportunities for children to observe the consequences for not attending (losing a turn).

As noted earlier in the discussion on facilitating group participation, peers may be taught to provide reinforcement. There are several advantages for teaching peers to praise and encourage one another. First, in many cases, peer attention and reinforcement are more powerful than adult attention. Second, when peers provide reinforcement, friendships develop (we tend to "like" individuals who reinforce us). Third, children often generalize the use of peer reinforcement beyond the group instruction setting. Fourth, children may imitate reinforcing behaviors, because such behaviors, in turn, earn reinforcement (reinforcement begets reinforcement).

Generalization Procedures. Group instruction can be used to enhance skill generalization. If group members are working on the same (or similar) objectives, use different materials and instructional stimuli for different children. This allows children to observe different stimuli associated with the target response and thus facilitates stimulus generalization. When different materials and stimuli are used to teach the same response, slightly different responses may be appropriate to accommodate the differences in the materials/stimuli. Observing the different appropriate responses assists children to learn the response class.

Most important, as young children participate in groups, they learn how to learn in a group. Much of the instruction provided to nondisabled children is large group instruction. Thus it is valuable to include children in more than one group, and in groups of various sizes (including groups of ten or more children, if possible). Variation across groups increases the likelihood that the children will generalize their group participation skills.

Summary

Group instruction is an important component in early intervention. It is particularly important for 2- through 5-year-olds who need group participation skills in regular early childhood settings. This chapter described strategies for facilitating participation in groups: quick pacing, selective attention, partial/adaptive participation, group interaction, and group responding. Techniques for using group arrangements to support the instructional process (assistance, encouragement, and generalization strategies) were also described.

Activities

1. Observe a preschool special education teacher and a kindergarten teacher conducting group instruction. In each case, note the following:
   a. Strategies used to maintain children's attention
   b. Strategies used to promote active child involvement
   c. Opportunities for interaction among the children
   d. Strategies used to avoid behavior problems

2. If you are teaching or in a practicum setting with infants or young children who have disabilities, have yourself videotaped conducting group instruction. Review the tape, and note your strengths and weaknesses. Refer to items a. through d. in activity 1.

3. Develop a script for group instruction using skill sequencing or embedded instruction. If you are not currently teaching or in a practicum situation, write a description of four young children with disabilities to serve as your group for this assignment. Place an asterisk next to each skill in the script that is an instructional objective.

4. Do assignment 3 for an integrated group of two nondisabled children and two young children with disabilities.

Review Questions

1. Define *group instruction*. Develop a rationale for group instruction in early intervention.
2. Describe and discuss considerations associated with the nature of groups: group composition, group interactions, and group content.
3. Brainstorm and write a list of group skills. Pick three of the skills, and list two instructional strategies that might be used to teach each skill.
4. Describe skill embedding and skill sequencing strategies for organizing group instruction.
5. Define and provide an example of the following strategies for promoting group participation:

   quick pacing
   selective attention
   partial/adaptive participation

group interaction
group responding
group contingencies

6. Describe ways in which the characteristics of group instruction can be used to enhance the instructional process in providing assistance, providing encouragement, and promoting generalization.

Environmental Arrangements to Promote Interaction

1. *Discuss methods to enhance and facilitate social and communication skills of children with disabilities.*

2. *Describe specific procedures for arranging the environment to increase and maintain appropriate peer interactions.*

*I*t has now been over two decades since the first arguments for educating preschool children with special needs in the same setting as their nondisabled peers (Bricker & Bricker, 1971). The many demonstrations of effective mainstreaming have led to broad consensus that young children with special needs and normally developing children derive substantial benefits from carefully planned integration (Guralnick, 1978, 1981; Guralnick & Groom, 1988; Odom & Strain, 1984).

The best arguments for providing young children with the benefits of mainstream settings as early as possible come from research showing that initial educational placements for children with disabilities are highly predictive of later placements (Edgar, Heggelund & Fischer, 1989; Edgar, McNulty, Gaetz & Maddox, 1984). This research found that children tend to get "stuck" in the special education system: the longer they are in special education classes, the more difficult it is to move them to regular classrooms.

As Vincent, Brown, and Getz-Sheftel (1981) put it: "The degree and type of integration needs to be individually determined for each young handicapped child, but whether integration is provided does not" (p. 23). It is difficult to imagine circumstances in which there could be justification for depriving a child of any opportunities for interactions with normally developing peers. Some children have dual placements: they receive services in a segregated early intervention program for part of the day in addition to placement in an integrated preschool or childcare program. Integrated environments are the best settings for promoting social and communicative competence because they provide (a) shared experiences, cooperative learning, and advanced play; (b) opportunities to practice social and communicative interactions; and (c) observational learning of appropriate social and communication behaviors. The challenge is how to maximize these benefits.

Intervention to facilitate social competence has two foci. One is the social interaction skills of children with disabilities. The other focus is the attitudes and values of nondisabled children. The goal where nondisabled children are concerned is to help them learn to respect and understand individual differences. The National Association for the Education of Young Children (NAEYC), in a description of developmentally appropriate practice, emphasizes the importance of providing many opportunities for children to develop social competence in the context of routine activities.

Social competence is a relative concept, in that there must be a defined context for the term to have meaning for a particular individual. A child's social competence can only be judged relative to that child's effectiveness with, or the outcome of, a specific well-defined social task. Examples of important social tasks for young children include gaining entry to a peer group, resolving conflicts with other children, acquiring a desired toy from another child, and making new friends on a playground (Guralnick, 1990b).

This chapter focuses on how to arrange the environment to increase and maintain peer interactions. Procedures for facilitating the social and communication competencies of young children with disabilities fall into four categories: (a) peer-

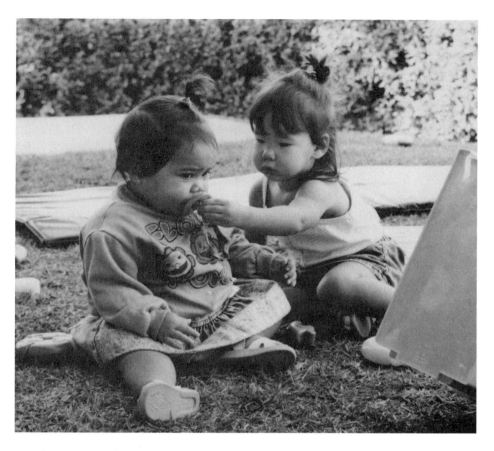

Interaction with a disabled peer helps nondisabled children learn respect and understanding.

mediated models, (b) adult-mediated models, (c) group models, and (d) direct instruction models. All of these models share a common goal: spontaneous interactions between children with disabilities and nondisabled peers. They can be implemented singly or in combination.

Peer-Mediated Models

Also called *confederate interventions*, peer-mediated models are based on the premise that socially competent peers naturally interact with one another in ways that promote development of social skills. Developmental research indicates that peer initiations *exert* a powerful influence over social behavior (Corsaro, 1979; 1981). The basic strategy of peer-mediated models is to teach socially competent young children to initiate interactions with less-competent peers as a means of enhancing their social skills. Most peer-mediated interventions require active peer-initiations (Odom and Strain, 1984). However, we will also discuss proximity.

Proximity Interventions

Proximity interventions do nothing more than just place children with disabilities in settings with their nondisabled peers. While simply placing children together in an early intervention setting is not a recommended method, there is at least one study with preschool children showing that proximity was enough to affect social interactions. Furman, Rahe, and Hartup (1979) randomly assigned preschool children identified as socially withdrawn to three treatments: (a) a small play group with same-age normally developing peers; (b) a small play group with younger, normally developing peers; or (c) a no-treatment control situation. Children assigned to the play group with younger, normally developing peers demonstrated significantly higher levels of social interaction than did children in either of the other groups. It would be helpful to know precisely what type of interactions occurred in the successful play group, but unfortunately this study did not provide this information.

The inclusion of proximity interventions here is not a recommendation for this type of interrvention. Mere physical integration may have some benefits as demonstrated in the Furman study, but it is generally considered to be insufficient to bring about the full range of possible benefits of integration (for preschoolers with disabilities or for their nondisabled peers).

Peer-Initiation Interventions

Strain and Odom (1986) emphasize that for peer-initiation interventions to be optimally effective, there must be:

1. Careful selection and teaching of specific peer initiations;
2. Arrangement of the physical environment in such a way as to promote interactions;
3. Training of peers to implement intervention; and
4. Implementation of daily intervention sessions.

Based on a series of naturalistic studies with both normally developing preschoolers and preschool children with disabilities, Strain (1983) and Strain and

Odom (1986) recommend teaching peers to initiate these specific behaviors: (a) play organizers, (b) shares, (c) physical assistance, and (d) affection. An example of a play organizer is "Let's play in the sandbox," or "You push it and I'll catch." An example of a share is offering to give or exchange an object with a peer or offering to use an object or toy mutually. Physical assistance is what the name implies—helping the child in some way. For example, the peer might help the child with disabilities climb on a stool to reach something on the counter. Examples of affection include patting, hugging, kissing, or holding hands.

Training for peer-initiation intervention begins with selection of socially competent peers. Strain and Odom (1986) suggest these peer selection criteria: (a) compliance with teacher requests, (b) regular attendance, (c) age-appropriate play skills, (d) either no history with the child with disabilities or a positive history, (e) enrollment in the same class as the child with disabilities, and (f) expressed willingness to participate. Daily lessons of 20 to 30 minutes are scheduled to teach the specific social initiations. Daily lessons follow this standard format:

1. Discussion of the importance of making new friends, sharing, playing cooperatively with others, and helping one another;
2. Description of the target social initiation (play organizing, sharing, physical assistance, or affection) for that day;
3. Teacher modeling of the target social initiation behavior with another adult playing the other child role (note that on about half of the occasions, the adult playing the child with disabilities is nonresponsive, so that the confederate has to persist in his or her initiations);
4. Practice opportunities where two or three children demonstrate the strategy with the second adult (with verbal feedback on their performance);
5. Role-playing examples of the incorrect use of the strategy with prompts to help the children identify the error and state the correct use of the strategy (choral responding is a good idea, as it ensures that all children rehearse the strategy).

Figure 10-1 provides a sample script for a daily training session. Strain and Odom (1986) note that confederate training typically requires four or five sessions. These are the steps for the daily intervention sessions:

1. Assemble the group (including the target child with disabilities and at least one confederate).
2. Introduce the scheduled activity and model specific ways to use the materials for that particular activity.
3. Tell all of the children (except the confederate) to begin the activity.
4. Take the confederate aside and remind him or her what to do ("Go and get _____ to play with you").
5. If the confederate does not make the appropriate initiation in 15 seconds, verbally prompt the initiation. Say "Remember, you need to get _____ to play with you." If the confederate does not come up with a good idea for an

---

Sample Script

Session 1: Introduction to System—Share Initiation—Persistence

Teacher: "Today you are going to learn how to be a good teacher. Sometimes your friends in your class do not know how to play with other children. You are going to learn how to teach them to play. What are you going to do?"

Child response: "Teach them to play."

Teacher: "One way you can get your friend to play with you is to share. How do you get your friend to play with you?"

Child response: "Share."

Teacher: "Right! You share. When you share you look at your friend and say, 'Here,' and put a toy in his hand. What do you do?" (Repeat this exercise until the child can repeat these three steps.)

Child response: "Look at friend and say, 'Here,' and put the toy in his hand."

Adult model with role player: "Now, watch me. I am going to share with ____. Tell me if I do it right." (Demonstrate sharing.) "Did I share with ____? What did I do?"

Child response: Yea! ____ looked at ____, said 'here ____' and put a toy in his hand."

Adult: "Right. I looked at ____ and said, 'here ____' and put a toy in his hand. Now watch me. See if I share with ____." (Move to the next activity in the classroom. This time provide a negative example of sharing by leaving out the "put in hand" component. Put the toy beside the role player). "Did I share?" (Correct if necessary and repeat this example if child got it wrong.) "Why not?"

Child response: "No.____You did not put the toy in ____'s hand."

Adult: "That's right. I did not put the toy in ____'s hand. When I have to look at ____ and say, 'here ' and put the toy in his hand." (Give the child two more positive and two more negative examples of sharing. When they answer incorrectly about sharing, repeat the example. Vary the negative examples by leaving out different components: looking, saying 'here,' putting in hand.)

Child practice with adults: "Now ____, I want you to get ____ to share with you. What do you do when you share?"

Child response: "Look at ____ and say, 'here ____,' and put a toy in his hand."

Adult: "Now, go get ____ to play with you." (For these practice examples, the role playing adult should be responsive to the child's sharing.) (To the other confederates:) "Did ____ share with ____? What did she/he do?"

Child response: "Yes/No. Looked at ____ and said, 'here ____' and put a toy in his hand."

Adult: (Move to the next activity.) "Now, ____ I want you to share with ____."

Figure 10-1 Sample script for confederate training session

initiation, be more explicit. For example, you might say "Tell _____to pour some tea in your cup."

Continue to prompt the confederate if he or she does not initiate an interaction every 15 to 20 seconds.

Sample Script — *(continued)*

Introduce Persistence

Teacher: "Sometimes when I play with ____, he/she does not want to play back. I have to keep on trying. What do I have to do?"

Child response: "Keep on trying."

Teacher: "Right, I have to keep on trying. Watch me. I am going to share with ____. Now I want you to see if I keep on trying." (Role player will be initially unresponsive.) (Teacher should be persistent until child finally responds.) "Did I get ____ to play with me?" *Child:* "Yes." "Did he want to play?" *Child:* "No." "What did I do?" *Child:* "Keep on trying." "Right, I kept on trying. Watch. See if I can get ____ to play with me this time." (Again, the role player should be unresponsive at first. Repeat above questions and correct if necessary. Repeat the example until the child responds correctly.)

SOURCE: From "Peer Social Initiations: Effective Intervention for Social Skills Development of Exceptional Children" by P. S. Strain, and S. L. Odom, *Exceptional Children,* 52 (6), 1986, p. 547. Copyright 1986 by The Council for Exceptional Children. Reprinted with permission.

Figure 10-1 — *(continued)*

Prompts are gradually reduced when it is obvious that they are no longer needed. If there is a noticeable reduction in initiations when prompts are reduced, they should be reinstated (and faded again at a later time).

Adult-Mediated Models

Adult-mediated models differ from peer-mediated models in that an adult (typically the teacher) works directly with the child with disabilities. Nondisabled peers are involved, of course, but the adult, rather than a peer, is the one responsible for affecting the social behavior of the child with disabilities. Three adult-mediated interventions are described: (a) prompt-praise interventions; (b) interventions that relies on rearranging the environment; and (c) incidental teaching interventions.

Prompt-Praise Interventions

The prompt-praise model relies on the teacher to provide encouragement in the form of instructions or another type of prompt and reinforcement (praise, attention, or other positive consequences) for social responses directed to peers (Hart, Reynolds, Baer, Browley & Harris, 1968). The systematic imitation approach is an example of this model. It comes from a series of studies by Apolloni and Cooke and colleagues (Apolloni & Cooke, 1978; Apolloni, Cooke & Cooke, 1977; Peck, Apolloni, Cooke & Raver, 1978). Children with disabilities are given verbal or physical prompts to imitate the behavior of a peer. The adult then praises the imitative behavior. Prompts are gradually faded. The premise is that children with disabilities will learn the more advanced skills if taught to imitate these skills.

Peck and colleagues (1978) investigated the effects of peer imitation training on three young children with Down syndrome. The children were placed in a free-play area with three nondisabled peers. Training periods were 4 minutes. This procedure was implemented when the child with disabilities was within 3 feet of a peer model:

> The teacher pointed to the peer model and said, "Look! See what he/she is doing? You do it."
> If the child imitated the behavior within 5 seconds, the teacher praised him and gave him a pat or a hug.
> If the child did not imitate, the teacher physically guided him through the behavior and then praised him.

Observations of the children's spontaneous imitation conducted for 3 minutes after each training period showed a significant increase in imitative behavior. Further and most significant, the effects of training generalized to the free-play situation when the teacher was not present.

Environment Rearrangement Interventions

The environment rearrangement model relies on adapting the physical context to encourage social interactions. The physical environment includes nonsocial dimensions of the environment. Environmental design, materials and equipment, and grouping and scheduling were discussed in Chapter 8. Here we will consider two aspects of the environment that have a high probability of increasing social interactions: (a) materials and equipment, and (b) activity structures.

Materials and Equipment. Some materials and equipment have a greater potential for promoting social interactions than others. Findings from research with nondisabled preschoolers indicate that there is more peer interaction with wagons, hollow blocks, dramatic-play materials, and games that require two players (Quilitch & Risley, 1973). There are similar findings with preschoolers with disabilities (Peterson & Haralick, 1977). Stoneman, Cantrell, and Hoover-Dempsey (1983) observed the play of six children at risk for special education placement and six nonhandicapped peers in an integrated setting. They found that play materials that require cooperative interaction (blocks and vehicles, water play, housekeeping, and music) were instrumental in facilitating peer interactions.

If sharing is increased, there is increased interaction and, very often, increased communication. Selection of materials that children are familiar with encourages

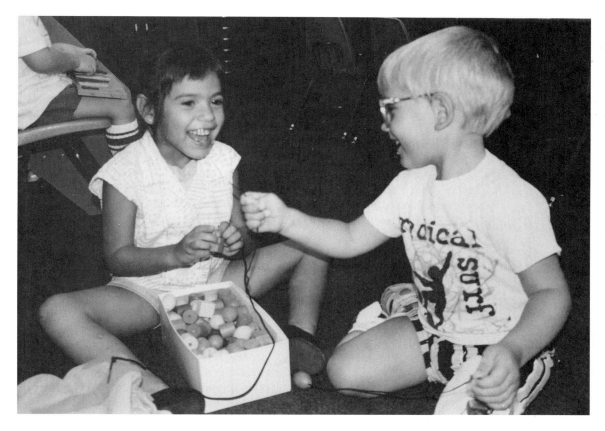

Certain types of play materials, such as blocks, have a greater potential to promote social interaction.

sharing and cooperative play. Limiting the amounts of materials is another way to encourage sharing (Montes & Risley, 1975; Quilitch & Risley, 1973). Besides sharing, some behaviors that are likely to increase positive interactions are (a) imitating peers, (b) assisting others in play or work, (c) physical affection, and (d) play-organizing statements.

Activity Structure.   Activity structure is another aspect of the physical context that has the potential to affect social and communication interaction. Activity structure has at least three dimensions: (a) the structure imposed by the activity itself, (b) the structure imposed on the activity by the toys and materials, and (c) the structure (or lack thereof) imposed by an adult's directions for the activity. Any one or some combination of these dimensions may affect children's peer interactions.

Shores, Hester, and Strain (1976) report the results of a study examining the influence of teacher-imposed structure on children's social interactions with peers. (Teacher-imposed structure is the degree to which the theme of play, roles of participants, and other rules governing play are stipulated by the teacher.) They observed the social interactions of nine preschool children with behavior disorders under three conditions. In the first condition the teacher was involved directly in the children's play activities. In the second condition there was no teacher involvement. In the third condition the teacher structured the play but was not otherwise involved. Children interacted most in the third, teacher structured, condition and least in the teacher-involvement condition.

Deklyen and Odom (1989) found similar results in their investigation of teacher-imposed structure. They hypothesized that the amount of peer interaction in various play activities would depend on the level of structure in that activity. This was, in fact, what occurred. Children interacted more frequently with each other in more-structured activities and less frequently in less-structured activities. The investigators in this study emphasize the importance of differentiating teacher involvement from teacher-imposed structure; teacher involvement was found to be negatively correlated with peer interactions. This suggests that teacher interactions in an activity may interfere with peer interactions.

Studies by McCormick (1987) and Spiegel-McGill, Zippiroli and Mistrett (1989) that consider the effectiveness of computer activities as a context for social interactions are also relevant here. These investigators describe the use of specific activities (in this case, computer activities) to facilitate social/communicative interactions. The Spiegel-McGill data come from a 3-year demonstration model using computers and related technology to promote the development of social skills in preschool children who are physically disabled or demonstrate severe speech-language delays.

The premise of both studies is that a toy or other activity with a single point of attention and a range of play options provides a rich environment for social and communication interactions. In both studies the teacher helped the children get started in the various activities, verbally instructed them to begin, and then withdrew. As there was no further involvement or teacher structuring of the activity, these would undoubtedly be classified as low-teacher-involvement activities. The results of these studies suggest that the environment can be arranged to promote and enhance social and communicative interactions.

Incidental Teaching Interventions

The incidental teaching model is the third type of adult-mediated intervention. As discussed in Chapter 8, incidental teaching is a well-validated procedure to promote language development (Hart, 1985; Rogers-Warren & Warren, 1980b). This intervention is equally applicable to teaching social and communication skills (Brown, McEvoy & Bishop, 1991).

As discussed in Chapter 8, incidental teaching is an umbrella term for a set of naturalistic instructional strategies. What makes these strategies unique is that they are (a) carried out in the natural environment, and (b) child-initiated. The incidental teaching sequence begins when the child initiates an interaction in the context of naturally occurring routines and activities. At that point the adult uses modeling or a prompt strategy to elicit an elaborated (more sophisticated) response.

The child with disabilities may initiate an interaction by showing an interest in an activity, another child, other children, or specific materials. The adult prompts an appropriate social or communicative response or encourages a peer to model the appropriate social/communication behavior for the child with disabilities. Table 10-1 provides examples of incidental teaching sequences.

Brown, McEvoy, and Bishop (1991) have compiled some suggestions for implementing incidental teaching interventions. The first step is to identify routine classroom activities that lend themselves to incidental teaching of social/communication behaviors. Keep in mind that incidental teaching episodes are most appropriate in unstructured activities (snack, transition times, free play, arriving at and leaving school). Then prepare a list of ways to encourage social interactions of target children during these activities (for example, at snack, give Taylor a double quantity of fruit or crackers and prompt him to share with a "friend"). When selecting these situations it is critical for the situation to be reinforcing to the child. The way to find out if a situation is reinforcing is to try implementing the planned episodes and observe whether the child is interested in the materials or peers that are involved. For example, if Taylor frequently watches Corey play with the Sesame Street® house and toys, he is probably interested in Corey, the toys, or both. Likewise, when a child grabs a toy or other object from another child, it is safe to say that he is interested in that toy or object. Both are excellent opportunities for an incidental teaching episode.

Groups Models

There are two validated approaches using dyadic or group activities as the context for promoting peer/peer social/communication skills: (a) cooperative learning, and (b) affection activities.

Cooperative Learning

There is now considerable research demonstrating that instruction in cooperative skills improves social interaction behaviors and promotes positive peer interactions among students who are disabled and those who are nondisabled (Putnam, Rynders, Johnson & Johnson, 1989). Drawing from the work of Johnson and Johnson (1975; 1981; 1983; 1986), the cooperative learning model structures activities to teach children to encourage one another, celebrate each other's successes, and work toward common goals.

TABLE 10-1
Examples of Possible Incidental Teaching of Social Behavior*

Activity	Incidental Teaching Direction by Teacher	Child Interactive Response	Anticipated Response from Peer(s)
Play			
Billy is playing with blocks and Susie (target child) is standing and watching.	"Susie, why don't you play with Billy?" "Billy, share the blocks with Susie."	Susie sits down next to Billy and says, "Me play too."	Susie begins to build a fort made of blocks with Billy.
Lunch			
David (target child) needs help opening a milk carton.	"David, ask Dana to help you open your milk carton."	"Dana, help me please."	Dana helps David open his milk, and David says, "Thanks, Dana."
Transition			
Bill (target child) needs his chair moved from table activities to large group.	"Susie, will you be a good friend and help Bill move his chair to large group?"	Susie says, "Bill, I'll help you. Where do you want to sit today?"	Bill walks to large group with his walker and points next to Susie's chair while Susie moves his chair next to hers.
Arrival			
Todd (target child) has trouble with the buttons on his coat when he comes to school.	"David, remember Todd has trouble unbuttoning his coat. Why don't you show him how you unbutton *your* coat?"	David approaches Todd and says, "Todd, you want to unbutton your coat? Watch me."	Todd nods his head yes and approaches David. Todd watches David unbutton his buttons and tries to do his own buttons the same way. David helps him if necessary.

A major difference between the confederate model and the cooperative learning model is the nature of the social behavior that is emphasized. The confederate model typically focuses on teaching peer initiations, responding positively, and sharing. The cooperative learning model, on the other hand, is concerned with fostering cooperative interactions. The premise is that peer relationships will develop from these interactions. Other goals of the cooperative model include facilitation of cooperative learning skills and enhanced self-esteem.

Cooperative learning groups are instructional situations in which children

TABLE 10-1 — (continued)

Activity	Incidental Teaching Direction by Teacher	Child Interactive Response	Anticipated Response from Peer(s)
Classtime Howard is walking from large group to the snack table and falls down.	"Oh, Mary (target child), look, Howard fell down. Let's give him a big hug, and make sure he's okay."	Mary and the teacher walk over to Howard. Mary hugs Howard and asks if he's okay.	Howard hugs Mary and says, "Let's go eat."
Fine Motor Activity Paul (target child), who is mute but can work complex connecting puzzles, is working a 20-piece puzzle.	"Look, Paul, Al needs help with his puzzle. Show him how to work it."	Paul shows Al where a piece of the puzzle goes and smiles.	Paul and Al take turns putting pieces of the puzzle in. After completing the puzzle, Al says, "We did it."

*Note that a target child or a peer can be used to initiate a social interaction, and that his or her prosocial behavior will vary with the child's level of developmental sophistication. Teachers' prompts for peer interaction should also vary with children's level of developmental sophistication and should allow for individual differences. Indeed, some children may not have the verbal repertoire of classmates and may need to indicate their preferences and requests nonverbally. For example, children who are nonambulatory and mute might indicate a desire for a prosocial interaction by smiling and nodding their heads yes. Initially, teachers may need to interpret children's communicative attempts, particularly if they are nonverbal and idiosyncratic. For example, teachers might inform nonhandicapped peers that when nonambulatory and nonverbal children look at a toy, they are indicating a desire to hold or play with that toy.

SOURCE: From "Incidental Teaching of Social Behavior—A Naturalistic Approach for Promoting Young Children's Peer Interactions" by W. H. Brown, M. A. McEvoy, and N. Bishop, *Teaching Exceptional Children,* 24 (1), 1991, p. 36. Copyright 1991 by The Council for Exceptional Children. Reprinted with permission.

perceive they can reach their learning goals if and only if peers in their group also reach their goals. The teacher's role is to teach the necessary cooperative skills so that groups function effectively. Cooperative learning (as a teaching strategy) has four basic elements: (a) positive interdependence, (b) face-to-face communication, (c) individual accountability, and (d) group process.

The first element, positive interdependence, requires group members to work together to accomplish a common goal. Methods for promoting positive interdependence are mutual goals; divisions of labor; dividing materials, resources, or information among group members; assigning students different roles; and giving joint rewards. The second element is face-to-face interaction with the requirement of verbal interaction (or another form of communication). The third element is individual accountability. Students are held individually accountable for mastering the assigned material and contributing to the group's efforts. Finally, the fourth element is group process. Students are expected to use appropriate interpersonal and small-group skills (for example, turn-taking).

Most research with cooperataive groups has been with school-age children. The youngest participant was in a study by Wilcox, Sbardellati and Nevin (1987) that applied the cooperative learning model to facilitate the social integration of an 8-year-old girl with severe disabilities into a regular first-grade class. There is some recent research using a cooperative activity structure at the preschool level with children with disabilities. Gackowski, Kobe, and McCormick (1991) increased the social/communication interactions of two children with disabilities who were placed in mainstream preschool settings. Five specific social/communication behaviors were targeted: (a) asking/offering help, (b) listening attentively to another's ideas, (c) sharing, (d) taking turns, and (e) showing someone how to do something. These skills were facilitated in the context of six to ten lessons that combined a story theme ("Stone Soup") with the curriculum unit (in one case, Christmas). Not only did positive social/communication initiations of the target children increase in the training context (during the lessons), but also both children demonstrated substantial increases in the rate of initiations at other times of the day in other contexts.

The following is an adaptation for preschool of the major strategies that Johnson and Johnson (1986) describe as promoting cooperative learning:

1. Select or develop a unit with clear cognitive/preacademic objectives and list the cooperative skills to be taught. Interpersonal and small-groups skills such as taking turns or assisting one another are examples of possible target skills.

2. Plan a series of lessons or activities. The objective is to teach cooperative skills in the context of cognitive/preacademic lessons and activities.

3. Assign children to dyads or three-member groups. Include one child with disabilities in each group. Maintain the same groups for all the lessons/activities in the unit.

4. Encourage cooperative effort by the way materials are distributed. There are many ways to do this in order to encourage group effort. For example, consider providing each group member with only part of the materials needed to complete the activity, or providing the group with only one set of materials.

5. Introduce the lessons/activities by providing a clear and specific description (and demonstrations if necessary) of what it means to be cooperative. Define cooperation operationally by specifying the behaviors that are appropriate and desirable within the groups. Beginning behavior might include "staying near one another," "using quiet voices," and "taking turns." Contrast "working with a friend" and "working alone" by showing pictures of each and asking the children what is happening in the pictures. Consider making a bulletin board with a "Friends help each other" theme. It may require more than one (or even two) sessions for the children to understand what it means to work with a partner to produce a single product. Stress that everybody is to have fun and that they will have lots of fun *and* be successful if they work together and help each other.

6. Assist and monitor. Monitor groups carefully to see where assistance is needed, either related to the activity or to cooperation. Publicly praise children when they share and help one another and prompt collaboration and cooperation as needed. Say, for example, "What does taking turns mean? It means doing it one at a time." Intervene if necessary to clarify instructions and/or answer questions related to the task.

7. Evaluate and provide feedback. Take time at the end of each lesson/activity to provide positive feedback on the qualitative and quantitative aspects of each group's product. It is particularly important to talk about cooperation efforts. Ask for examples of cooperation and comment on how well group members worked together. Ask questions such as "Did you enjoy working together?" "What did you like best about it?" "What was the hardest part?" "How does it feel when you help someone?" "How do you think your group could cooperate better next time?"

The basic premise of the cooperative learning model is that accomplishing some goal together leads children to invest in each other's learning. In turn, this helps children build more realistic and multifaceted views of each other, and encourages acceptance and positive feelings. The cooperative learning model uses the social dynamics of the group as a means of encouraging social interactions and friendships (Johnson & Johnson, 1982).

Affection Activities

Tremblay, Strain, Hendrickson, and Shores (1981) identified physical affection as one of several categories of behavior that are likely to be responded to positively by preschool-age peers. Several researchers have developed and evaluated the effects of group affection activities on social interactions (Brown, Ragland & Fox, 1988; Twardosz, Nordquist, Simon & Botkin, 1983).

Affection activities are incorporated into typical group games and songs such as "Simon Says," "The Farmer in the Dell," and "If You're Happy and You Know It." At the beginning of the activity the children are instructed to exchange some form of physical affection such as a hug, pat on the back, high five, or handshake. Then they participate in the song/game as usual. For example, after "The Farmer in the Dell," they are told "we are going to play/sing this a little differently this time. Instead of singing 'the farmer takes a wife' or 'the wife takes a child' we will sing 'the farmer hugs a wife' or 'the wife hugs a child' and then *do it.*"

Twardosz and others (1983) suggest three reasons why modification of well-known games and songs to include affection activities is effective. There is pairing of peers with pleasurable experiences, desensitization to peer interaction, and/or opportunities to practice affectionate behavior in a nonthreatening situation.

Direct Instruction

Direct instruction is different from adult-mediated interventions in that training is more structured and systematic. Haring and Lovinger (1989) demonstrated the effectiveness of direct instruction with preschool children with severe disabilities (autism). Children with disabilities are taught initiations and play behaviors. Same-age nondisabled peers participate in training, as in the confederate model, but they are not directly responsible for *initiating* social interactions.

These are direct-instruction procedures suggested by Haring and Lovinger (1989):

1. Prepare nondisabled peers. Set aside a time (at least one 20-minute session) to prepare the nondisabled children. Center the discussion on what children have in common (for example, *all* children like to play, *all* children like to have friends) and how they are different (for example, some point when they want something instead of asking). Show slides or pictures of children with disabilities interacting with nondisabled peers. Ask the children to describe the children in the picture and talk about what is occurring. Use a praise statement that includes positive descriptions of the children with disabilities. Give children a chance to ask questions.

2. Arrange training conditions. Identify nondisabled peers who are highly interactive and responsive to adult direction. Two or three peers should be selected to participate during each training session and should be available as playmates at other times of the day. Plan on training sessions varying in length from 3 to 13 minutes, depending on the length of time the children play together after a play episode is prompted.

3. Select training contexts. Select three or four activities as contexts for initiation and play training. Possibilities might include (a) toy cars and garages, (b) trains and tracks, (c) blocks, (d) puzzles, (e) coloring, and so on.

4. Perform task analyses. Perform a task analysis for each play activity. As an example, this is the task analysis for blocks done by Haring and Lovinger (1989):

1. Take a block.
2. Place the block in proximity to peers.
3. Place a second block next to the first.
4. Find a peer.
5. If peer refuses, find another peer. If peer accepts, stack blocks together for at least 10 seconds.
6. Knock over blocks when peers do.

5. Provide training sessions. Prior to each training session coach the two or three nondisabled peers. Tell them to play with the materials that are arranged in the play area and wait for the target child to initiate an interaction. Once an interaction is initiated, the nondisabled peers should respond naturally to the play attempt (for example, "Act as you would with any friend"). Instruct nondisabled peers how to refuse some interactions by saying "No, thanks" or "I don't want that toy," or by handing the toy back without playing with it. (This is to teach the child who is disabled to persist when an initiation is refused.)

6. Begin the play session. Wait for the child who is disabled to approach the toys and initiate an interaction. If this does not occur within 5 seconds, prompt the behavior by pointing to the play area. Then teach each step of the task analysis using a constant 5-second time delay to give the child the opportunity to respond. If there is no response, provide an unintrusive prompt. Praise each independent initiation of a step from the sequence.

After the initiation sequence is completed, allow the children to play together with minimal teacher intervention for 2 to 6 minutes. Then provide another trial of the same activity initiation sequence with another nondisabled peer or another activity initiation sequence with the same peer. A modification of this procedure is possible. The child who is disabled may be taught to first observe the toys being played with by the nondisabled partner and then initiate an interaction by handing the peer an item that is the same as the one being played with.

Summary

This chapter has described procedures for enhancing peer-related social/ communication skills. Peer social and communication skills have significant implications for success in both academic and social domains (Guralnick, 1990b). This makes them especially important instructional targets for young children with disabilities.

Activities

1. Visit a special education preschool class and an integrated preschool class. Compare the quantity and quality of peer social and communication interactions in the two settings. Select a child with special needs and a nondisabled peer in the integrated preschool setting, and a child with special needs in the special education setting. Specifically observe how they (a) gain entry to a peer group, (b) resolve conflicts with other children, (c) acquire a desired toy from another child, and (d) make new friends on the playground. Also observe and list the toys or other materials in these environments that seem most conducive to social interactions.

2. Talk with a special education preschool teacher and a professional trained in regular early childhood. Ask each teacher to describe what methods they use to increase and promote peer interactions.

3. Expand the incidental teaching examples presented in Table 10-1 by adding these examples: morning circle, a field trip to the zoo, a picnic, and recess.

Review Questions

1. Discuss the basic premises underlying extant models to promote and enhance social and communication skills.
2. Describe target behaviors and specific procedures that peer-mediated models use to encourage and facilitate peer interactions.
3. Compare and contrast the three adult-mediated interventions.
4. Describe how the two group models (cooperative learning and affection activities) could be implemented in a childcare setting.

Environmental Arrangements to Promote Independence

1. *Define independent behavior and describe teaching strategies to promote independence.*

2. *Define functional independence and describe adaptations for accomplishing it.*

3. *Describe adaptations for promoting functional independence in gross motor, fine motor, and communication.*

4. *Discuss considerations for promoting independence in the design of instructional programs.*

I ndependent behavior is behavior performed without the assistance of others (Bailey, Harms & Clifford, 1983). It may be *initiated* by the infant/young child to address personal needs, wants, or desires, or it may be in *response* to the requests, suggestions, or demands of others. Independence is the "criterion of ultimate functioning" (Brown, Nietupski & Hamre-Nietupski, 1976). As a standard for skill acquisition, it allows for meaningful participation in integrated social and physical environments.

There are many reasons why infants and young children with disabilities may not develop age-appropriate independent behaviors. Teachers, infant specialists, or family members who provide various forms of assistance to children with disabilities and fail to fade instructional prompts may inadvertantly teach "always wait for assistance." Seligman (1975) labeled the tendency to wait for assistance "learned helplessness." Another name for it is *prompt dependence.* A second reason why many children with disabilities do not develop age-appropriate independent skills is the low expectations of adults. They may not provide opportunities to learn independence (Foster, Schmidt & Sabatino, 1976; Foster, Ysseldyke & Reese, 1974). Third, physical, sensory, or communication disabilities may interfere with independence. Infant specialists and early childhood teachers must systematically plan and implement procedures and adaptations that teach independence.

Teaching Independent Behaviors

Independent behavior goals for infants/young children with disabilities must be chronologically age-appropriate. For example, "independent play" could be a goal for a 1-year-old (for example, for 5 minutes upon awakening from nap; for 5 to 10 minutes when placed on a blanket with some toys, or for 5 to 10 minutes when sitting on the kitchen floor and given pots, pans, and plastic containers). "Independent requesting" might be an appropriate goal for a toddler. The toddler could be taught to point to request desired objects, locations, and people.

A caution is in order: when independence is the goal, avoid stating performance conditions in which the behavior is initiated or prompted by an adult. Such conditions lead to dependence rather than independence. Instead, the conditions specified in the objective should be the natural conditions under which the skill is needed (Baine, 1982). Some examples of objectives stating natural conditions under which children have opportunities to make a choice are "when getting dressed in the morning, Sarah will choose a T-shirt from the drawer," or "When playing with a friend in the free-play area, Tommy will choose a toy from the shelves." These are more natural conditions than "given two T-shirts" or "when presented with three toys."

In addition to teaching independent behavior as generalized skills, independence can be incorporated into objectives in other domains as performance criteria. For example, when teaching a child to hold a spoon, the criterion might state that the child independently picks up the spoon if it drops on the tray. Criterion levels for independent behaviors should correspond to the standards or requirements of independence in the natural environment (Snell & Zirpoli, 1987). Ask: How accurately or how fluently must the skill be performed to be functional (to accomplish the intended result)? Must the child get every bit of food into her mouth to feed herself? Is it acceptable for her to spill a little? How much? Can she feed herself well enough to meet her nutritional needs and satisfy her hunger? How quickly must she feed herself? Once objectives have been formulated, the next step is to plan instruction.

Least Intrusive Procedures

Most of the learning experiences of nondisabled infants/young children occur in the daily routines and interactions of family life. Generally, these experiences are not specific procedures to teach skills and concepts, but they function that way. Family members let young children attempt adaptive skills, such as washing hands, providing assistance only when needed to teach handwashing. When children begin to speak, family members expand and elaborate on what the children say (Slobin, 1968) to teach language. And when parents feed their children, they provide the children with extra spoons to feed themselves; this teaches self-feeding.

The more similar instructional procedures are to the experiences provided for normally developing infants/young children, the less intrusive they are (Sulzer-Azaroff & Mayer, 1977). The more a procedure or teaching strategy differs from typical learning experiences, the more intrusive it is. Also, if an instructional strategy interferes with ordinary routines, it is intrusive.

Least intrusive procedures have two advantages in teaching independent behavior. First, they are easily eliminated through fading. Instructional strategies must be faded, because independence means that behaviors are demonstrated *without* assistance from others. The second advantage is that they are easy for other persons to implement across different settings. Implementing instructional procedures in different places by different persons increases the amount of instruction a child receives and promotes generalization. Most infants/young children with disabilities will require special instruction for independence. Least intrusive instructional procedures, however, are the procedures of choice.

Naturalistic Procedures

Naturalistic instruction, particularly incidental teaching, was described at length in previous chapters. Naturalistic procedures promote independence because the child's behavior is self-initiated rather than adult-prompted. When planning incidental teaching, a specific child behavior is identified as an "occasion for instruction." An occasion for instruction may be child behaviors as subtle as the child's looking at the object, or as obvious as reaching for a desired object, or vocalizing for attention (for example, "Watch me"). For example, Andrea and her father are playing with a mechanical toy. The toy stops moving and Andrea looks at her father expectantly. Instead of reactivating the toy, however, he looks at Andrea and waits. When she vocalizes, he says "Oh, you want to see it go again," and activates the toy. If Andrea had not vocalized, her father could model the desired response (as by saying "ahhh") and wait for her to imitate all or some part of the response before activating the toy, or he might say "Tell me what you want."

Daily Routines and Environmental Modifications

Daily routines provide infants/young children with predictable sequences of events so they learn to anticipate what comes next. They also provide an ideal context for teaching independent behaviors. For example, a young child's morning routine with a babysitter always begins with the child selecting some toys or books, playing with the sitter for a while, putting the toys/books away, and having a snack. After days or weeks of the routine, the sitter might arrive and be greeted by the child with a book for their playtime. When the sitter stops playing and goes to the kitchen to prepare a snack, the child might put the book away, anticipating the snack.

An instructional procedure, such as time delay, may be inserted into a routine to facilitate learning. The first step is to obtain a list of typical daily routines (through observation or interview). A listing of a toddler's early morning routines might include the following:

1. Wake up
2. Diaper change
3. Feeding
4. Play with sibling
5. Diaper change
6. Dressing
7. Sitter arrives/family departs
8. Play with sitter
9. Snack
10. Diaper change
11. Morning nap

Instruction may be planned *within* any of the routines, or in the *transition* from one routine to the next (transitions should also be considered as routines). Using the above list, the babysitter could wait at transitions (*after* putting away toys/books, *after* snack) for the child to indicate what is supposed to occur next (pointing toward the kitchen or vocalizing "ba ba" for "book"). Any behavior indicating anticipation can be reinforced by beginning the activity immediately.

In the natural course of events, relatively few behaviors occur in isolation; they occur sequentially, one right after another (Holvoet, Guess, Mulligan & Brown, 1980). For example, a toddler walks up to his parent, requests a drink of water, says "Thank you," drinks the water, and puts the cup in the sink. This chain of behavior includes a physical skill (walking), two communication skills (requesting a drink and saying "Thank you"), and two adaptive skills (drinking and putting the cup in the sink). In skill sequences, each skill is a stimulus for the next skill and a consequence for the previous one (Ferster, Culbertson & Boren, 1975; Staats & Staats, 1963). Routines are natural skill sequences.

Recall from Chapter 6 that skill sequences may be comprised of two or more new skills or a combination of new skills and previously acquired skills (Guess et al., 1978; Holvoet, Guess, Mulligan & Brown, 1980). Skill sequences are formed by reviewing a child's objectives and listing a few of the objectives in a logical order (for example, "point to desired object," "vocalize," and "grasp"). Skill sequences may also be constructed by inserting objectives into daily activities. For example, "pointing" and "verbal imitation" could be inserted into the activity of reading a book.

Regardless of how many skills are being taught, it is important to focus the child's attention on the natural prompts and consequences inherent in the skill sequence. The instructional objective is the *sequence*, not just the skills. For example, in teaching a young child the sequence of grasping a brush and brushing her hair, nudging her hand toward her hair might be a more effective prompt to teach the relationship between the two skills than a verbal prompt such as "Good, you got the brush, now brush your hair." The nudge is more subtle (less intrusive) than the verbal prompt, it partially assists the child to begin the second skill, and it does not interrupt the natural flow of the performance.

Environmental modifications provide reminders to help children respond independently. Achieved by physically altering the environment, modifications can range from very intrusive to nonintrusive (or minimally intrusive). Consider this example: a toddler is learning to distribute napkins and cups at snacktime. She does fine once started, but always has to be told to begin. Providing the napkins and cups at the child's place setting is a natural, nonintrusive prompt for the child to begin passing out the napkins and cups.

Materials or equipment can be arranged to prompt independent behavior. For example, placing materials in the sequence of task steps (a toothbrush, the toothpaste, and a cup, in that order on the bathroom counter) prompts each step of the skill. It is simple to fade the environmental prompts by gradually moving the materials closer and closer to their original locations. Other examples of materials prompting independent behavior include stools to promote independent handwashing, low shelves to promote putting toys away, and modifications to switches (color codes on a tape recorder "on" button).

Generalization Techniques

As noted in the introduction to this chapter, independent behaviors are behaviors that are performed without the assistance of others. Generalization procedures described in Chapter 6 facilitate independence. However, generalization strategies may not be necessary when naturalistic instruction is used because they are inherent in the procedures (Bailey & Wolery, 1984; Hart & Risley, 1980). When generalization does not occur with naturalistic teaching, there must be specific planning for generalization. Several of the generalization procedures described by Stokes and Baer (1977) are well-suited to promoting independence: use natural maintaining contingencies, train sufficient exemplars, program common stimuli, mediate generalization, and train to generalize.

Use Natural Maintaining Contingencies. Natural contingencies may be paired with instructional ones to assist the infant/young child. For example, when an infant grasps a toy and experiences the natural consequence of playing with it, the sibling who is playing with the infant hugs him and provides social praise. The hug and praise are faded gradually as the child shows increasing enjoyment in the toy play, the natural consequence.

Train Sufficient Exemplars. Sufficient exemplar training promotes independence because it teaches a stimulus class (the group of stimuli that are typically associated with the response). If a preschooler who uses a wheelchair is taught to ask a peer for assistance in maneuvering through a doorway, getting materials that are out of reach, and carrying his lunch tray, then he is likely to generalize and ask a peer for assistance when he needs help to retrieve a dropped toy. The preschooler who has learned to ask for assistance in three different types of situations (maneuvering his wheelchair, accessing materials that are out of reach, carrying a lunchtray), is likely to ask for assistance in a new situation (for example, retrieving a dropped material).

Program Common Stimuli. Encountering material from the instructional setting in natural environments may prompt a new behavior. An example is teaching a toddler to place her hands on her knees to support herself in a sitting position when in a corner chair. Once she learns this she is likely to support herself with her hands on her knees whenever she sits in a corner chair.

Mediate Generalization. Self-prompting, a common mediation technique, facilitates independence across settings/situations because a child can take self-prompting techniques with him wherever he goes. For example, a preschooler is taught to wash his face by learning a song that directs him to first wash his forehead, one cheek, then the other, his nose, mouth, and chin. When the teacher or parent is not present, the preschooler sings the facewashing song and washes his face.

Train to Generalize. Instructional techniques that promote generalization (for example, incidental teaching, training sufficient exemplars, programming common stimuli) are "train to generalize" strategies that facilitate independence. For example, through sufficient exemplar training Lea learns to take turns playing the game of peek-a-boo with Mom and Dad, stacking blocks with a friend at preschool, and using the swing when she and her brother are at the park. This generalized response is in contrast to learning turn-taking with one type of game, person, and situation. When an infant/young child does not generalize a skill, independence is impossible.

Adaptations for Functional Independence

White (1980) uses the term *critical function* to distinguish the purpose of a behavior from the behavior or action used to accomplish it. Crawling, for example, serves the purpose of getting from one place to another—the critical function of mobility. Reaching and vocalizing may serve the purpose of requesting more food—the critical function of expressive communication. A *functionally equivalent response* is a response that accomplishes the same critical function (purpose) as the target behavior, but by another means (Carr & Durand, 1985; Helmstetter & Durand, 1991). For example, *pointing* is a functionally equivalent response for *grasping* if a child who is unable to reach for and grasp a toy is taught to request it by pointing. The responses are functionally equivalent because both result in obtaining a toy. Functionally equivalent responses provide alternative means of accomplishing important outcomes (for example, teaching a child to scoop food *away* from his body to eliminate spillage, whereas most children would scoop *toward* their body) or environmental adaptations (such as placing nonskid rubber under a child's dish to keep it from sliding, whereas most children would be able to scoop from their dish without the nonskid rubber).

When an infant/young child uses functionally equivalent responses to a task without assistance, this is *functional independence.* The following strategies teach an infant or young child to be functionally independent: (a) individualized participation,(b) environmental prompts, (c) peer assistance, and (d) prosthetic devices and adaptive equipment.

Individualized Participation

Recall the discussion of group instruction from Chapter 9. Many activities in childcare, preschool settings, and early intervention programs are conducted in small- or large-group situations. However, there is no requirement that all children in a group activity participate at the same level or in the same way; participation can be individualized (Bailey & McWilliam, 1990; Salisbury & Vincent, 1990). Consider, for example, using a puppet activity to teach turn-taking. The activity requirement to manipulate and speak for the puppets is a problem for Jason, a preschooler with a language delay and hearing impairment. (Jason uses mostly single words and a few two-word phrases.) This activity is individualized by assigning some children to manipulate the puppets (an assignment that Jason could fulfill) and others to speak for the puppets. When a child performs part of a task, it is *partial participation* (Brown et al., 1976). Thus, functional independence can be achieved by allowing children to use partial participation.

Environmental Prompts

Another way to help an infant or young child achieve independence is to modify the environment or materials to provide extra clues or reminders (Bailey et al., 1983). When teaching a child to wash her hands after toileting, a parent places a photograph of washing hands on the wall next to the toilet. A series of pictures illustrating task steps can be posted to remind a child how to perform a complex task (Snell & Browder, 1987; Spellman, DeBriere, Jarboe, Campbell & Harris, 1978). Color coding (for example, cubbies, chairs, coats, rug squares, crayon boxes, toothbrushes) is another example of an environmental prompt that allows children to perform independently.

An environmental prompt may be a permanent prompt (one that remains in place) or a temporary prompt (one that will be faded). There are a number of possible fading techniques to eliminate temporary environmental prompts (Sulzer-Azaroff & Mayer, 1977). The prompt can be made less noticeable by moving it farther and farther away from the situation (a photograph placed next to a child's name may gradually be moved away from the name). Or the prompt can be made smaller and smaller in size, or lighter and lighter in color. An auditory prompt can be made softer and softer. Environmental prompts enable an infant/young child to acquire functional independence immediately or very quickly in a task that would otherwise take a long time to learn.

Learning Centers

Recall from Chapter 8 that activity centers are intended to teach children to play without adult assistance. For example, a childcare center may have a learning center that includes various types of blocks and other building materials, or a preschool may have a learning center that includes science materials that change from week to week (for example, "dinosaur week" might include coloring pictures, plastic dinosaur figures, a dictionary of dinosaurs, and story books of dinosaurs).

Learning centers provide opportunities for functional independence because children decide how they want to participate, interacting with the learning center materials in whatever manner suits their interests and skills. Because play in learning centers tends to be child-directed, children can repeat activities when they need practice on a skill. For example, a learning center might have an activity in which children pick up small items with a tweezer and place them in tall, narrow containers. This activity is appropriate for children at different levels. Children with disabilities may work more slowly and need more practice to feel competent with the task. The ideas on peer assistance presented next may also be used in conjunction with learning centers.

Peer Assistance

In many situations, peer assistance can help a child be independent (Guralnick, 1984; Strain & Odom, 1986). Peer assistance may be provided by a sibling, cousin, or neighborhood friend. Peers can assist in a wide range of tasks, such as helping a child balance while walking, picking up items that a child drops, reminding a child what should be done next, and so on. Although we should be careful not to burden a sibling or young child with too much responsibility for another child, providing assistance in certain situations teaches children to be helpful. It also encourages nurturing, an important attitude for children to develop. At the same time, it helps children with disabilities to be independent of adults.

Prosthetic Devices and Adaptive Equipment

Infants/young children with physical or sensory disabilities sometimes need special equipment to compensate for their disabilities. One type of equipment is a *prosthetic device*. A prosthetic device is a replacement for a missing or nonfunctional limb (Dykes & Venn, 1983). An artificial leg is a prosthesis for a child who is missing a leg. A hand splint with a Velcro® band that secures a crayon in a child's hand is a prosthesis for a child who is otherwise unable to hold a crayon. With the use of a prosthesis, the child may be independent. If a child is not able to achieve functional independence immediately, independence may be possible relatively quickly with practice.

Adaptive equipment refers to specialized furniture and other materials designed to meet the needs of individuals with disabilities, usually physical disabilities (Bergen & Colangelo, 1982). Wheelchairs, walkers, positioning chairs, standers, adjustable tables, modified bicycles, and feeding equipment are examples of adaptive equipment. For many infants/young children with special needs, physical support and therapeutically beneficial physical responses obtained with the use of appropriately selected and fitted adaptive equipment result in functional independence (Bailey et al., 1983).

Functional Independence in Basic Skills

Disabilities or delays associated with basic skills (physical development and communication skills) may interfere with an infant/young child's development of independence in home, community, play, and daycare/preschool activities. When significant basic skill needs are present, objectives may need to be formulated as functionally equivalent responses to provide opportunities for functional independence.

Independence in Gross Motor Skills

Children with physical delays, impairments, or neuromotor disabilities may not progress through the normal sequence of physical development. Motor skill development may be splintered (i.e., skills in the normal sequence may be skipped), skills may be acquired partially, or they may develop in an atypical fashion (Illingworth, 1980). For example, a child with cerebral palsy may not crawl, but may learn to sit and scoot backward. Similarly, a child who cannot crawl may roll in order to move independently to desired locations. When motor delays/impairments preclude or interfere with independence, functionally equivalent gross motor objectives may be targeted. In the previous examples of children scooting and rolling instead of crawling, scooting and rolling could be instructional objectives to accomplish independent mobility.

Several gross motor functions are critical for social and physical independence in home, community, childcare, and preschool environments. These include postural and movement functions. Table 11-1 presents a list of gross motor responses needed by infants/young children and some of the critical functions achieved by the motor responses. Suggestions for responses or adaptations that are functionally equivalent are also indicated (the list is not exhaustive). An ecological inventory may yield other gross motor functions critical to participation in present or future environments or activities.

Therapeutic positioning and handling techniques are included in Table 11-1 among the suggestions for functionally equivalent responses. These techniques are special adaptations that allow infants/young children with gross motor delays or disabilities to achieve postures and movements that might otherwise be impossible or nonfunctional (Copeland & Kimmel, 1989). For example, a preschooler who is unable to sit is not able to see his peers during circle time if he is lying on the floor. If positioned or held in a sitting posture at the same level as his peers, he can be involved in the activity from the same perspective as his peers.

Adaptive equipment considerations are also included in the suggestions for functionally equivalent responses in Table 11-1. Adaptive equipment is used to maintain therapeutically beneficial positions or to facilitate normalized movement for children who have motor delays or disabilities (Copeland & Kimmel, 1989). The preschooler who needs to be at the same level as his peers during a group activity may achieve functional independence by sitting in a special chair. With adequate trunk support provided by the special chair, the child may be able to move his head freely to observe and participate in the activity. Gross motor delays and disabilities do not need to preclude the achievement of functional independence among infants/young children. Identifying functionally equivalent responses,

TABLE 11-1

Gross Motor Responses Important for Independence, Their Critical Functions, and Suggestions for Achieving Functionally Equivalent Responses

Gross Motor Responses	Critical Functions	Functional Equivalents
Head erect in midline	Visual orientation	Head rest on chairback
	Visual attending	Physical assistance/prompts
	Visual scanning	Verbal reminders
	Oral-motor control	Momentary head erect
		Foam neck brace
		Head rest with strap
		Mirror
Floor and chair sitting	Arms free for fine motor tasks	Physical assistance/prompts
	Access to materials and toys	Adaptive chair/wheelchair
	Upright posture for eating & drinking	Side-lying or prone posture for floor sitting
	Upright posture for adaptive, daily living, and other functional skills	Propped sitting against wall or other surface for floor sitting
	Participate at same level as peers	Kneeling (with/without support or adaptive equipment)
		Communication of need for access or participation
Standing	Hands free for fine motor tasks	Physical assistance/prompts
	Access to materials and toys	Adaptive chair/wheelchair
	Upright posture for adaptive, daily living, and other functional skills	Prone stander or tilt table
		Standing table
	Participate at same level as peers	Walker
		Leaning against furniture or wall
		Sitting
		Kneeling
		Use of basket/bag if hands not free for handling materials
		Communication of need for access or participation

(continued)

TABLE 11-1—*(continued)*

Gross Motor Responses	Critical Functions	Functional Equivalents
Walking	Access to areas in the environment	Physical assistance/prompts
		Wheelchair
	Access to materials and toys	Walker or cane(s)
	Arms free for handling materials	Knee-walking
	Upright posture for adaptive, daily living, and other functional skills	Crawling or creeping
		Scooting in sitting posture
	Participate with peers in mobility activities	Rolling
		Scooter board
		Use of basket/bag if hands not free for handling materials
		Communication of need for access or participation

using positioning and handling techniques, and adaptive equipment can promote independent behavior when gross motor delays or disabilities are present.

Independence in Fine Motor Skills

In the sequence of normal physical development, fine motor skills are refined following accomplishment of gross motor skills (Illingworth, 1980). Consistent with the developmental relationship of fine motor to gross motor, delays in gross motor are almost always accompanied by fine motor delays (Illingworth, 1980). Additionally, when neuromotor disabilities are present, fine motor and gross motor skills are usually affected.

Fine motor skills are critical for independence in most daily living, adaptive, play, and school skills. If fine motor performance is delayed or impaired, functionally equivalent responses may provide alternatives for accomplishing independence. Important fine motor responses, the critical functions they accomplish, and ideas for functionally equivalent responses are presented in Table 11-2.

Positioning and handling techniques that facilitate normalized gross motor responding provide an essential foundation for facilitating fine motor behavior. For example, an infant who has not yet learned to reach for objects, or an infant with low muscle tone, is unable to reach for a toy when lying supine. If positioned side-lying, however, the infant's shoulder falls forward in a position that facilitates reaching. Similarly, an infant with cerebral palsy lying on his back will not be able to reach for a toy when his high muscle tone causes stiffness and inhibits movement. Lying on his back also results in an abnormal reflex (for example, asymmetrical tonic neck reflex or the tonic labyrinthine reflex) that interferes with voluntary movement. Positioning this infant in side-lying decreases his abnormally high tone, inhibits the abnormal reflexes, and brings his shoulder forward for reaching.

Trunk, shoulder, and upper arm stability ("postural" and "proximal" stability)

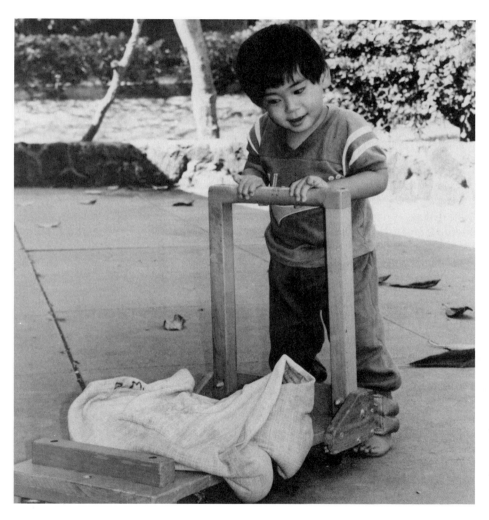

Mobility is a critical function that can often be accomplished with the use of adaptive equipment.

are necessary for fine motor control (Ford, 1975; Illingworth, 1980). Stability does not mean that body parts are completely stationary; it means that postural support is adequate to allow for controlled movement (Bly, 1983). When postural stability is lacking, positioning and handling techniques help to achieve postural stability. A young child leaning against a sink and struggling to maintain standing is not able to perform the fine motor skills necessary for toothbrushing; the child must be in a secure position that frees her arms and hands for movement.

Several of the suggestions in Table 11-2 involve the use of positioning and handling techniques to achieve functionally equivalent responses for fine motor skills. Adaptive equipment suggestions are also included. Most of the adaptive equipment suggestions provide positioning to achieve normalized tone and postural stability in lieu of positioning provided by an adult. For example, an adaptive chair or prone stander provides body alignment and trunk stability. A tray or tabletop at mid-chest level attached to a chair or stander provides stability to the shoulders and upper arms.

Independence in Communication Skills

Communication involves sending and receiving messages, verbally or gesturally (McCormick, 1990d). Infants communicate effectively long before they are able to speak. For example, they spit, purse their lips, gurgle, and smile to indicate their distaste or preference for foods, or they smile and coo to urge a sibling to continue playing. When they begin approximating words, their communication increases in effectiveness and efficiency. Communication becomes a critical tool to meet needs and desires, control environmental events, establish social relationships, participate in family activities, and learn new skills and concepts.

As with gross and fine motor skills, functionally equivalent responses can provide alternatives for accomplishing communication behaviors when communication delays or impairments are present. Table 11-3 lists key communication responses, some of the functions accomplished by the responses, and suggestions for functionally equivalent responses. Most of the functionally equivalent responses are skill approximations or communication responses accomplished through *augmentative communication systems.*

Augmentative communication includes gestural, pictorial, or symbolic communication systems. According to McCormick and Shane (1990), augmentative communication supplements and enhances communication; it is not intended to replace oral communication. Examples of augmentative systems include American Sign Language, common gestures (for example, waving to someone as a request to "come"); pictures, symbols, or words displayed in a book or on a large surface ("communication board"); pictures, symbols, or words displayed on an elevated plexiglass grid for eye-pointing (eye-gaze system); or electronic communication boards, some of which "talk" using voice-synthesizer microcomputer technology.

TABLE 11-2

Fine Motor Responses Important for Independence, Their Critical Functions, and Suggestions for Achieving Functionally Equivalent Responses

Fine Motor Responses	Critical Functions	Functional Equivalents
Reach	Touch and exploration of toys and materials Access to materials and locations	Toys/materials within close proximity Stabilize proximal areas through positioning, handling, or adaptive equipment Position to facilitate normal movement and tone, and inhibit interfering reflexes Attachments (e.g., strings) to eliminate need to reach Prosthetic reaching stick Communication of need/desire to obtain toys or materials that are out of reach
Grasp	Access to materials Hold and carry materials Play with toys Engage in adaptive, daily living, and other functional skills Indicate choice of objects or materials	Stabilize proximal areas through positioning, handling, or adaptive equipment Position to facilitate normal movement and tone, and inhibit interfering reflexes Adaptive feeding utensils Use of shoulder bag or adaptive tray to hold and carry materials Strap materials to hand(s) (e.g., Velcro® strap on pen) Physical modifications to materials to allow for easier grasp (wider handles, etc.) Use of stabilization peg to facilitate controlled grasp and release Secure materials to surface when holding or stabilizing is necessary Physical assistance/prompts Verbal reminders Two-handed grasp when one-handed grasp is typical Use of arms, mouth, or feet to hold materials Communication of need/desire to grasp Use of visual fixation (eye-pointing) to indicate choice

TABLE 11-2—(continued)

Fine Motor Responses	Critical Functions	Functional Equivalents
Manipulation or transfer	Explore materials Play with toys Engage in adaptive, daily living, and other functional skills	Stabilize proximal areas through positioning, handling, and adaptive equipment Position to facilitate normal movement and tone, and to inhibit interfering reflexes Physical modifications to materials to allow for easier manipulation or transfer Physical assistance/prompts Verbal cues Two-handed manipulation when one-handed manipulation is typical Use of stabilization peg to facilitate controlled manipulation Use of arms, mouth, or feet to manipulate or transfer materials Communication of need/desire to manipulate or transfer
Release	Terminate use of materials Explore materials Play with toys Engage in adaptive, daily living, and other functional skills	Stabilize proximal areas through positioning, handling, or adaptive equipment Position to facilitate normal movement and tone, and to inhibit interfering reflexes Physical assistance/prompts Verbal reminders Use of stabilization peg to facilitate controlled grasp and release Communication of need/desire to release
Point	Indicate focus of interest Clarify object of communication Indicate desired object or event	Stabilize proximal areas through positioning, handling, and adaptive equipment Position to facilitate normal movement and tone, and to inhibit interfering reflexes Use whole hand/fist to indicate/clarify Eye-point Use augmentative communication to indicate/clarify (using hand/fist, eye-pointing, hand or head switch, etc.) Indicate "yes" when focus of interest/desired object is named

Anything that augments speech or accomplishes communication functions may be considered augmentative communication. Very often the best solution is to combine systems (McCormick & Shane, 1990). For example, a child hits a bell attached to her wheelchair to call for attention. When someone responds, she points to the picture for "drink" on her communication board, and nods yes when asked

---

TABLE 11-3

Communication Responses Important for Independence, Their Critical Functions, and Suggestions for Achieving Functionally Equivalent Responses

Communication Responses	Critical Functions	Functional Equivalents
Cry or smile	Request/maintain attention of others	Visual or gestural signal for attention, greeting, or to indicate feelings
	Greet others	Eye contact to maintain attention of others
	Express feelings and emotions	Touch or hug to express emotion
	Maintain pleasant social interactions	Activate a switch attached to a light or call device
	Terminate/rectify uncomfortable or unpleasant situations	
Point or gesture	Request/maintain attention of others	Whole hand/fist used to indicate/clarify
		Eye-point
	Indicate focus of interest	Augmentative communication to indicate/clarify (using hand/fist, eye-pointing, hand or head switch, etc.)
	Clarify communication	
	Indicate desired object or event	
	Engage in social and conversational interactions	Indication of "yes" with head nod when focus of interest/desired object or event is named
	Demonstrate understanding of communication	
Babble	"Experiment" or practice elements of speech, language, and oral-motor skills	Visual or gestural signal for attention or to indicate feelings
	Request/maintain attention of others	Eye contact to maintain attention of others
	Greet others	Gestural/physical turn-taking during interactional play
	Engage in social and conversational interactions	Activate a switch attached to a light or call device

(continued)

TABLE 11-3—*(continued)*

Communication Responses	Critical Functions	Functional Equivalents
Imitate words, phrases, and sentences	"Experiment" or practice elements of speech, language, and oral-motor skills	Approximations of words, phrases, and/or sentences
	Build expressive and receptive language skills	Imitation of gestures, symbols and/or signs (when gestures, symbols, or signs are paired with models)
	Request/maintain attention of others	Touch or hug to express emotion
	Engage in social and conversational interactions	Activate a switch to indicate words, drawings, pictures, or symbols on a communication board
Talk with single words, phrases, or sentences	Practice elements of speech, language, and oral-motor skills	Approximations of words, phrases, or sentences
	Request/maintain attention of others	Use of gestures, symbols, and/or signs
	Send specific messages	Visual or gestural signal to gain attention or indicate feelings
	Fulfill needs and desires	Eye contact to maintain attention of others
	Express feelings and emotions	
	Terminate/rectify uncomfortable or unpleasant situations	"Yes" signaled with head nod when focus of interest/desired object or event is named
	Engage in social and conversational interactions	Activate a switch to indicate words, drawings, pictures, or symbols on a communication board
	Demonstrate understanding of communication	

if she wants a drink of juice. Infants/young children with communication delays or disabilities should be provided with functionally equivalent skills that accomplish independence in communication.

 Designing Instructional Programs to Promote Independence

This chapter has described environmental arrangements that promote independence among infants and young children with special needs. The next step is to apply these recommendations to plan instruction. Figure 11-1 provides a form that an infant specialist or teacher might use for instruction. This final section of the chapter describes where and how to incorporate environmental arrangements that promote independence into each component of the instructional plan. Refer to the program plan examples in Figures 11-2 and 11-3 as you read through this section.

Section I: Objective

This is a short-term objective that corresponds to a goal on an IFSP or IEP. Short-term objectives usually describe behaviors that can be accomplished within 3 or 4 months (Sailor & Guess, 1983). As discussed in Chapter 5, objectives are stated in behavioral terms and specify the conditions, response, and criterion. In developing objectives that promote independence, remember the following pointers:

1. The performance conditions of the objective should be stated as *independent performance conditions*. If adult reminders or prompts do not typically precede the behavior, they should not be included in the conditions of the objective.

2. Whenever possible, the response specified in the objective should be stated as a *general case response*.

3. If the desired response is too difficult for the child to perform independently, consider targeting a *functionally equivalent response* or a response that requires *partial participation*.

4. State the criterion for the objective at a level that allows or results in independent performance. It may be necessary to observe others performing the skill to determine the accuracy, fluency, or whatever, that represents the *independent performance criterion*.

Section II: Instructional Context

The instructional context section includes descriptions of environmental variables that support and facilitate the development of independent behaviors. As discussed throughout this chapter, the decisions of where, when, and under what conditions instruction occurs play a major role in promoting independence. The following situational variables should be considered in formulating the instructional context of the instructional plan:

1. Conduct instruction in *natural settings* where the skill would typically occur, and preferably in *more than one natural setting*. This will facilitate generalization and independent performance.

	Date begun: _____
Infant/Child: _____	Date completed: _____
Objective: _____	Interventionist: _____
Conditions: _____	
Response: _____	
Criterion: _____	

Intervention Context	*Prompting/Facilitation Techniques*	*Consequences*
Setting(s):	*Positioning and Handling; Special Equipment/Materials:*	*Reinforcement:*
Routine(s)/Activity(ies):		
	Environmental Modifications:	*Corrections:*
Skill Sequence(s):		
	Prompting/Facilitation:	
Occasions for Incidental Intervention:		

Figure 11-1 Instructional plan

	Date begun:	4/1/92

Infant/Child: **Sarah B.**

Date completed: _____

Objective: **Turn-taking**

Interventionist: **Casey Kealoha**

Conditions: **When an adult or child begins a game and pauses, or passes the material/toy to Sarah**

Response: **Sarah will take a turn by playing for a few moments, and pausing or passing the material/toy back to the adult or child.**

Criterion: **Plays for 10-60 seconds; pauses or passes material/toy 3 of 4 times.**

Intervention Context	*Prompting/Facilitation Techniques*	*Consequences*
Setting(s): ◆ In the morning at the sitter's ◆ After school with her brother ◆ After dinner with Mom, Dad or Grandpa *Routine(s)/Activity(ies):* ◆ Clapping games, rocking or "dancing" to music, playing with toys that shake	*Positioning and Handling; Special Equipment/Materials:* ◆ Supported sitting in high chair, propped against couch or in corner of couch, or on someone's lap; a table top (lap tray or high chair tray) will help her to manipulate and shake toys	*Reinforcement:* ◆ Verbally praise Sarah, laugh and show lots of excitement as she takes her turn ◆ Immediately take a turn when Sarah stops (play for about 30 seconds)
	Environmental Modifications: n/a	
Skill Sequence(s): 1. Vocalizes to request attention 2. Turn-taking 3. Requests "more" Occasions for Incidental Intervention: n/a	*Prompting/Facilitation:* ◆ Start a turn-taking game and play for about 30 seconds ◆ Then implement time delay: Physically assist Sarah to take her turn 2 times For all additional turns, wait 4 seconds If Sarah takes her turn within the 4-second delay, reinforce If Sarah does not take her turn within 4 seconds, implement correction 1.	*Corrections:* 1. (If Sarah waits beyond the 4-second delay) Physically assist Sarah to take her turn 2. (If Sarah starts doing something else) Start the turn-taking game again. If she doesn't attend and does something else again, stop the intervention and try again later

Figure 11-2 Instructional plan

	Date begun:	2/25/92

Infant/Child: Joseph K.

Objective: Says "Please"

Interventionist: Janet Yim

Conditions: When Joseph wants something that is out of reach

Response: He will say "Please"

Criterion: So that it is clearly audible, 5 times within 3 days

Intervention Context	Prompting/Facilitation Techniques	Consequences
Setting(s): ♦ At home, at preschool, and in stores or restaurants	*Positioning and Handling; Special Equipment/Materials:* n/a	*Reinforcement:* ♦ Tell Joseph that he can see/have what he asks for when he says "Please." Give him the item immediately; assist him in exploring or playing with the item if he does not interact with it
Routine(s)/Activity(ies): ♦ During play times at home or preschool, during mealtimes, and while shopping	*Environmental Modifications:* ♦ Place several desired items or toys out of reach, but within sight (leave a cup at the edge of the counter; toys on top shelf of toy shelf, and books on top of end table)	
Skill Sequence(s): n/a		*Corrections:* 1. Say "Please," wait 5 seconds; reinforce if correct 2. If still incorrect or no response, say "Please" and give Joseph the item; do not praise him or interact further
Occasions for Incidental Intervention: ♦ Whenever Joseph focuses on an item for 5 seconds, or whenever Joseph reaches for an item that is beyond his reach	*Prompting/Facilitation:* ♦ Approach Joseph, make eye contact, and say, "What do you say, Joseph?" (wait 5 seconds for a response). If he says "Please," reinforce; if not, proceed to the correction	

Figure 11-3 Instructional plan

2. Use *naturally occurring routines and activities* as instructional situations, rather than setting aside a particular time for instruction. Teaching during naturally occurring routines and activities will assist the infant/young child to recognize when the skill is needed and what purpose it serves.

3. Construct *skill sequences* and conduct instruction with more than one skill at a time. Skill sequences teach relationships between behaviors.

4. Identify infant/child responses that signal the *occasion for instruction* if using incidental teaching procedures. Using child-determined occasions for instruction is responsive to the interests of the infant/young child and provides a meaningful and motivating situation for teaching.

Section III: Prompting and Facilitation Techniques

A wide array of effective prompting and facilitation techniques have been demonstrated to assist infants/young children in acquiring or improving skills. Some techniques, however, are more effective than others in accomplishing independent performance of skills. The following considerations should be addressed in instructional plans designed to promote independence:

1. Use *least intrusive procedures,* that is, procedures that do not interfere any more than necessary with the naturally occurring events or interactions. The more instruction interferes with the natural situation, the less likely the infant/young child is to generalize the response.

2. Select *naturalistic teaching procedures* such as incidental teaching and time delay. These procedures help infants/young children respond independently to the natural prompts provided by the environment.

3. Include *generalization techniques,* such as sufficient exemplars, common stimuli, or mediational strategies among the prompting/facilitation techniques. In addition to naturalistic teaching procedures, instructional plans should include multiple approaches to facilitate generalization. Independence is greatly enhanced when responses are generalized.

4. If independent performance of the response seems too difficult for the infant/young child (the skill is complex, or the skill includes physical responses beyond the child's present abilities), develop *environmental prompts or modifications* to make independence a realistic goal. The environmental prompts or modifications may be "permanent" additions to the environment, or they may be faded as part of the instructional plan.

5. Use *prosthetic devices, special equipment, or therapeutic positioning and handling techniques* to facilitate independent responding when the infant/young child has physical or sensory disabilities. Sometimes these accommodations alone will result in independent responding.

6. Consider the use of *peer assistance* to help the infant/young child with

special needs respond independent of adult assistance. Peer assistance is well-suited to group activities and free-play situations.

Section IV: Reinforcement and Corrections

After the prompting and facilitation techniques are implemented, the infant/young child is given an opportunity to respond. If the response is the desired one, a reinforcing consequence is provided. If the response is not correct, or if the infant/young child does not respond, the instructional plan specifies further instruction that assists the infant/young child to learn the response. There are two specific recommendations for promoting independence that apply to this section of the instructional plan:

1. Develop *minimally intrusive* corrections, that is, use corrections that interfere as little as possible. As in the recommendations for prompting and facilitation techniques, the less the instruction interferes with the situation, the more likely it is that the infant/young child will generalize and perform the skill independently.

2. Use *naturally occurring reinforcers and corrections* whenever possible. If infants/young children learn to recognize and use natural contingencies, they will rely less on instructional support and adult assistance. Pairing artificial consequences with the natural ones, or exaggerating the natural ones, are simple ways to highlight natural consequences.

These recommendations summarize teaching strategies to consider in formulating an individualized instructional plan to promote independence. Figures 11-2 and 11-3 are examples of instructional plans illustrating these recommendations. As emphasized in the strategies described throughout this chapter, independence is not a goal to *hope* for—it is a goal to actively address through intervention strategies that promote independence effectively.

 Summary

This chapter discusses independent skills for meaningful participation in natural settings. Instructional procedures should be least intrusive, naturalistic, incorporated into daily routines, and designed to facilitate generalization. When a young child's age or disability limits the extent to which independence can be achieved, goals for functional independence need to be developed. Functional independence is accomplished by teaching the child equivalent responses or by providing adaptive strategies.

Activities

1. Observe a nondisabled 2-year-old at home. List at least ten skills that the child is able to do independently. Fill in a chart (like the one below) identifying adaptations that would allow a child with a disability to perform the same skills independently.

Independent skills of a 2-year-old	Adaptations if the child has . . .		
	a physical disability	a visual disability	a hearing disability

2. Using the instructional plan form presented in the chapter (Figure 11-1), write two instructional plans to teach independent behaviors. In one plan, use a naturalistic teaching procedure; in the other plan, use an adaptation. If you are presently in contact with infants and young children with disabilities, the plans should be designed for a specific infant or young child.

3. Observe a special education preschool class and identify independent behaviors performed in response to consistent routines. Based on your observations, suggest other routines that could be implemented consistently in the classroom you are observing to promote independence.

Review Questions

1. Describe how the following procedures promote independence: (a) least intrusive procedures, (b) naturalistic procedures, (c) daily routines and environmental modifications, and (d) generalization techniques.
2. Define *functional independence.*
3. Describe each of the following adaptations for promoting independence,

and provide an example of each type that is appropriate for a 2-year-old and a 5-year-old.

1. Individualized participation
2. Environmental prompts
3. Learning centers
4. Peer assistance
5. Prosthetic devices and adaptive equipment

4. Describe adaptations to promote independence in physical (gross and fine motor) and communication skills.
5. Describe strategies for promoting independence in the four major sections of instructional plans (objective, intervention context, prompting/facilitation techniques, reinforcement and corrections).

Program Organization and Management

Objectives

1. *Describe programmatic variables associated with early intervention service delivery.*

2. *Discuss program management concerns in early intervention.*

*T*he various program models that characterize early intervention for infants and young children with disabilities were described in Chapter 1 (home-based, center-based, integrated preschool, and so on). Although the models differ in where, how, and when early intervention services are provided, all early intervention services (a) offer service delivery options to meet individual child and family needs, (b) demonstrate a commitment to integration, and (c) provide normalized experiences. Management involves planning, implementing, and monitoring the programmatic variables of service delivery models. That service delivery models and programmatic variables can be combined in various ways to create options for infants, young children, and their families.

Programmatic Variables

Programmatic variables in early intervention include (a) setting, (b) schedule, (c) curriculum, and (d) staffing pattern. For example, a center-based service delivery model is an early intervention program that is conducted at a specialized location rather than in an infant's home. The center-based model may have 1-hour per week intervention sessions (schedule); a Montessori program (curriculum); and a one-to-one child-staff arrangement. The alternatives associated with each of these variables create a broad range of service delivery models.

Providing Options

Whatever the primary service delivery model for an early intervention program, alternatives must be available to meet individual child/family characteristics and needs. For infants and toddlers, the guidelines for the Individualized Family Services Plan (IFSP) specify that families must have service options. For 3- to 5-year olds, the least restrictive environment (LRE) requirement of IDEA also requires availability of service delivery options. McLean and Hanline (1990) stress that early intervention service delivery alternatives must truly be options, and not be limited to a restricted set of alternatives based on traditional concepts of the LRE. Providing only the alternatives of a self-contained preschool special education class or a Head Start classroom, and no other alternatives, does not truly provide options for preschoolers. Neither option may be appropriate. A 3-year-old may need to spend a portion of her day socializing with nondisabled peers, and neither the special education preschool classroom nor the Head Start classroom permits this (the special education classroom does not include nondisabled peers, and the Head Start program does not serve 3-year-olds). Also, combinations of options should be an alternative, such as a center-based program *and* community childcare, or childcare *plus* consultation with parents.

While some alternatives associated with a particular programmatic variable may be considered theoretically, philosophically, or empirically "superior", most alternatives cannot be judged on their merit alone. There must be a match between the program variable and child/family characteristics and needs. For example, a home-based infant program (delivery of services in the infant's home) may be more personalized, individualized, and sensitive to family culture, style, and resources, than a center-based model. However, it does not provide opportunities for parents or caregivers to meet other parents or caregivers. A center-based program that affords opportunities to meet other families and develop a community support system may be a better match for some families. The nature of services should only be determined *after* child and family goals have been established.

Integration Opportunities

There is a professional and legal preference for settings that serve primarily children who are not disabled. This preference is based on the belief that infants and young children with disabilities need specialized instruction, *not* specialized settings (Bricker, Bruder & Bailey, 1982; Carta, Schwartz, Atwater & McConnell, 1991; McLean & Hanline, 1990; Taylor, 1988). It would be useful to reconceptualize the LRE as a commitment to integration, and replace the LRE continuum with a focus on creating options for integration (McLean & Hanline, 1990; Taylor, 1988). Furthermore, integration options beyond the scope of intervention/education settings should be included in developing alternatives: child and family activities available in the community (babysitting, childcare, parenting classes, play groups) should be available to *all* families, including those with children who have disabilities (Hanline & Hanson, 1989).

Normalized Experiences

In addition to a commitment to providing service delivery options and integration opportunities, early intervention should provide services that are as "normalized" as possible even in a segregated setting (Bailey & McWilliam, 1990). Bailey and McWilliam note that the normalization principle (Nirje, 1985; Wolfensberger, 1972) encompasses variables in addition to the physical setting: it requires settings, freedom within settings, and that the instruction, and social interaction opportunities available to nondisabled infants/young children be made available to those with disabilities.

Studies comparing early childhood programs that serve infants and young children with disabilities to programs that serve nondisabled children indicate that the programs vary on factors such as physical arrangement, schedule of activities, types of activities, staff-to-child ratio, adult and child interactions, children's play and interactions, and so on (Bailey, Clifford & Harms, 1982; Beckman & Kohl, 1984; Esposito & Koorland, 1989; Guralnick & Groom, 1987). Participating in atypical environments will not afford infants and young children with disabilities opportunities to learn skills associated with natural environments or to share the experiences available to nondisabled infants/young children. Normalized experiences increase the likelihood of learning and generalizing new skills (Bailey & McWilliam, 1990).

Program Management

A wide range of service delivery options for infants, toddlers, preschoolers, and 5-year-olds with disabilities was described in Chapter 1. The options range from models of services used primarily by infants and young children who are not disabled, to segregated and specialized service delivery models that only serve children with disabilities. Early intervention service delivery models are expanding to include a greater variety of models and combinations of models, and further increasing options to include models that have traditionally served only nondisabled infants and young children. The management of each service delivery component (setting and materials, staffing, scheduling, curriculum, and family support and participation) must balance the goals of providing environments that are nonrestrictive, normalized, safe, and healthy, with meeting the special needs of infants and young children with disabilities. In this section, program management goals (nonrestrictiveness, normalization, safety, and health) are addressed for each of the major components of service delivery models.

Settings and Materials

As discussed in Chapter 8, the physical environment of early intervention includes the setting and materials. The setting is the service delivery model's location and its physical space. Materials include furniture, therapeutic equipment, toys, and other instructional supplies or items. A setting and materials that are attractive, engaging, and safe can create an enjoyable environment.

The first program management goal, nonrestrictiveness, is significantly affected by the service delivery model's setting and materials. The setting and materials can prevent or support the inclusion of infants and young children in the routines and activities of an early intervention service delivery model. If a child cannot reach materials because of her physical disabilities, for example, the location of materials creates a restrictive environment.

Service delivery models that serve primarily nondisabled infants/young children are the most natural early intervention environments. They may be restrictive, however, if environmental modifications or arrangements necessary to the inclusion of a child with disabilities are not implemented. The value of placement in a natural environment is lost if the environment is unduly restrictive. Alternatively, although segregated settings are not the most natural instructional settings, they can be designed to be minimally restrictive and thus worthwhile instructional environments (materials can be stored at "child-level" to allow for independence in selecting and returning materials).

Four factors that affect restrictiveness should be considered in the design/ selection and evaluation of a setting and materials: (a) availability (Does the program have adequate space and materials to conduct appropriate programs and meet the needs of infants/young children?); (b) accessibility (Do all children have an equal opportunity to obtain materials and engage in activities regardless of where the materials are located or the activities are conducted?); (c) organization (Are activity boundaries clearly indicated? Are there designated locations for the storage/display of materials?); and (d) scheduling and use (Are environmental areas and materials designed or selected because they are important to the program and, if so, are there opportunities to use them in the program?) (Bailey & McWilliam, 1990).

When applied to the service delivery model's setting and materials, the program management goal of normalization involves the extent to which the physical environment appears and functions like the environments serving nondisabled age peers. Program location is one aspect of the setting that influences normalization. Services that share the same space or are located in close proximity to natural service delivery models, are potentially more normalized than specialized services that are physically isolated. Research has shown that settings and materials of early intervention environments for infants/young children with disabilities differ significantly from those serving primarily nondisabled infants/young children (Bailey et al., 1982). When nondisabled infants/young children do not participate in a program, or when program staff are not in frequent contact with natural settings, the environment is usually designed around therapy and instructional needs (a clinical environment), with very little consideration for arrangements that focus on children's play, activity preferences, and independence (a child-centered environment).

A concerted effort should be made to locate services for infants/young children within or near programs serving same-age peers to increase the likelihood that infants/young children receive services in normalized environments. When the service delivery model is a segregated program, the setting and materials should be as similar as possible to the setting and materials for nondisabled age peers. Characteristics of settings and materials in natural early intervention environments that are frequently absent from segregated specialized settings include activity centers (for example, water and sand play, house play, dramatic play, art/paint), book area, gross-motor area, outdoor playground, rest area, group play materials (such as large blocks), age-appropriate toys, and displays of children's work.

The third program management goal is to ensure the safety and health of the infants/young children in the program. Most of the safety and health concerns related to the setting and materials are concerns for all young children. However, some of the concerns are of particular importance for young children with disabilities. They may be more susceptible to infections (due to a heart condition, poor immune system, or chronic illness) or more apt to fall (due to poor motor

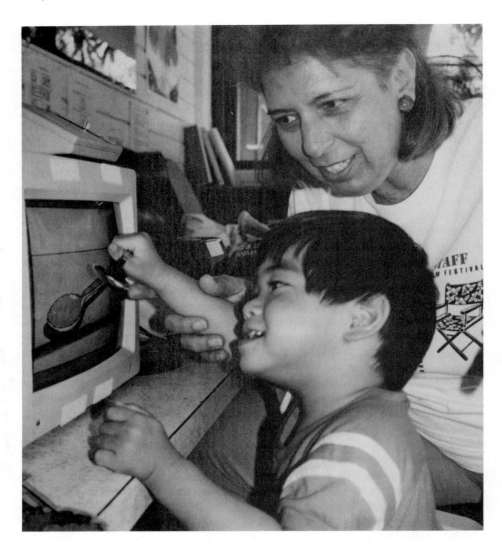

Activity centers are commonly found in early childhood programs.

coordination). Hanson and Lynch (1989, p. 195) provide suggestions for "childproofing" early intervention environments:

1. Modify or pad sharp edges on furniture and materials.
2. Supervise play involving materials with small parts.
3. Be certain that paint on walls, toys, and so on, is lead free.
4. Cover electrical outlets with commercially available protectors.

5. Keep medical and cleaning supplies in locked cabinets.
6. Cover hot water faucet outlets with protectors.
7. Supervise play at water tables and when using gross motor play equipment.
8. Use floor play (on clean, carpeted floors) for most activities. Use sturdy standing and climbing equipment under close supervision.

In addition to childproofing the environment, good hygiene practices will prevent the spread of infectious diseases. Infectious diseases of particular concern among infants and young children with special needs include cytomegalovirus (CMV), hepatitis B, herpes, and AIDS (Lehr & Noonan, 1989). CMV is a virus characterized by mild flu-like symptoms and frequently goes unnoticed. The virus is shed in body fluids, and is commonly transmitted through coughing and sneezing (Pass & Kinney, 1985). Although CMV is often undetected in children and adults, if a woman contracts CMV in her first trimester of pregnancy, the virus can have devastating effects on her unborn child (spontaneous abortion, mental retardation, central nervous system damage, and hearing loss). Children with CMV pose a risk in early childhood settings because the virus may be spread directly, or through others, to a pregnant woman (early intervention staff member, parent).

Hepatitis B, a disease that affects the liver, is a major public health problem affecting over 200,000 Americans each year (Immunization Practices Advisory Committee, 1985). Hepatitis B is incurable and can be contagious even when symptoms are not present. It is transmitted through blood and other body fluids and can live on environmental surfaces, such as changing tables, toys, and utensils.

Herpes is another incurable infectious disease of concern to early intervention professionals (American Academy of Pediatrics, 1982). Herpes simplex virus Type 1 (HSV-1, also known as oral herpes) generally affects the individual above the waist. It is characterized by sores in the oral areas and eye infections. The brain and skin may also be affected. The virus is usually transmitted through saliva or respiratory droplets. Herpes simplex virus Type 2 (HSV-2, also known as genital herpes) usually affects the individual in the area of the genitals. Symptoms associated with HSV-2 include sores and or swelling in the genital area, rectal pain, frequent urination, and fever. HSV-2 is usually transmitted through skin contact (touching the infected area). Although there is no cure for HSV-1 and HSV-2, there are medications that minimize or alleviate the symptoms.

AIDS, the acronym for Acquired Immune Deficiency Syndrome, is a disease caused by the human immunodeficiency virus (HIV), and is characterized by a breakdown of the body's natural immunity system. Not all individuals who test positive for HIV have AIDS (or develop AIDS). An individual with AIDS cannot ward off diseases and infections, and therefore is vulnerable to contracting life-threatening illnesses.

AIDS is transmitted through the mixing of blood or body fluids (through sexual contact, breast milk, amniotic fluids, or the introduction of infected blood into the bloodstream through blood transfusions or contaminated hypodermic needles). Children are most at risk for contracting AIDS if their mother is infected: Most children with AIDS have contracted the virus from their infected mothers through the amniotic fluid or the mother's blood system prenatally, or in the birth canal at the time of delivery. A few children have become infected after birth, possibly from the mother's breast milk.

AIDS is a frightening disease because there is no known cure. Although the prevalence of AIDS is increasing, it is not easily spread among children or from children to adults. At the end of March 1992 there were 3692 children under the age of 13 with AIDS in the United States (U.S. Department of Health and Human Services, Public Health Services, Center for Disease Control, April, 1992). Teachers and infant specialists should not be afraid to hold and touch children with AIDS in normal play and interactions—there has not been a single instance of AIDS transmission in an early childhood or school setting (even when children have been bitten), nor among family members in the absence of sexual contact (Hawaii State Department of Health, 1986).

The spread of infectious diseases can be prevented through good hygiene practices. Some bacteria and viruses can live on the surfaces of equipment and materials (for example, hepatitis B); many are passed through body fluids such as saliva and blood (such as CMV, AIDS). Materials and equipment should be cleaned daily with a disinfectant wash. This is particularly important for positioning equipment, floor mats, changing tables, toilet chairs and seats, food preparation surfaces, and play materials. Staff should wash their hands after assisting a child who needs special positioning or handling techniques before they touch other children. If children or staff have any cuts or open sores, the cuts or sores should be covered with bandages to protect themselves and the children/adults with whom they have physical contact. The use of disposable gloves when changing diapers or washing children following toileting or toileting accidents should be a program policy that is strictly enforced. Soiled diapers should be disposed of in lined and covered receptacles. Local departments of health can provide information on obtaining disinfectants for handwashing and cleaning materials for equipment.

Environmental safety and health concerns also require that early intervention programs meet the requirements of fire safety codes (such as having regularly maintained and tested fire alarms, more than one accessible exit, unobstructed pathways to exits, and pre-planned emergency exit routes).

Staffing

The staffing component of program management involves adult:child ratios and the scheduling and utilization of personnel, including family members, professionals, paraprofessionals, and volunteers. The concern that staffing arrangements be nonrestrictive and normalized suggests that personnel be utilized in a manner similar to settings serving primarily nondisabled infants/young children. In a home-based program, it may be disruptive to the family's routines for more than one interventionist to visit. There is a greater chance that a single interventionist will be successful in encouraging the family to maintain their typical activities. If the interventionist arrives during an infant's feeding, for example, the interventionist observes the meal, talks to the parents about feeding or related concerns, comments on gains that the infant or family are demonstrating, and guides the family in trying out new strategies to address specific feeding concerns. In some situations, the interventionist participates in (rather than observes) the family's activity, and is less intrusive by virtue of fitting into the environment. In the feeding example, if a big sister were feeding the infant, and the parents were sitting at the kitchen table having coffee, the interventionist could join the parents and discuss feeding accomplishments and concerns over coffee.

In home-based service delivery models, the staff member who visits the family on a regular basis is called the *primary interventionist.* Sometimes primary interventionists are assigned to families by matching the most significant disability or intervention need of the child to staff members' disciplines (for example, a speech therapist would be primary interventionist for a young child with a cleft palate and hearing impairment). Other programs assign infants/young children randomly or by geographic area; and still other programs assign only paraprofessionals as primary interventionists (with professionals as consultants).

Regardless of how primary interventionists are matched to the infants and young children, using primary interventionists in the home-based model requires role release and joint staff development, activities characteristic of transdisciplinary teaming. As described in Chapter 2, role release and joint staff development ..."require that"... professionals in various disciplines be willing to work across traditional boundaries and train one another. As a result of role release and joint staff development, all members of the transdisciplinary team learn to approach the needs of infants/young children from a holistic perspective. Implementing a home-based intervention program in which staff members practice role release and joint staff development necessitates flexible staff schedules.

The primary interventionist may also fill the role of service coordinator. (This also addresses the issue of limiting the numbers of staff involved with a family so that intervention is nonintrusive and normalized). As discussed in Chapter 2, however, there are some advantages to separating the role of interventionist from service coordinator (for example, the family might be more apt to express dissatisfaction with an early intervention service if the service coordinator is not the same person as their primary interventionist). Programs serving 0- to 3-year-olds must decide whether to combine or separate the roles of primary interventionist and service coordinator by considering the pros and cons of each relative to the number and type of personnel in their program, as well as the needs of the families they serve.

In a program serving primarily nondisabled infants/young children, staff:child ratios may need to be reduced if a child with special needs requires support that places extra demands on staff time. A child may need monitoring because of a behavioral problem, or an infant with special feeding needs may take longer to eat or need more frequent feedings. When additional staff are required to meet the needs of a particular infant/young child, the extra assistance should be used in a manner that is nonintrusive and normalized. Assigning one adult to work exclusively with one infant or child should be avoided. Instead, if a preschooler needs assistance to participate in an activity (such as blockbuilding with three other children), a volunteer may be assigned to monitor and play with *all* the children involved in the activity. The volunteer reinforces all children for playing appropriately, assists the child with disabilities to watch and imitate her more competent peers, and supports cooperation and helping among the children by reinforcement, modeling, and guidance (for example, "Sean, look how Marie is trying to lift that big block. Can you help her? . . . Wow, look at the big block that Sean and Marie put on top of the pile!"). When staff assist a child with special needs by assisting a group of children, the children learn to play, work, and socialize together. The child with disabilities learns to participate independently and is not stigmatized by being singled out with continual adult attention.

A second staffing issue associated with nonrestrictiveness and normalization is the use of specialized staff (for example, early interventionists, special education consultants, therapists). When specialized staff are needed, scheduling and instructional arrangements should not interfere with the typical schedule and activities of the setting. Specialists should incorporate their instruction into the natural activities (Vandercook & York, 1990). This is integrated therapy model described earlier in this chapter (in contrast to "pull-out" models in which children are removed from their classroom to receive a related service). In addition to being nonintrusive and normalizing, the integrated therapy approach ensures that specialized interventions are designed to be practical and immediately useful in natural settings.

Early interventionists can also provide support to infants/young children with special needs in natural early childhood settings through consultation and collaboration with program staff. The specialists work as team members with the regular program staff and assist problem solving and designing instructional strategies. For example, if a speech therapist is consulting with a Head Start teacher who is teaching a hearing-impaired student, the therapist may meet with the teacher after school hours to train him in sign language and methods to encourage the spontaneous use of signs.

In segregated early childhood settings, concerns for nonintrusiveness and normalization suggest that staffing patterns should be as similar as possible to those of early childhood settings serving primarily nondisabled children. The differences in staffing between the two types of programs are that segregated programs will often have more highly trained professionals and a smaller staff: child ratio than the early childhood program serving primarily nondisabled children. Segregated programs should see that young children with disabilities do not come to rely on 1:1 or small-group arrangements. Providing young children with frequent experiences in large groups may require team-teaching arrangements (perhaps with a nearby program serving nondisabled children). Specialists serving infants/young children in segregated settings should follow the integrated therapy model to minimize intrusiveness and promote normalization.

There are four safety and health concerns related to the program management component of staffing. First, all program staff should have detailed job descriptions and schedules that clearly identify their responsibilities. Detailed job descriptions provide a mechanism for establishing accountability and ensuring that *someone* has responsibility for the various tasks related to the safety and health of the children. Staff members, for example, should have assignments for monitoring specific children, activities and/or physical areas of the program, assisting children during fire drills, implementing interventions that involve specialized training, and maintaining a safe and healthy physical environment.

The second safety and health concern is that staff members must be trained to implement specialized interventions and instructional techniques. This is a particularly serious matter in therapeutic or behavioral interventions, because incorrect procedures may be harmful. For example, if a paraprofessional staff member is expected to implement range-of-motion exercises, the childcare worker should be trained directly by a physical therapist and should demonstrate proficiency in implementing the prescribed exercises. Paraprofessionals, volunteers, or professionals from other disciplines should receive training for *each* specialized intervention program they are expected to implement. In other words, if a paraprofessional is trained to implement range-of-motion exercises for Tommy, she must receive additional training to provide range-of-motion exercises for Sally.

The third major safety and health concern related to staffing is monitoring children. This is particularly important when there are large groups of children. Staff can monitor children by being assigned to specific physical areas of a program (a "zone" approach). An alternative is to assign staff to monitor specific groups of children (a "person to person" approach; for example, each staff member monitors six children). In either case, frequent child counts should be taken on a regular schedule throughout the day. In childcare settings where children sometimes arrive and depart at many different times , and attendance may vary significantly from day to day, it is imperative that there is staff responsibility for documenting children's arrivals and departures.

The fourth and final staffing concern related to safety and health is practicing good hygiene. The importance of good hygiene to prevent the spread of infectious diseases was discussed earlier in this chapter. All staff should be trained in specific practices: washing all dishes and utensils with hot soapy water, washing hands after each diaper change with disinfectant soap, wiping surfaces and toys with disinfectant cleaner on a daily basis, and so forth. Staff should be assigned duties for maintaining a clean and healthy environment to ensure that all essential tasks are done on a regular basis.

Scheduling

Schedules of service delivery pertain to the frequency and duration of services, as well as the ordering and organization of activities and instruction. As stated repeatedly, options are essential to addressing individual family/child needs and preferences. Scheduling options should be available to families and children. How often services should be scheduled will depend on family preferences and a variety of other factors, including the child's age; the child's health; instructional needs; and family support needs. For example, the family of an infant recently released from a neonatal intensive-care unit may want consultative services for one hour, once every two weeks. A family with a 2-year-old may prefer half-day childcare on a daily basis because the child does not have siblings and needs opportunities for socialization and modeling.

In determining the schedule within a service delivery model (the selection and organization of activities), the program management goals of nonrestrictiveness, normalization, and safety and health are key considerations. A schedule that is nonrestrictive has the following characteristics:

1. Allows ample time for meaningful participation in activities,
2. Enables all children to have access to the same scope of activities,
3. Provides sufficient instructional time to address goals,
4. Integrates instructional strategies addressing goals into a schedule of age-appropriate activities,
5. Is implemented consistently to allow infants/young children to learn routines and expectations, and
6. Allows for integration with nondisabled age peers if the program is conducted in a segregated setting.

Nonrestrictive schedules support infants'/young children's participation and independence (refer to strategies for promoting functional independence in Chapter 11). Schedules that include adequate time and are implemented consistently facilitate learning and responding (Krantz & Risley, 1977; LeLaurin & Risley, 1972; Rogers-Warren, 1982).

Normalized schedules are those that are similar to the schedules of service delivery models serving primarily nondisabled infants and young children. Children with disabilities should be provided with normalized schedules so that they have the same opportunities as their nondisabled peers to learn the routines and behaviors expected in natural settings. In the home, the normalized schedule is the family's typical schedule of activities. Rather than suggesting that families set aside specific times for instruction, home-based service delivery models should provide instructional programs that fit into the family's routines. For example, if an infant has an instructional program to encourage babbling, the program is incorporated into diapering, dressing, and play routines. This provides many natural opportunities for instruction and allows the family to maintain their typical lifestyle. Furthermore, the normalized schedule supports family members in maintaining normalized roles and relationships with their children as parents, siblings, and grandparents, without pressuring them to become their children's therapists or teachers. The recommendation to incorporate instruction into typical home routines and activities is also true when families who participate in center-based programs ask for suggestions to carry through with instructional programs at home.

Typical schedules of early intervention programs serving primarily nondisabled children are organized by play and care times for infants and toddlers; structured activity times, free play, independent and group activity/play times, outdoor play, and care routines (for example, toileting, eating, brushing teeth, napping) for preschoolers; and a school-like schedule for 5-year-olds (academic time, large group instruction/activities, recess). The schedules of segregated early intervention service delivery models usually have more 1:1 and small-group situations, and fewer large-group situations than programs serving primarily nondisabled infants/ young children (refer to Chapter 9 for strategies for implementing group instruction). Segregated preschool models have also been found to have less play time than segregated models (Bailey et al., 1982). Segregated preschool models should attempt to mirror the schedules of early childhood programs that serve primarily nondisabled children.

As noted in the description of service delivery models in Chapter 1, activity-based curriculum is a recent recommendation for segregated programs (Bricker, 1989, Ch. 12; Bricker & Cripe, 1992). When instructional schedules are structured around activities rather than the objectives of each infant/young child, instruction is scheduled within the context of the age-appropriate activities. This instructional arrangement was described as part of the ecological curriculum model in Chapter 5. The scheduling matrix illustrated in Chapter 5 (see Figure 5-2) is a useful tool for embedding instruction in an activity-based schedule.

The concern for normalization also suggests that opportunities for integration with nondisabled peers should be scheduled for infants/young children who are provided services through segregated programs. For infants, families might participate in an infant play group for support in learning to play with their child. The infant play group experiences may assist the parents of the infant with disabilities to provide their child with same types of experiences provided to the nondisabled infants. This is particularly helpful for infants with disabilities who have subtle or inconsistent responses, or have difficulty sustaining interactions. For children who attend segregated toddler, preschool, or kindergarten programs, reverse mainstreaming can be scheduled with nearby programs that serve nondisabled age peers to provide integration opportunities. Similarly, siblings of the children with disabilities can be invited to participate in the program on a routine basis.

Joint enrollment in programs provides a valuable scheduling option. Some children need the intensive services provided in segregated settings and yet also need ongoing opportunities for interaction with their nondisabled peers. Joint enrollment addresses both of these needs. Additionally, the time spent in the natural service delivery model provides them with the opportunity to learn the routines and activities of a normalized schedule.

There are three safety concerns in scheduling. First, the schedule should allow for continual monitoring and supervision of the infants/young children. It is unsafe, for example, to schedule one group of children for outdoor play while another group is scheduled for an art activity indoors if there are not sufficient staff to monitor both groups. The second safety concern relates to the scheduling of groups of children in activity areas. If an activity area is overcrowded, children may inadvertantly knock each other over, or worse yet, fight over an insufficient number of materials. Research on preschool environments indicates that overcrowding results in an increase in disruptions (Loo, 1972; McGrew, 1970). And third, adequate time should be allowed for transitions between activities. This allows children to return equipment and materials to their appropriate place, and thereby assist in maintaining an organized and clean environment (this also addresses a health concern). Furthermore, if children do not need to rush from one activity to the next, they will be less likely to fall or drop things, and less likely to push and shove each other. The only other scheduling consideration related to health concerns is that children's instructional schedules should be appropriate to their health status. For example, it may be appropriate for some children to be scheduled for services less frequently than others if their health conditions are fragile, or they may be scheduled for in-home services if their immune systems are not strong enough to tolerate the germs present among a group of children.

Early intervention programs have scheduling needs in addition to those associated with direct services to infants/young children. Schedules must include time for meetings with new families and children, child evaluations, team meetings, staff development, evaluation and report writing, consultation and collaboration to support integration. Daily or weekly blocks of time should be scheduled so that these activities occur in a timely manner (for example, an infant program may schedule Monday afternoons for evaluations, and for report writing if no evaluations are needed).

Curriculum

The program management goals of nonrestrictiveness and normalization are pertinent to curriculum development/selection in early intervention. To be nonrestrictive, curriculum must be comprehensive and employ the most effective instructional strategies available. Given the "state of the art" in early intervention (McDonnell & Hardman, 1988), a nonrestrictive curriculum has the following characteristics:

1. **Comprehensive**—the curriculum has an adequate scope and includes all relevant domains and skills.
2. **Individualized**—curriculum is individually tailored to address child/family needs, preferences, and cultural styles.

3. **Developmentally appropriate**—curricular content and instructional strategies are age appropriate; instruction capitalizes on opportunities for child-initiated and child-directed activities.
4. **Community-referenced**—individually tailored curriculum addresses skills needed for participation within the family, with peers, and in the community.
5. **Functional**—curriculum includes skills that are immediately useful; there is an emphasis on the purpose of objectives rather than on specific response forms.
6. **Generalized**—curriculum emphasizes generalized skill rather than discrete skills; and
7. **Preparatory**—curriculum addresses skill needs for future environments and more normalized settings.

If these characteristics are not present in an early intervention curriculum, infants/young children with disabilities are at risk for being excluded from adequate instruction. A service delivery model that fails to provide adequate instruction denies access to appropriate services, and therefore is restrictive.

The characteristics of a curriculum that determine if it is nonrestrictive overlap with many of the characteristics associated with a normalized curriculum. The nonrestrictive characteristics of comprehensiveness and developmental appropriateness, for example, are also characteristics of a normalized early intervention curriculum. At least four additional characteristics are associated with a normalized curriculum: First, curricula should be structured so that instruction takes place in context. Instruction in context assists children to learn the purpose of the skills they are acquiring, as well as the relationship of the skills to other behaviors. Second, normalized curricula fosters independence and self-initiated behavior. This requires that children be taught to demonstrate skills without adult prompting. Third, instructional reinforcement procedures should only be used when absolutely necessary and, when they are used, they should be systematically faded as the children begin to acquire skills. Finally, curricula should address children's needs related to social interaction with nondisabled peers. Early intervention curricula/program goals for infants/young children who are nondisabled without exception prioritize socialization skills over other objectives.

Family Support and Participation

The overall program management concern for families in early intervention is supporting families to meet the needs of themselves and their children. Restrictive family involvement practices are those that foster family reliance on program staff (for example, program staff offer to find the family a physician, program staff conduct their evaluations and then explain their findings to the family). Family support is nonrestrictive if it enables families to advocate for themselves, make decisions for themselves and their children, determine the services that they will access, and develop a feeling of competence as to their abilities to meet their own needs. As noted in Chapter 2, family support should not be "doing" for families; instead, support is enablement that assists families to identify their needs and available resources to meet their needs.

Normalization in family support and involvement is addressed by enabling families to have a typical lifestyle, encouraging and providing opportunities for families to participate in early intervention and early childhood programs, and assuming that families of children with disabilities are competent to make decisions in the best interest of themselves and their children. Supporting families in having a lifestyle typical of their culture requires that each family's needs for work, socialization, and relaxation be respected. Some parents may not choose to implement specialized interventions in their homes because of their own needs or the needs of other family members. Family decisions and choices should be honored nonjudgmentally.

If a child has severe disabilities, a family may need assistance in developing adaptations or other strategies that will allow them to maintain highly valued activities. For example, a parent who is a dedicated jogger might be assisted in locating a source for purchasing a stroller designed for outdoor use and rough terrains. Normalized family participation in early intervention and early childhood programs may include informal communication with program staff, and parents as volunteers or members of parent groups.

Parents of infants/young children must be recognized and supported in their roles as parents (McDonnell & Hardman, 1988), and thus should be encouraged to participate in typical early childhood family involvement activities (for example, preschool board of directors). Bailey and McWilliam (1990), however, caution that we must be sensitive to the feelings of parents who have disabled children who are integrated into natural early intervention programs. The integrated setting provides reminders that their children have special needs and challenges, and this reminder may cause some to feel sadness and pain. Although there may be benefits to families for participating in normalized family activities, parents' wishes with respect to such participation should be honored.

The third concern for normalization in family support is assuming family competence. Unfortunately, there is a long history of professionals treating families of children with disabilities as though they too were disabled. The traditional approach to family support was "family counseling" (implying that families needed help). If families are treated as though they need help or are unable to make decisions for themselves and their families, some will begin to view themselves as incompetent. A powerful way to support families is to assume family competence, and treat families accordingly. Supporting competence will involve, among other things, accepting family choices without making judgments, listening to family concerns, and constructing IFSPs/IEPs on the basis of family priorities and preferences.

Summary

Programmatic variables and the major components of service delivery models (settings and materials, staffing, scheduling, curriculum, and parent involvement) have been described in this chapter. Each component of service delivery models was reviewed with respect to the program management goals of nonrestrictiveness, normalization, and safety and health (as applicable). Other program management concerns, such as budget and record keeping, were not included in this chapter because they are primarily administrative concerns rather than substantive program concerns. There is not one best way of developing each component of service delivery models; instead, there must be options and flexibility. What is "best" will ultimately be determined by how the components meet the needs of each infant, young child, and their family for nonrestrictiveness, normalization, safety, and health.

Activities

1. Interview a staff member of a program for infants with disabilities. Find out what service delivery options are available through the infant program. If options are limited, ask the staff member if he or she is knowledgeable about options available within your community. Discuss integration opportunities and the range of normalizing experiences in the infant program.

2. Interview a preschool special education teacher and a preschool teacher who teaches primarily nondisabled children. Ask them to describe the following characteristics of their class: settings and materials, staffing, scheduling, curriculum, and family support and participation. Compare the results of the two interviews.

3. Contact the Department of Health in your community and obtain a copy of health care and hygiene guidelines for childcare and early childhood programs.

Review Questions

1. Discuss the range of service delivery options that should be available in early intervention services.

2. Discuss the concerns for integration and normalization in early intervention service delivery.
3. Discuss the concerns of (a) nonrestrictiveness, (b) normalization, and (c) safety and health as they relate to the following program management variables:
    1. settings and materials
    2. staffing
    3. scheduling
    4. curriculum
    5. family support and participation
4. Identify infectious diseases that are of concern in early intervention programs. Discuss good hygiene practices for early intervention settings to prevent the spread of infectious diseases.
5. Discuss ways that parents of infants and young children with disabilities can be supported in their roles as parents.

13

Transitions

1. Discuss the important transitions in early childhood.

2. Present procedures to promote smooth transitions.

*T*ransitions involve change. Thus they are turning points. During transitions there is greater than usual vulnerability *and* the potential for problems. Change and stress go together. Even when change is positive—when the transition represents achievement of a long-awaited goal—stress is unavoidable.

The concept of transition was popularized initially as a response to the need to facilitate movement of secondary students in special education from school into postschool environments. It was soon evident that the concerns and processes associated with the phenomenon of transition have far broader application than postsecondary adjustment. Actually, an individual's entire lifespan is a sequence of transitions.

Recall that the IDEA makes a major distinction between services for infants and toddlers (birth to age 3) and services for preschoolers (3- to 5-year-olds). Similarly, there is a distinction between services for preschoolers and those for school-age children. However, in both cases there is clearly an intent to ensure continuity of services. The legislation and accompanying rules and regulations of PL 102-119 are most specific about transitions. Part H requires that the Individualized Family Service Plan (IFSP) include steps to support the transition from infant services to services for preschool-age children, and the preschool component of the law also stresses the importance of carefully planned transitions. Interagency coordination and written agreements are recommended to help clarify local options, identify funds within each program to cover transition planning expenses, and develop guidelines for exchange of records, so that parent and child rights to privacy are protected.

The stress inherent in transitions may not be avoidable but it can certainly be minimized. Planning can break down (a) the arbitrary boundaries among agencies and programs, and (b) the differences between settings and expectations. Planning translates to "being there" now and continuing to be there for as long as assistance is needed.

Among the general issues associated with all transitions are concerns related to transfer of skills from one environment to another to questions about how to help parents adjust to new routines. Additionally, there are specific issues related to (a) the unique needs and requirements of individual children and their families, (b) the nature of the intervention (whether from home or infant program to preschool or preschool to kindergarten), and (c) cultural and community contexts.

This chapter is organized around these questions:

1. What are the important transitions for infants and young children with special needs and their families?
2. Who should be responsible for planning and implementing of the transition process?
3. How can we promote a smooth transition process for the child and the family?

Important Transitions in Early Childhood

As brief as it is, the early childhood period is a time of many transitions for infants and young children with disabilities and their families. They transition across all or some subset of the following programs and services: neonatal intensive care unit, follow-up clinic, public or private health care services, infant intervention services, private therapies, public or private childcare, preschool, and kindergarten. Most of the transition literature deals with the transitions from infant services to a preschool program and from a preschool program to kindergarten. The transition from the hospital to the home for premature infants or infants with special health care needs deserves equal attention, as it is particularly stressful.

Hospital-to-Home and Infant Services

Assuming responsibility for the day-to-day care of a newborn requires adjustments in any family. Required adjustments are many times multiplied when the infant is at risk and in need of special health care. Transition of the infant with established or biological risk from the hospital's Neonatal Intensive Care Unit (NICU) to home care is particularly stressful because it comes when the family is most vulnerable and most anxious.

Hanline and Deppe (1990) identify four issues that parents of premature infants face with this first transition. These issues have direct application to all families who must deal with their infant's basic survival as a primary concern when they leave the hospital. They fall into four categories: (a) understanding their infant's condition, (b) basic caregiving responsibilities, (c) self-esteem and confidence, and (d) decisions about services. Each has specific implications for intervention.

Understanding the Infant's Condition.   First the parents must cope with issues related to their infant's condition (for example, prematurity, sensory impairment, motor impairment). Their nervousness and apprehension are compounded by the fact that they are living with uncertainty about the survival and future development of their infant and, at the same time, dealing with feelings of shock, sadness, anger, grief, disappointment, and guilt. Feelings of being alone and isolated intensify when the infant is discharged from the NICU. When the parents lose contact with hospital staff and other parents, they lose what are often their primary emotional supports. This leaves them on their own, trying to understand what caused their infant's condition, trying to get information regarding their infant's chances for survival, and trying to find someone willing to give them a definitive statement as to the developmental prognosis for their child.

Every family has unique resources and needs, as well as a distinctive coping style. These will determine the best type of support for that family when the parents are beginning to deal with the birth of an infant with special needs. Early interventionists must be sensitive and nonjudgmental; accepting and trying to understand the family's reality. Most important is to focus on the family's strengths and what parents and other family members see as important. The one predictable variable across families is the desire for accurate, honest, and complete information about the baby's condition.

Early intervention personnel should determine if parents or caregivers want assistance (a) establishing and maintaining contacts with a parent support group or parents whom they met in the hospital, (b) obtaining respite care or locating other childcare services, and (c) locating and joining community-based family activities (for example, parenting classes). Whatever supports the parents/caregivers want should be arranged or provided without delay.

Caregiving Responsibilities.   Infants with special needs are often fussy and irritable. Many are still dependent on a ventilator, gastrointestinal tube feeding, or an apnea monitor when they are discharged from the hospital. Parents leave the hospital with misgivings about their ability to care for their infant, particularly when the infant with special needs is their first child.

It is certainly not difficult to understand parents feeling incompetent. To feel confident about necessary caregiving responsibilities, parents need substantial preparation prior to the infant's discharge. The professional who will support the transition process participates in this training with the parents or caregivers. The pre-discharge hospital training typically focuses on the infant's special nutritional needs, operation of specific equipment, and/or proper positioning.

The hospital-to-home model developed by Bruder and Walker (1990) suggests a discharge planning process that includes a NICU discharge summary form. This form is designed to enhance the communication process between families and professionals by providing details of the infants' current and future care needs to those individuals who will be providing community- and home-based services. The type of discharge summary form suggested by Bruder and Walker is markedly different from the nursing discharge summary provided by most NICUs. The traditional nursing discharge summary tends to be a progress report in a narrative format. What information is included depends on the style of the writer. Much of the language and most symbols are difficult for nonmedical professionals to interpret. Moreover, parents may not be among the persons who receive a copy of the summary.

The Bruder and Walker discharge summary form is intended to ensure that all community service providers receive the same information. It is also designed to facilitate continual sharing of information and needs between parents and professionals in the NICU. The form provides space for information in these areas: maternal and infant history, the infant's current medical needs, the infant's needs for growth and development, assessment of family function, cultural considerations, assessment of family needs, and linking families with community services.

Once the infant is home, the focus of early intervention support services shifts to (a) helping the parents implement the recommended techniques, (b) answering questions not answered prior to discharge, (c) assisting parents to understand and respond to the infant's social and communicative cues, and (d) monitoring the infant's developmental progress. In addition, personnel supporting the transition may collaborate with the primary care pediatrician and other health professionals to assure that the infant's health care needs are met.

Self-Esteem and Confidence.   A third issue for parents of infants with special needs is the feeling of lack of control. Premature birth shatters any assumption of controlling the outcomes of pregnancy. The sense of having lost control is heightened during the infant's stay in the NICU because parents are not able to make decisions about the day-to-day care of their child. Understandably, they lose confidence in themselves as caregivers.

The first and most important response for someone who wants to help parents at this stage is to understand and acknowledge the parents' need to regain some control in their lives. The enablement and empowerment approaches to professional/parent interactions described in Chapters 2 and 3 provide specific guidelines for helping parents regain confidence in their ability to make decisions regarding their family and their child.

Decisions about Services.   Finally, parents of infants with special needs must locate community-based early intervention services and make some decisions about how they want to participate in these programs. While this may appear to be straightforward, it is not: the problem is more basic and more involved than locating and accessing services. This is the point at which the parents must "go public." They must come to terms with two very difficult matters—the possibility of developmental delay *and* the need to allow unfamiliar professionals to enter their lives. If a service coordinator has established a relationship with the family prior to the infant's discharge and supported the transition process, he or she is in a good position to help parents with these decisions. An understanding and supportive attitude is essential.

Transition planning is only one component of the IFSP, but it can serve an important function in focusing attention on the child's future. Every goal and objective for the child can (and should) address independence in future (as well as present) environments. Periodic review and updating with parents will keep planning current and responsive.

Infant Program to Preschool

There are some similarities and many differences in the transition from the hospital to home and infant program, and the transition from infant program to preschool. Both involve locating and making decisions about services and in both processes the family's need for information is foremost. However, there are also significant differences. The most salient issues associated with transitioning from an infant program to a preschool setting are continuity of services, adapting to change, and adjusting to new program expectations.

Kilgo, Richard, and Noonan (1989) describe a model to assist families and infants with special needs in dealing with these issues. The model was developed in a demonstration project called Preschool Preparation and Transition (PPT) funded by the Handicapped Children's Early Education Program (HCEEP). (Recall that this federal program [HCEEP] is now called the Early Education Program for Children with Disabilities [EEPCD].)

Parent Needs Assessment.   The first step in the PPT transition process is determining the parents' or caregivers' preferences, strengths, and need for support in the transition from infant program (home-based, center-based, or mixed) to a private or public preschool program. The PPT project uses a form called the Parent Needs Assessment (PNA) to structure the interview when this information is collected. The person who will support the family during the transition process, typically the service coordinator, and the parents or caregivers schedule a meeting to assemble information about:

1. **Future planning:** Parents are asked if they have thought about what they want for their child when he or she reaches age 3 and leaves the infant program.
2. **Need or desire for assistance:** If the parents have considered some future options, they are asked more about these (such as whether they have made any contacts with possible programs, what portion of the transition activities they want to do themselves, and what they would like assistance with).
3. **Need for information:** Parents are asked if they need more information about their child's needs in any area (medical care, independent play skills, social skills, motor development, nutrition). This is a means of highlighting concerns that need to be addressed by the infant program staff.
4. **Need for support:** Parents are asked if they would like to meet parents of an older child with special needs, one who is similar to their child. Some parents prefer to meet and talk with other parents individually, while others want to join a group. Still others may want written materials (suggesting a desire to learn in privacy).
5. **Transition issues:** Here again parents are asked what types of information would make it easier for them to plan for particular aspects of transition. They are asked how important the following issues are to them (whether each is "not important at all," "somewhat important," or "very important").
   a. The skills my child will need in preschool
   b. What kinds of preschools are available
   c. My child's legal rights relative to attending a private or a public preschool

d. The types of assessments and records needed to apply for different preschools

e. Planning the transition with infant program staff

f. How to decide what type of preschool is best for my child

6. **Parent awareness/knowledge:** There is an effort to determine how much the parents know about their legal rights and about the least restrictive environment (LRE) concept.

When should an interview be conducted to assemble this information and begin the transition planning process? Who should administer an interview concerned with future planning? When the PPT project investigated these issues, it became clear that there is a specific readiness period for parents and that readiness for transition planning varies among families. While most are ready to plan around the time of their child's second birthday, some families indicate readiness for planning prior to age 2. Others are not yet ready when their child's third birthday is approaching. When characteristics of the families and children were compared with the time they indicated readiness for transition planning, PPT staff found that the readiness period was related to the severity of the child's disability. Parents of more severely disabled children seem less likely to look ahead to future programming (unless actively encouraged to do so).

As to who should administer a future planning interview, the PPT staff found that the roles and responsibilities associated with transition may be assumed by any professional or paraprofessional who is sensitive to parents' or caregivers' signals and able to coordinate future planning.

Parent Education. The second step in the PPT transition process is providing parents or caregivers with information that will facilitate smooth adaptations to change. When parents express an interest in the transition process they are provided with the information contained in five short modules, each with a short, easy-to-read booklet. These modules/booklets are entitled:

What's in a transition?
Legal rights for children with special needs
Preparing my child for independence
Who is the transition coordinator?
Parents and the IEP

Transition Planning and Support. The third step in the PPT transition process is the actual transition planning and support. Transition planning is flexible and responsive to the individual family. It begins by addressing needs identified during the family needs assessment process, recognizing that these needs are continually changing. The parents or caregivers, the transition coordinator, and others on the team as appropriate, work to develop a transition timeline. These are the steps that are included on a typical timeline: (a) complete evaluations, (b) discuss future program possibilities, (c) visit future program possibilities, (d) select a program and verify eligibility, (e) apply for enrollment, (f) prepare the child and the receiving program.

Preschool to Kindergarten

The transition from a special education preschool program to the regular education kindergarten classroom also places special demands on professionals, the family, the child, and the system. Faculty at the University of Vermont have developed a model for planning this transition (Conn-Powers, Ross-Allen & Holburn, 1990). This model was developed and field-tested through Project TEEM (Transitioning into the Elementary Education Mainstream) which, like PPT, was a demonstration project funded by the HCEEP.

Project TEEM lists the following requirements for the transition from preschool to kindergarten to be successful: a transition planning process must (a) be individualized for each child and family; (b) be initiated well before the child enters the classroom (at least 1 year ahead of time for most children); and (c) reflect the collaborative efforts of the family and all involved professionals.

Both the child and the setting must be prepared for a transition. Preparation of the entering child is discussed later in the sections dealing with teacher expectation and peer standards. Preparation of the kindergarten setting for the entering child may include any one or all of these activities: (a) identifying and removing boundaries to physical access, (b) identifying and obtaining inservice training and technical assistance for the staff, (c) identifying and obtaining special materials and equipment, and (d) developing a workable plan. The plan should specify goals, adaptations, strategies, how peers will be prepared, and what resources will be needed to ensure that the child will have a successful educational experience.

The transition plan does not end when the child enters the new setting; the transition planning process is ongoing. The planning team continues to serve as a resource after the child's transition so that, if problems arise, they can be addressed quickly and positively.

There are many opportunities to smooth the way for transitions when preschool and kindergarten programs share the same building or the same campus. Some communities have sought classroom space for kindergartens in community facilities that house preschool programs, and some Head Start and childcare programs are physically housed in public schools. Teachers in these settings tend to combine their classes for celebrations, children's performances, field trips, and special audiovisual presentations. Some even exchange instructional materials and visual aids. Proximity does not guarantee cooperative or collaborative interactions between programs, but it can help to narrow the gap.

Communication is enhanced by familiarity. Individuals who respect and are comfortable with one another are more likely to exchange information about themselves and their programs. The key requirement for successful transition is exchange of accurate information. Planning that includes appropriate exchange of information increases a child's chance for a successful transition.

How to Promote Smooth Transitions

In the transition from infant services to preschool and preschool to kindergarten, the onus for initiating the transition process typically falls on parents or staff of the sending program. Parents are the most essential participants. At the very least, subsequent planning efforts should include the family and staff of both the sending and receiving agencies.

For the transition from infant services to a preschool program, participants from the infant program may include the service coordinator, program director, and auxiliary staff. Participants from the receiving preschool may include the director or coordinator, teaching staff, and auxiliary staff. For the transition from preschool to kindergarten, participants from the preschool may include the director or coordinator, teachers, teacher aides and assistants, and auxiliary personnel. Kindergarten representatives in the planning process may include principals, kindergarten and primary teachers, teacher aides and assistants, district personnel, and auxiliary personnel. In the process of developing and implementing transition plans, the staff of both sending and receiving agencies must work to understand one another's goals and procedures.

Steps in Planning Transition

Table 13-1 shows the steps to follow in planning a transition. These steps provide an outline for transition from infant program to preschool and preschool to a kindergarten setting. There are other less formal activities in the larger community arena that facilitate these steps. Most important is to make others aware of transition concepts and goals. Communication at the level of awareness can occur at professional meetings, workshops, or social functions. Networking is useful to help individuals get acquainted, share ideas and concerns about transitions, and brainstorm transition strategies.

Family Involvement

In a 1986 study, Johnson, Chandler, Kerns, and Fowler interviewed families whose children had experienced a recent transition from an early childhood special education program to a public school program. Questions mentioned by parents most often as concerns *before* transition were:

1. When should transition planning begin?
2. How should transition planning proceed?

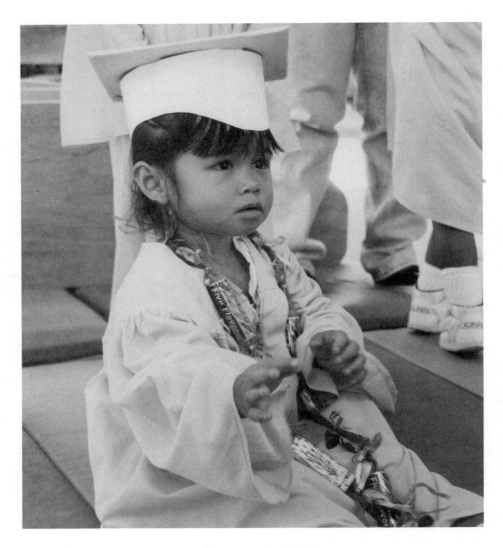

Transition planning focuses attention on the child's future.

3. Who is responsible for interaction between the preschool and the new program?
4. How can parents prepare themselves, their families, and their child for the transition?
5. What characteristics should parents look for in a new program that will meet their child's (and family's) special needs?

Johnson and the others emphasize that parents have much to offer, as well as much to gain, by being active in the transition process. They can (a) provide

---

TABLE 13-1

Steps in Transition

---

1. Form a transition team—including parents, current program staff, and staff of the most likely receiving programs.
2. Schedule meetings—the first meeting will be to develop an initial written plan; the later meetings will consider specific transition tasks.
3. Identify possible receiving settings.
4. Identify basic transition tasks—What will be necessary to implement the transition?
5. Agree on assignments—specifically, who will perform each of the different transition tasks?
6. Establish timelines—including the referral date and dates for pre-placement activities.
7. Decide communication procedures—including transfer of records and other information.
8. Agree on pre-placement activities—such as (a) parent visits to potential receiving environments, (b) information sharing between teaching staff in sending and receiving agencies, (c) observations in the receiving setting to determine needed adaptations, (d) arrangements for whatever family support will be provided, (e) therapy and other special services, and (f) future consultative interactions.
9. Plan for follow-up activities—should be planned and carried out between the family and the agencies involved.
10. Place the child—after needed environmental adaptations have been completed.
11. Provide consultation and therapy services.
12. Follow up and evaluate.

---

valuable information, (b) teach their child skills at home that can generalize to the new setting, (c) act as advocates for their child and the program, and (d) provide social and emotional support for other parents. Communication and planning between families and professionals supplements the program's knowledge of a family's concerns, desires, and resources.

Transitions require the family to alter familiar routines and initiate new behaviors, experiences, and expectations. Among the changes required of the family are different schedules, new relationships to establish, relinquishing of time with familiar staff in the old program or agency, and helping to set new goals and objectives for their child.

Participation in the transition process can lessen the negative effects of change. Several studies offer suggestions for helping families address their concerns (Brinckerhoff & Vincent, 1986; Diamond, Spiegel-McGill & Hanrahan, 1988; Fowler, Chandler, Johnson & Stella, 1988). Diamond and colleagues (1988) assisted parents through these activities:

1. Identifying survival skills their children would need for the receiving (new) placement
2. Assembling information about community services and the parents' legal rights

3. Presenting their concerns to the school system
4. Participating in meetings to develop an IEP and plan for transition
5. Monitoring their children's progress
6. Assessing the success of the transition

Teacher Expectations

Undoubtedly the most critical ingredient for successful transition is information about the demands of the new setting. Increased class size and very different daily routines may place much greater emphasis on functioning independently, skills for large-group functioning, learning new rules and routines, and getting along with new adults and peers. The child's adjustment depends in part on demonstrating the necessary survival skills to respond to these new demands.

One source of critical information about requirements of the receiving program is the teacher. Interviewing the teacher can yield valuable information about the schedule of activities, the type of instruction, the grouping of children, and setting demands. Sainato and Lyon (1989) suggest interviews to collect this information from teacher(s) in the receiving program:

- ◆ The number of children and staff in the setting
- ◆ The amount of time allocated to various activities
- ◆ The level of teacher involvement in the various activities
- ◆ Number of children participating in each activity
- ◆ Type of seating provided
- ◆ Typical response demands of the activity

This information can then be used as the basis for observations in the receiving setting.

Another type of information that will be helpful in preparing the entering child is information about teacher expectations related to independent work behaviors. Where interviews or observations to define survival skills are not possible, teachers can adopt (with or without modification) one of a number of available survival skills checklists.

The first application of the notion that teachers should look to the next education environment to identify skills, and use these skills to set goals and objectives for current programming for preschoolers, was by Vincent and her colleagues (Vincent et al., 1980). Experienced kindergarten and early childhood special education teachers were asked to generate a list of classroom skills necessary for students to succeed in mainstream kindergarten settings. Hains, Fowler, Schwartz, Kottwitz, and Rosenkoetter (1989) used a different approach (a structured teacher interview format) to identify essential kindergarten skills, but the results were very similar.

Noonan and colleagues (1992) developed a *preschool* survival skills checklist as part of the PPT project described earlier. Again there is considerable overlap. The skills validated by Noonan and the others as preschool survival skills in Hawaii are similar to the survival skills identified for 18- to 36-month-olds in daycare centers in Wisconsin (Murphy & Vincent, 1989), and kindergarten survival skills in Wisconsin (Vincent et al., 1980; Walters & Vincent, 1982) and Hawaii (McCormick & Kawate, 1982). The ethnic and cultural differences between the two states make these commonalities especially interesting. The 11 skills that appear on the PPT preschool survival skills list and also appear on at least two or three other kindergarten checklists are:

1. Follows general rules and routines
2. Expresses wants and needs
3. Cooperates with/helps others
4. Complies with directions given by adult
5. Shares materials/toys with peers
6. Socializes with peers
7. Takes turns
8. Interacts verbally with adults
9. Interacts verbally with peers
10. Focuses attention on speaker
11. Makes own decisions

These skills are primarily social/communication and adaptive skills. That these skills seem to be important for both preschool *and* kindergarten suggests there may be different competence levels. For example, presumably the 5-year-old is expected to "express wants and needs" at a more sophisticated level than the 3-year-old.

Figure 13-1 presents the preschool survival skills checklist developed by the PPT project at the University of Hawaii. (Behavior definitions are included in Table 13-2.) Instructions for using the checklist are available from the PPT project. Figure 13-2 is a kindergarten checklist adapted from McCormick and Kawate (1982).

Discussion of survival skills is not complete without reiterating this caveat: *Survival skills are optimum goals, not behavioral prerequisites* (Salisbury & Vincent, 1990). A child's failure to demonstrate any one or all of the skills on a survival skills checklist should not prevent that child's transition to, and placement in, mainstream early childhood settings. Moreover, while it is helpful to have a list of behaviors that will facilitate successful transition and maintenance in the next environment, this is not sufficient. As Fowler, Schwartz, and Atwater (1991) point out, each child's success in the future environment will be based not only on *having* the essential skills but also actually *using* them when and where they should be used *and* using them appropriately (Anderson-Inman, Paine, & Deutchman, 1984).

Preparation of the Child

Adjustment in the new setting will depend in large part on whether the child demonstrates the necessary survival skills to meet teacher expectations. Assessment

Hawaii Preparing for Integrated Preschool (PIP) Assessment

Preschool Preparation and Transition Project   University of Hawaii at Manoa

IS THE SKILL MASTERED?
+   YES
/   PARTIALLY
-   NO
O   NO OPPORTUNITY
     TO OBSERVE

Child's Name: _____   Date of Birth: _____

Assessor: _____

		Date	Comments	Date	Comments
Self-Help	1. Grasps objects				
	2. Drinks independently				
	3. Eats independently				
	4. Cares for toileting needs				
	5. Cares for personal hygiene				
	6. Moves about independently				
Classroom routines	7. Makes transitions from one activity to another				
	8. Complies with directions				
	9. Follows rules and routines				
	10. Knows and recognizes name				
	11. Focuses on task				
	12. Uses materials appropriately				
	13. Throws rubbish in wastebasket				
	14. Puts materials away when finished				
Communication/Socialization	15. Focuses attention on speaker				
	16. Expresses wants/needs				
	17. Socializes with others				
	18. Problem-solves with words				
	19. Makes own decisions				
	20. Communicates with peers				
	21. Communicates with adults				
	22. Takes turns				
	23. Shares materials/toys with peers				
	24. Responds when spoken to				
	25. Cooperates with/helps others				
	26. Does not disturb peers				
	27. Uses voice appropriate to activity				

Figure 13-1

TABLE 13-2
Hawaii Preparing for Integrated Preschool (PIP) Skill Definitions

	Skill	Definition
Self-Help	1. Grasps objects	Child grasps and holds objects such as fat pencils, crayons, manipulative toys, and other small objects (typical response of 3-year-old: without assistance)
	2. Drinks independently	Given a cup, juice box, or thermos, child picks up cup, juice box, or thermos and sips from cup, straw, or thermos spout without assistance (typical response of 3-year-old: without assistance)
	3. Eats independently	During snack or lunch, child completes meal within 30 minutes, feeding himself finger foods with his hands and other foods with a spoon and a fork (typical response of 3-year-old: without assistance)
	4. Cares for toileting needs	Child performs all aspects of toileting independently: communicating need to go to the bathroom, independence in managing clothing, toileting, washing/drying hands. Some assistance with clothing fasteners may be required (typical response of 3-year-old: independently)
	5. Cares for personal hygiene	Child covers nose or mouth when sneezing/coughing when reminded by an adult; washes hands, cleans face, and wipes nose at routine times, e.g., before/after snack, cooking, outdoor play, etc., (typical response of 3-year-old: with one or no reminders)
	6. Moves about independently	Child moves independently either walking or with the use of adaptive aids, e.g., wheelchair, scooterboard, walker, etc., (typical response of 3-year-old: long duration, independently)
Classroom Routines	7. Makes transitions from one activity to another	At transition points between any activity, child responds to a familiar signal. Child's response includes completion of one activity and movement to area for next activity within the allotted time (typical response of 3-year-old: with one announcement)
	8. Complies with directions	Child complies to teacher's verbal request to perform routine activities or change behavior (typical response of 3-year-old: immediately)
	9. Follows rules and routines	Child complies to teacher's verbal request, participates with group, and adheres to safety rules (typical response of 3-year-old: with one verbal reminder)
	10. Knows and recognizes name	In classroom areas (e.g., on cubby) or during activities (e.g., circle), child recognizes his/her printed name by finding correct flashcard or labelled cubby (typical response of 3-year-old: first and last name without prompts)

(continued)

TABLE 13-2—*(continued)*
Hawaii Preparing for Integrated Preschool (PIP) Skill Definitions

	Skill	*Definition*
Classroom Routines	11. Focuses on task	Child attends to any activity that requires concentration (e.g., story time, art, or music) until task is complete. Child appears "tuned into task," sitting, gazing, manipulating, and performing task (typical response of 3-year-old: looks, manipulates, performs more than once)
	12. Uses materials appropriately	Child manipulates toys, art supplies, games, blocks, and/or outdoor equipment in manner that each is intended to be used (typical response of 3-year-old: without reminder)
	13. Throws rubbish in wastebasket	After any activity that creates rubbish, child picks up all rubbish, takes it to wastebasket, and places it in wastebasket (typical response of 3-year-old: without reminder)
	14. Puts material away when finished	At the signaled end of an activity, child places classroom materials, personal belongings, and rubbish in the correct places (typical response of 3-year-old: with one verbal reminder)
Communication/Socialization	15. Focuses attention on speaker	When one adult talks to child or group of children, child listens attentively: looking at speaker, sitting or standing quietly, and not interrupting, for an appropriate length of time (typical response of 3-year-old: not interrupting, quiet, looks at speaker intermittently)
	16. Expresses wants/needs	When a child wants or needs something such as a toy or a drink of water, the child asks for it (typical response of 3-year-old: verbally)
	17. Socializes with others	Child solicits attention of another child or responds to a child's bid for attention either positively or negatively (typical response of 3-year-old: talks)
	18. Problem solves with words	In a situation involving physical or verbal conflict, child uses words to resolve the conflict so that play either continues or ends (typical response of 3-year-old: independently)
	19. Makes own decisions	Child chooses materials/activity, location, or person when a choice is presented (typical response of 3-year-old: immediately)
	20. Communicates with peers	Child initiates or responds, either verbally or through alternative means (e.g., sign language, communication board), to peer about different topics (typical response of 3-year-old: single turns)
	21. Communicates with adults	Child initiates or responds, either verbally or through alternative means (e.g., sign language, communication board), to adults about different topics (typical response of 3-year-old: single turns)

TABLE 13-2—*(continued)*
Hawaii Preparing for Integrated Preschool (PIP) Skill Definitions

	Skill	Definition
Communication/Socialization	22. Takes turns	In group activities that require taking turns (e.g., using outdoor equipment, playing circle games, etc.), child waits without protest for his/her turn, participates, and gives up his/her turn without protest (typical response of 3-year-old: with one or no reminders)
	23. Shares materials/toys with peers	When two children are playing with same materials, child releases material to another child even briefly (typical response of 3-year-old: independently)
	24. Responds when spoken to	When individually addressed by adult or peer throughout the day, child shifts attention to speaker: turning toward, looking at, talking to, or stopping ongoing activity (typical response of 3-year-old: immediately)
	25. Cooperates with/helps others	When engaged in an activity, child participates without protest or struggle, or offers help to another person (typical response of 3-year-old: independently)
	26. Does not disturb others	Child does not use hands or feet to distract or hurt another child, refrains from making loud or inappropriate noises and does not talk out of turn (typical response of 3-year-old: independently)
	27. Uses voice appropriate to activity	When engaged in indoor activity, child talks in conversational tones. When requested to use softer/louder volume, child responds accordingly (typical response of 3-year-old: without reminder)

with future environment surveys, which describe behaviors essential to the next classroom, is a first step. Then children must be taught the identified skills.

The PPT project has developed a curriculum to prepare children for regular preschool placement. This curriculum is based on the PIP checklist shown in Figure 13-1. The curriculum includes suggestions for adapting each skill to accommodate a child with physical or sensory impairments. Five instructional strategies are described for each skill: model, prompt, guide, practice, and reinforce. (Figure 13-3 shows PPT curriculum guidelines for one skill: ''complies with directions.'')

Several research programs have developed and validated curriculum to teach survival skills to children entering kindergarten (Carta, Atwater, Schwartz & Miller, 1990; Rule, Fiechtl & Innocenti, 1990). Rule and colleagues provide data showing that children who were taught the nine activities in their Skills for School Success curriculum while in daycare centers actually demonstrated the survival skills when they transitioned into the kindergarten classroom.

Hawaii Kindergarten Survival Skills Checklist

Teacher: _____   Dates of Observation: _____

Observer: _____   Child's Name: _____

Skills	Never		Sometimes		Consistently		
	1	2	3	4	5	6	7
Independent Task Work							
1. Begins work within an appropriate time without extra teacher direction							
2. Stays on task without extra teacher direction							
3. Completes tasks within allotted time							
4. Completes task at criterion							
5. Follows routine at end of work session							
Group Attending/Participation							
1. Sits appropriately							
2. Does not disrupt peers							
3. Focuses visual attention on speaker(s)							
4. Participates and/or follows task directions in a small group							
5. Participates and/or follows task directions in a large group							
6. Participates at appropriate time							
Following Class Routine							
1. Locates *own* possessions and returns them to appropriate locations							
2. Locates materials and replaces or puts them in order when finished							
3. Goes to various areas in the room when requested and/or directed							
4. Makes transitions with general group verbal cue							
5. Makes transitions from one activity to the next using contextual cues							
6. Follows general rules and routines established in classroom							

Figure 13-2 Survival skills checklist

Hawaii Kindergarten Survival Skills Checklist

Teacher: _____   Dates of Observation: _____

Observer: _____   Child's Name: _____

Skills	Never		Sometimes		Consistently		
	1	2	3	4	5	6	7
Appropriate Classroom Behavior							
1. Works/plays without disrupting or bothering peers							
2. Waits appropriately							
3. Modifies behavior when provided with verbal direction							
4. Reacts appropriately to changes in the routine							
5. Uses time between activities appropriately							
Self-Care							
1. Takes care of own toileting needs without supervision							
2. Washes hands without supervision							
3. Undresses without supervision (except for help with fasteners)							
4. Dresses without supervision (except for help with fasteners)							
Direction Following							
1. Complies with simple directions provided by adult to the child							
2. Complies with simple directions by an adult to the group							
3. Follows two-step directions							
Social/Play Skills							
1. Spontaneously begins play activities during play time							
2. Maintains play activity for an appropriate length of time							
3. Interacts verbally with peers							
4. Maintains play with peers for an appropriate length of time							
5. Participates appropriately, performing game actions according to rules							
Functional Communication							
1. Asks for information							
2. States needs							

SOURCE: Adapted from ''Kindergarten Survival Skills: New Directions For Preschool Special Education'' by L. McCormick and J. Kawate, 1982, *Education and Training of the Mentally Retarded, 17,* 247-251.

Figure 13-2—(continued)

SKILL 8: Complies with directions.

DEFINITION: Child complies to teacher's verbal request to perform routine activities or change behavior (typical response of 3-year-old: immediately).

Adaptations to Make the Skill Easier for Me	Adaptations to Accommodate Physical or Sensory Impairments
a) Start small Keep your directions simple, clear, and specific. Give me one direction at a time (e.g., after story-time, tell me to put the book back on the shelf).	a) If I have fine motor difficulties... I may need a little extra time to perform the activity or change my behavior.
b) Limit the skill Give me the direction only after storytime.	b) If I have gross motor difficulties... Give me enough time so I can comply to your request.
c) Teach part of the skill Teach me to stop what I am doing and look at you when you give me a direction.	c) If I have a hearing impairment... Stand in front of me and look at me when giving me a direction. Show me the sign and/or use a gesture when making a request.
d) Teach a related skill Play "Follow-the-Leader" during music time.	d) If I have a visual impairment... Make sure supplies and furniture are always in the same place. Speak slowly and allow me extra time to follow your request.

How to Help Me Learn the Skill...

In My Infant/Preschool Program	At Home	In the Community
a) model After I've colored a picture, tell me, "It's time to put the crayons back in the box." Show me how to do it.	a) model Have Daddy show me how to go and sit at the table when Mommy says, "It's dinnertime."	a) model Let me watch other children holding their mommy's hand as they cross the street.
b) prompt Place the crayon box in front of me when it's time to put the crayons away.	b) prompt You may have to remind me, "Come to the table, it's time for dinner."	b) prompt Tell me, "It's time to cross the street," and put your hand out so I can hold it.
c) guide Help me put a few crayons in the box and let me put the rest away.	c) guide Take my hand and lead me to the table when I'm told it's dinnertime.	c) guide Take my hand as we get ready to cross the street.

(continued)

Figure 13-3 Example of one skill from the Hawaii Preparing for Integrated Preschool Curriculum (1991)

In My Infant/Preschool Program	At Home	In the Community
d) practice Play "Simon Says" during a coloring activity, directing me to choose another color and color a different part of my paper. e) reinforce Direct and assist me to hang my finished work on the bulletin board where all can see it. Praise me for good work and for following directions.	d) practice Let me play with you and help you with your chores. e) reinforce Let me have my favorite dessert since I followed the directions.	d) practice Take me on lots of outings so I can learn the rules outside of our home and school. e) reinforce Let me pick a fun outing to go on since I held your hand while crossing the street.

SOURCE: University of Hawaii, Department of Special Education and University Affiliated Program.

Figure 13-3—(continued)

The findings reported by Carta and colleagues (Carta et al., 1990) are equally impressive. Their curriculum addresses three kindergarten survival skills: (a) completing within-classroom transitions, (b) participating in large instructional groups, and (c) working independently. Classroom survival skills were rated by teachers before and after implementation of the curriculum. After the intervention, participating children responded more frequently to group instructions and demonstrated higher rates of task engagement, with fewer teacher prompts during independent activities. Sixty-one percent of the children with disabilities who received the survival skills curriculum in special education preschool programs were subsequently placed in mainstreamed kindergarten classrooms. Only 48% of the children in the control group classrooms were placed in mainstreamed classrooms.

As Fowler and others (1991) point out, at present there are no published data to answer the question of whether children who have received instruction in survival skills continue to use their new skills in appropriate contexts in the next environment. Nor are there data indicating whether children who have had instruction in survival skills are successful in their mainstreamed placements. However, the findings cited above are certainly a promising first step in this direction.

Toward the end of the pretransition year, everything possible should be done to lessen differences between the sending and receiving settings. When feasible, the transition from one program to the next should occur gradually. Some procedures that sending teachers can begin to make transition to the new program easier for young children include:

1. **Field trips to the "new" school.** Ideally such tours would include lunch in the cafeteria, some time for play on the playground, and participation in a few kindergarten activities.

2. **Reading stories about the fun of new adventures and new friends.** Read (or make up) stories about new experiences.

3. **Helping the children create a scrapbook about kindergarten.** Each child's scrapbook could include photos taken during the field trip, as well as pictures of kindergarten activities created by the child.

4. **Role playing "going to the new school."** In the course of role-play sessions, encourage the children to express their feeling about the new experiences.

5. **Invite kindergarten teachers to visit the class.** Try to arrange for each receiving kindergarten teacher to visit the preschool class. The goal is for kindergarten teachers to get to know the children in a familiar setting.

Children in transition need time to adjust to the different (and often increased) demands of the new environment and changes in child/teacher ratio, rules, routines, and social experiences.

Program Differences

There are many differences among early childhood programs and many differences among kindergarten programs. However, the differences *between* the two types of programs are most salient (and problematic) where transitions are concerned. A kindergarten class is very different from a childcare center, a Head Start program, a special education program, or a regular preschool program that a child may have attended. There are differences related to:

1. **Group sizes.** It is common to find relatively small group sizes in preschool and childcare centers. The latter may have groups of 15 to 20 with two or three adults. Kindergarten classes rarely have more than one teacher and the class typically includes 25 or more children.

2. **Schedules.** Preschool scheduling is relatively flexible. Kindergarten schedules are often set by the school administration to facilitate cooperative use of playgrounds, cafeterias, transportation, and so on.

3. **Structure.** In Head Start programs, preschools and childcare centers, children are encouraged to play together cooperatively and to select their own activities. There is typically some emphasis on arranging activities that promote communication and other social interactions. Kindergarten activities are more structured; the emphasis is on developing independent work habits and such preacademic behaviors as following directions.

4. **Goals.** Preschool programs and kindergarten programs have different

purposes. Many kindergartens emphasize preacademic goals, whereas the emphasis in preschools is typically on developmental curriculum.

5. **Parent involvement.** Regular, informal communications between parents and teachers (or other school personnel) are less common in kindergartens than in Head Start, childcare, or preschool programs. Moreover, participation in daily activities seems less feasible at the kindergarten level. Also, medical, dental, and social services may be less readily available in the kindergarten setting.

6. **Behavioral expectations.** The expectations of kindergarten teachers are very different than those of most teachers in programs for preschoolers.

An individual's behavior in a given environment is a function of two variables: (a) the demands and expectations of that environment, and (b) the skills of the individual. To understand the requirements for independent functioning in mainstream environments, Sainato and Lyon (1989) first observed how children in the mainstream setting spent their time. Second, they examined the similarities and differences in grouping arrangements between the special education preschool and the mainstream setting. Finally, they explored the level of teacher involvement during instruction in the two settings.

Although the two programs were similar in terms of scheduled activities, there were significant differences in the way time was spent. The potential matching of future setting to students requires comparison of how much time is spent in different activities in the two settings. This requires careful examination of child goals, competencies, and environmental demands. Among the most important questions to ask about potential mainstream classrooms are:

How is instruction delivered?
Will the instruction meet the needs of the child?

Sainato and Lyon (1989) found distinct differences between the special preschool and the mainstream classrooms in teaching formats. In the special preschool, the child spends very little time (only 3%) in child-guided activities, compared to 69% in teacher-directed and 28% in teacher-guided activities. In one of the mainstream settings, child-guided activities occurred for 22% of the time. In the other mainstream setting, child-guided activities occurred for 50% of the time. With regard to teacher-directed activities, the first mainstream setting had a high level of teacher-directed activities (42%), while the other mainstream setting had only 6% of teacher-directed activities.

Barriers to Transition Planning

The most frequently cited barrier to transition planning is lack of time and money resources (Fowler et al., 1991; Peterson, 1991). Staff need to meet with families, visit program sites with families, communicate with receiving teachers, collect data concerning teacher expectations, and evaluate the success of the placement.

Moreover, the transition process does not end when the child has begun attending the new program; there must be an ongoing commitment to serve as a resource to the family and the receiving program. These activities require considerable time. The most obvious financial barrier is associated with staffing. Providing teachers with release time to participate in the activities listed above generally means hiring a substitute.

Lack of commitment to the goals of the transition process is also a barrier to successful transitions (Conn-Powers et al., 1990). For the transition process to be effective requires system-wide commitment and support.

 Summary

This chapter has considered the three major transitions in the early childhood period. We have specifically described processes for transition planning and implementation. Careful attention to these activities will facilitate smooth and successful movement from one set of circumstances to another and accommodation to new and different environments.

Activities

1. Talk with a parent or parents whose child was born prematurely. Ask what supports were most helpful to them when they brought their newborn home from the hospital. What were the most difficult adjustments? How long was it before the parent felt confident and in control? What suggestions would they offer to professionals concerned with supporting this transition?

2. Talk with a parent or parents whose child has made the transition from an infant intervention program to a preschool program. Ask if the transition went smoothly. When did planning begin? Who was involved in the planning? What suggestions would they offer to professionals concerned with supporting this transition?

3. Talk with a parent or parents whose child has made the transition from preschool to kindergarten. Ask when planning began and who was involved. How was the child prepared for the transition? How was the receiving preschool prepared for the transition?

4. Visit a regular preschool class and a kindergarten class. Show the PIP Assessment (Figure 13-1) to the teaching staff in the preschool and ask if these behaviors match their expectations for 3-year-olds entering their program. Show

the Kindergarten Survival Skills Checklist (Figure 13-2) to the teaching staff in the kindergarten class and ask if the behaviors on that checklist match their expectations for children entering their kindergarten. Get their ideas for individualizing the lists and make the indicated modifications to the two instruments. Then give each program a modified instrument.

Review Questions

1. Compare similarities and differences in the three important transitions in early childhood: hospital to home and infant services, infant program to preschool, preschool to kindergarten.
2. Describe the four issues that parents of premature infants face when they bring their infant home from the hospital.
3. Describe the transition process as developed and demonstrated in the Preschool Preparation and Transition (PPT) program.
4. Describe the transition process as developed and demonstrated in Project TEEM (Transitioning into the Elementary Education Mainstream).
5. List and discuss the 12 steps in the transition process.
6. Explain the rationale for identifying skills that have the potential to promote participation and success in the next education environment and discuss how knowing survival skills can smooth the transition process.
7. Describe procedures (other than teaching survival skills) that sending teachers can undertake to make transition to a new program smoother.
8. Discuss differences between programs that can cause problems in the transition process.

References

ABLE-BOONE, H., SANDALL, S. R., LOUGHRY, A., & FREDERICK, L. L. (1990). An informed, family-centered approach to Public Law 99-457: Parental views. *Topics in Early Childhood Special Education, 10*(1), 100–111.

AINSWORTH, M. D. S., & BELL, S. M. (1970). Attachment, exploration, and separation: Illustrated by the behavior of one-year-olds in a strange situation. *Child Development, 41,* 49–67.

ALBERTO, P., JOBES, N., SIZEMORE, A., & DORAN, D. (1980). A comparison of individual and group instruction across response tasks. *Journal of the Association for Persons with Severe Handicaps, 5,* 285–293.

ALEXANDER, R. (1990). Oral-motor and respiratory-phonatory assessment. In E. D. Gibbs & D. M. Teti (Eds.), *Interdisciplinary assessment of infants* (pp. 63–90). Baltimore, MD: Brookes.

ALS, H., LESTER, B. M., & BRAZELTON, T. B. (1979). Dynamics of the behavioral organization of the premature infant. In T. M. Field, A. M. Sostek, S. Goldberg, & H. H. Shuman (Eds.), *Infants born at risk* (pp. 173–192). New York: Spectrum.

AMERICAN ACADEMY OF PEDIATRICS. (1982). *Report on the committee on infectious diseases.* Elk Grove Village, IL: Author.

ANDERSON, L. W. (1976). An empirical investigation of individual differences in time to learn. *Journal of Educational Psychology, 68,* 226–233.

ANDERSON, S. R., & SPRADLIN, J. E. (1980). The generalized effects of productive labeling training involving common object classes. *Journal of the Association for the Severely Handicapped, 5,* 143–157.

ANDERSON-INMAN, L., PAINE, S. C., & DEUTCHMAN, L. (1984). Neatness counts: Effects of direct instruction and self-monitoring on the transfer of neat-paper skills to non-training settings. *Analysis and Intervention in Developmental Disabilities, 4,* 137–155.

APOLLONI, T., & COOKE, T. P. (1978). Integrated programming at the infant, toddler, and preschool levels. In M. J. Guralnick (Ed.), *Early intervention and the integration of handicapped and nonhandicapped children* (pp. 147–166). Baltimore: University Park Press.

APOLLONI, T., COOKE, S. A., & COOKE, T. P. (1977). Establishing a normal peer as behavioral model for developmentally delayed toddlers. *Perceptual and Motor Skills, 44,* 231–241.

ASHER, S. R., SINGLETON, L. C., TINSLEY, B. R., & HYMEL, S. (1979). The reliability of a rating scale sociometric method with preschool children. *Developmental Psychology, 15,* 443–444.

AYLLON, T., & AZRIN, N. (1968). *The token economy: A motivational system for therapy and rehabilitation.* New York: Appleton-Century-Crofts.

AZRIN, N. H., & BESALEL, V. A. (1979). *A parent's guide to bedwetting control: A step-by-step method.* New York: Simon & Schuster.

AZRIN, N. H., & FOXX, R. M. (1974). *Toilet training in less than a day.* New York: Simon & Schuster.

AZRIN, N., & HOLZ, W. C. (1966). Punishment. In W. R. Honig (Ed.), *Operant behavior: Areas of research and application* (pp. 380–447). New Jersey: Prentice-Hall.

AZRIN, N. H., SNEED, T. J., & FOXX, R. M. (1973). Dry bed: A rapid method of eliminating bedwetting (enuresis) of the retarded. *Behavior Research and Therapy, 11,* 427–434.

AZRIN, N. H., SNEED, T. J., & FOXX, R. M. (1974). Dry-bed training: Rapid elimination of childhood enuresis. *Behavior Research and Therapy, 12,* 147–156.

BAER, D. M. (1970). An age-irrelevant concept of development. *Merrill-Palmer Quarterly, 16,* 238–245.

BAER, D. M., & WOLF, M. M. (1970). The entry into natural communities of reinforcement. In R. Ulrich, T. Stachnik & M. Mabry (Eds.), *Control of human behavior* (Vol. 2) (pp. 319–324). Glenview, IL: Scott, Foresman.

BAGNATO, S., KONTOS, S., & NEISWORTH, J. (1987). Integrated day care as special education: Profiles of programs and children. *Topics in Early Childhood Special Education, 7*(1), 28–47.

BAGNATO, S. J., NEISWORTH, J. T., & CAPONE, A. (1986). Curriculum-based assessment for the young exceptional child: Rationale and review. *Topics in Early Childhood Special Education, 6*(2), 97–110.

BAILEY, D. B. (1984). A triaxial model of the interdisciplinary team and group process. *Exceptional Children, 51,* 17–25.

BAILEY, D. B. (1984). *Teaching infants and preschoolers with handicaps.* Columbus, OH: Merrill.

BAILEY, D. B. (1987). Collaborative goal setting with families: Resolving differences in values and priorities for services. *Topics in Early Childhood Special Education, 7*(2), 59–71.

BAILEY, D. B. (1989). Assessment and its importance in early intervention. In D. B. Bailey & M. Wolery (Eds.), *Assessing infants and preschoolers with handicaps* (pp. 1–22). Columbus, OH: Merrill.

BAILEY, D. B. (1989). Case management in early intervention. *Journal of Early Intervention, 13*(2), 120–134.

BAILEY, D. B., & BROCHIN, H. A. (1989). Tests and test development. In D. B. Bailey & M. Wolery (Eds.), *Assessing infants and preschoolers with handicaps* (pp. 22–46). Columbus: Merrill.

BAILEY, D. B., CLIFFORD, R. M., & HARMS, T. (1982). Comparison of preschool environments for handicapped and nonhandicapped preschoolers. *Topics in Early Childhood Special Education, 2*(1), 9–20.

BAILEY, D. B., HARMS, T., & CLIFFORD, R. M. (1983). Matching changes in preschool environments to desired changes in child behavior. *Journal of the Division for Early Childhood, 7,* 61–68.

BAILEY, D. B., JENS, K. G., & JOHNSON, N. (1983). Curricula for handicapped infants. In S. G. Garwood & R. R. Fewell (Eds.), *Educating handicapped infants: Issues in development and intervention* (pp. 387–415). Rockville, MD: Aspen.

BAILEY, D. B., & McWILLIAM, R. A. (1990). Normalizing early intervention. *Topics in Early Childhood Special Education, 10,* 33–47.

BAILEY, D. B., & WOLERY, M. (1984). *Teaching infants and preschoolers with handicaps.* Columbus, OH: Merrill.

BAILEY, D. B., & WOLERY, M. (1989). *Assessing infants and preschoolers with handicaps.* Columbus: Merrill.

BAINE, D. (1982). *Instructional design for special education.* Englewood Cliffs, NJ: Educational Technology Publications.

BALTHAZAR, E. E. (1976). *Balthazar Scales of Adaptive Behavior, I.* Palo Alto, CA: Consulting Psychologists Press.

BANDURA, A. (1969). *Principles of behavior modification.* New York: Holt, Rinehart, and Winston.

BANDURA, A. (1986). *Social foundations of thought and action: A social cognitive theory.* Englewood Cliffs, NJ: Prentice-Hall.

BARNES, M. R., CRUTCHFIELD, C. A., & HEZRA, C. B. (1978). *The neurological basis of patient treatment—Vol. II: Reflexes in motor development.* Atlanta: Stokesville.

BAYLEY, N. (1969). *Bayley scales of infant development.* New York: Psychological Corp.

BECKER, W., ENGELMANN, S., & THOMAS, D. (1975). *Teaching 2: Cognitive learning and instruction.* Chicago: Science Research Associates.

BECKMAN, P. J., & BRISTOL, M. M. (1991). Issues in developing the IFSP: A framework for establishing family outcomes. *Topics in Early Childhood Special Education, 11*(3), 19–31.

BECKMAN, P. J., & KOHL, F. L. (1984). The effects of social and isolate toys on the interactions and play of integrated and nonintegrated groups of preschoolers. *Education and Training of the Mentally Retarded, 19,* 169–174.

BECKMAN, P. J., ROBINSON, C. C., JACKSON, B., & ROSENBERG, S. A. (1986). Translating developmental findings into teaching strategies for young handicapped children. *Journal of the Division for Early Childhood, 10,* 45–52.

BENNER, S. M. (1992). *Assessing young children with special needs.* New York: Longman.

BENNETT, T., LINGERFELT, B. V., & NELSON, D. E. (1990). *Developing individualized family support plans.* Cambridge, MA: Brookline.

BEREITER, C., & ENGELMANN, S. (1966). *Teaching disadvantaged children in the preschool.* Englewood Cliffs, NJ: Prentice-Hall.

BERGEN, A. F., & COLANGELO, C. (1982). *Positioning the client with central nervous system deficits: The wheelchair and other adapted equipment.* Valhalla, NY: Valhalla Rehabilitation Publications, Ltd.

BERKELEY, T. R., & LUDLOW, B. L. (1989). Toward a reconceptualization of the developmental model. *Topics in Early Childhood Special Education, 9*(3), 51–66.

BERNSTEIN, B. (Ed.) (1989). *Day by day: 300 calendar-related activities, crafts, and bulletin boards for the elementary grades.* Carthage, IL: Fearon.

BLANK, M., ROSE, S., & BERLIN, L. (1978). *Preschool Language Assessment Instrument.* New York: Grune & Stratton.

BLECK, E. E., & NAGEL, D. A. (1983). *Physically handicapped children: A medical atlas for teachers* (2nd ed.). New York: Grune & Stratton.

BLOOM, B. (1964). *Stability and change in human characteristics.* New York: Wiley.

BLUMA, S. M., SHEARER, M. S., FROHMAN, D., & HILLARD, J. M. (1976). *Portage Guide to Early Education.* Portage, WI: The Portage Project.

BLY, L. (1983). *The components of normal movement during the first year of life and abnormal motor development.* Chicago: Neurodevelopmental Treatment Association.

BOBATH, B. (1967). The very early treatment of cerebral palsy. *Developmental Medicine and Child Neurology, 9,* 373–390.

BOBATH, K., & BOBATH, B. (1972). Cerebral palsy. In P. H. Pearson & C. E. Williams (Eds.), *Physical therapy services in the developmental disabilities* (pp. 31–185). Springfield, IL: Charles C Thomas.

BOEHM, A. (1986). *Boehm Test of Basic Concepts.* New York: The Psychological Corp.

BRACKEN, B. A. (1986). *Bracken Concept Development Series.* New York: The Psychological Corp.

BRAZELTON, T. B. (1973). *Neonatal behavioral assessment scale.* (Clinics in Developmental Medicine No. 50). Philadelphia: Lippincott.

BRAZELTON, T. B. (1982). Early intervention: What does it mean? In H. E. Fitzgerald, B. M. Lester, & M. W. Yogman (Eds.), *Theory and research in behavioral pediatrics* (Vol. 1) (pp. 1–34). New York: Plenum.

BRAZELTON, T. B. (1984). *Neonatal behavioral assessment scale* (2nd ed.) (Clinics in Developmental Medicine No. 88). Philadelphia: Lippincott.

BREDEKAMP, S. (Ed.). (1987). *Developmentally appropriate practice in early childhood programs serving children from birth through age 8.* Washington, D.C.: NAEYC.

BREDEKAMP, S., & SHEPARD, L. (1989). How best to protect children from inappropriate school expectations, practices, and policies. *Young Children, 44,* 14–42.

BRICKER, D. (1978). A rationale for the integration of handicapped and nonhandicapped children. In M. F. Guralnick (Ed.), *Early intervention and the integration of handicapped and nonhandicapped children* (pp. 3–26). Baltimore: University Park Press.

BRICKER, D. (1989). *Early intervention for at-risk and handicapped infants, toddlers, and preschool children* (2nd ed.). Palo Alto, CA: VORT.

BRICKER, D., & BRICKER, W. (1971). *Toddler research and intervention project report: Year I* (IMRID Behavioral Science Monograph No. 20). Nashville, TN: Institute on Mental Retardation and Intellectual Development, George Peabody College.

BRICKER, D. D., & BRICKER, W. A. (1973). *Infant, toddler, and preschool research and intervention project report: Year III* (IMRID Behavioral Science Monograph No. 23). Nashville, TN: Institute on Mental Retardation and Intellectual Development, George Peabody College.

BRICKER, D. D., BRUDER, M. B., & BAILEY, D. B.(1982). Developmental integration of preschool children. *Analysis and Intervention in Developmental Disabilities, 2,* 207–222.

BRICKER, D. & CRIPE, J. J. (1992). *An activity-based approach to early intervention.* Baltimore: Brookes.

BRICKER, D., CRIPE, J., & NORSTAD, S. (1990, October). *Activity-based intervention.* Paper presented at Post Conference Workshop, Council for Exceptional Children Conference, Albuquerque, New Mexico.

BRICKER, W. A., & BRICKER, D. D. (1976). The infant, toddler, and research and intervention project. In T. D. Tjossem (Ed.), *Intervention strategies for high-risk infants and young children* (pp. 545–572). Baltimore: University Park Press.

BRIGANCE, A. H. (1978). *Brigance Diagnostic Inventory of Early Development.* Woburn, MA: Curriculum Associates.

BRINCKERHOFF, J. L., & VINCENT, L. J. (1986). Increasing parental decision-making at the individualized educational program meeting. *Journal of the Division for Early Childhood,* 11, 46–58.

BROWDER, D., DEMCHACK, M. A., HELLER, M., & KING, D. (1989). An in vivo evaluation of the use of data-based rules to guide instructional decisions. *Journal of the Association for Persons with Severe Handicaps, 14,* 234–240.

BROWN, F., & HOLVOET, J. (1982). Effects of systematic peer interaction on the incidental learning of two severely handicapped students. *Journal of the Association for Persons with Severe Handicaps, 7*(4), 19–28.

BROWN, F., HOLVOET, J., GUESS, D., & MULLIGAN, M. (1980). The individualized curriculum sequencing model (III): Small group instruction. *Journal of the Association for the Severely Handicapped, 5*(4), 352–367.

BROWN, L., NIETUPSKI, J., HAMRE-NIETUPSKI, S. (1976). The criterion of ultimate functioning. In M. A. Thomas (Ed.), *Hey, don't forget about me!* (pp. 2–15). Reston, VA: Council for Exceptional Children.

BROWN, W. H., McEVOY, M. A., & BISHOP, N. (1991). Incidental teaching of social behavior. *Teaching Exceptional Children, 24*(1), 35–38.

BROWN, W. H., RAGLAND, E. V., & FOX, J. J. (1988). Effects of group socialization procedures on the social interactions of preschool children. *Research in Developmental Disabilities, 9,* 359–376.

BRUDER, M. B., DEINER, P., & SACHS, S. (1990). Models of integration through early intervention/child care collaborations. *Zero to Three, X*(3), 14–17.

BRUDER, M. B., & WALKER, L. (1990). Discharge planning: Hospital to home transitions for infants. *Topics in Early Childhood Special Education, 9*(4), 26–42.

BRUNER, J. (1975). The ontogenesis of speech acts. *Journal of Child Language. 2,* 1–19.

BRUNER, J. (1977). Early social interaction and language acquisition. In H. Schaffer (Ed.), *Studies in mother-infant interaction* (pp. 271–289). New York: Academic Press.

BZOCH, K., & LEAGUE, R. (1971). *Receptive-Expressive Emergent Language Scale.* Baltimore: University Park Press.

CALDWELL, B. M., & BRADLEY, R. H. (1972). *Home observation and measurement of the environment inventory.* Center for Child Development and Education, University of Arkansas at Little Rock, 33rd and University Avenues, Little Rock, AR 72204.

CALIFORNIA STATE DEPARTMENT OF EDUCATION. (1980). *Guidelines and procedures for meeting the specialized health care needs of students.* Sacramento: California State Department of Education.

CAMPBELL, P. H. (1987). Programming for students with dysfunction in posture and movement. In M. E. Snell (Ed.), *Systematic instruction of persons with severe handicaps* (3rd ed.; pp. 174–211). Columbus, OH: Merrill.

CAMPBELL, P. H. (1989). Students with physical disabilities. In R. Gaylord-Ross (Ed.). *Integration strategies for persons with handicaps* (pp. 53–76). Baltimore, MD: Brookes.

CAMPBELL, P. H., & STEWART, B. (1986). Measuring changes in movement skills with infants and young children with handicaps. *Journal of the Association of Persons with Severe Handicaps, 11*(3), 153–161.

CAPUTE, A. J., ACCARDO, P. J., VINING, E. P., RUBENSTEIN, J. E., WALCHER, J. R., HARRYMAN, S., & ROSS, A. (1978). Primitive reflex profile. *Physical Therapy, 58,* 1061–1065.

CAREY, W. B., & McDEVITT, S. C. (1978). Revision of the Infant Temperament Questionnaire. *Pediatrics, 61*(5), 735–738.

CARR, E. G., & DURAND, V. M. (1985). Reducing behavior problems through functional communication training. *Journal of Applied Behavior Analysis, 18,* 111–126.

CARTA, J. J., ATWATER, J. B., SCHWARTZ, I. S., & MILLER, P. A. (1990). Applications of ecobehavioral analysis to the study of transitions across early education settings. *Education and Treatment of Children, 13,* 298–315.

CARTA, J. J., SCHWARTZ, I. S., ATWATER, J. B., & McCONNELL, S. R. (1991). Developmentally appropriate practice: Appraising its usefulness for young children with disabilities. *Topics in Early Childhood Special Education, 11*(1), 1–20.

CAVALLARO, C. C., & POULSON, C. L. (1985). Teaching language to handicapped children in natural settings. *Education and Treatment of Children, 8,* 1–24.

CHANDLER, L., ANDREWS, M., & SWANSON, M. (1981). *The Movement Assessment of Infants.* Rolling Bay, WA: Infant Movement Research.

CHESS, S., & THOMAS, A. (1986). *Temperament in clinical practice.* New York: The Guilford Press.

CHRISTOPHERSEN, E. R. (1988). *Little people: Guidelines for common sense child rearing* (3rd ed.). Kansas City, MO: Westport.

CLARK, P. N., & ALLEN, A. S. (1985). *Occupational therapy for children.* St. Louis: Mosby.

COLLINS, B. C., GAST, D. L., AULT, M. J., & WOLERY, M. (1991). Small group instruction: Guidelines for teachers of students with moderate to severe handicaps. *Education and Training in Mental Retardation, 26,* 18–32.

CONN-POWERS, M. C., ROSS-ALLEN, J., & HOLBURN, S. (1990). Transition of young children in the elementary education mainstream. *Topics in Early Childhood Special Education, 9*(4), 91–105.

COPELAND, M. E., & KIMMEL, J. R. (1989). *Evaluation and management of infants and young children with developmental disabilities.* Baltimore: Brookes.

CORSARO, W. A. (1979). "We're friends, right?": Children's use of access rituals in a nursery school. *Language in Society, 8,* 315–336.

CORSARO, W. A. (1981). Friendship in the nursery school: Social organization in a peer environment. In S. R. Ahser & J. M. Gottman (Eds.), *The development of children's friendships* (pp. 207–241). New York: Cambridge University Press.

CSAPO, M. (1981). Comparison of two prompting procedures to increase response fluency among severely handicapped learners. *Journal of the Association for the Severely Handicapped, 6*(1), 39–47.

CULATTA, B., & HORN, D. (1981). Systematic modification of parental input to train language symbols. *Language, Speech, and Hearing Services in the Schools, 12,* 4–12.

DANILOFF, J., NOLL, J., FRISTOE, M., & LLOYD, L. (1982). Gesture recognition in patients with aphasia. *Journal of Speech and Hearing Disorders, 47,* 43–49.

DAY, H. M. (1987). Comparison of two prompting procedures to facilitate skill acquisition among severely mentally retarded adolescents. *American Journal of Mental Deficiency, 91,* 366–372.

DEAL, A. G., DUNST, C. J., & TRIVETTE, C. M. (1989). A flexible and functional approach to developing Individualized Family Service Plans. *Infants and Young Children, 1*(4), 32–43.

DEC COMMUNICATOR. (1991, May/June). Developmental delay: Questions and answers. *Newsletter of the Division for Early Childhood of CEC,* Vol. 17, No. 4.

DEKLYEN, M., & ODOM, S. L. (1989). Activity structure and social interactions with peers in developmentally integrated play groups. *Journal of Early Intervention, 13*(4), 342–352.

DIAMOND, K. E., SPIEGEL-MCGILL, P., & HANRAHAN, P. (1988). Planning for school transition: An ecological-developmental approach. *Journal of the Division of Early Childhood, 12,* 245–252.

DODGE, D. T., & COLKER, L. J. (1992). *The creative curriculum for early childhood.* Washington, DC: Teaching Strategies.

DOUGHTY, P. (1985). *The coordination of handicap services in Head Start.* Chapel Hill, NC: University of North Carolina, Chapel Hill Outreach Training Project.

DUNST, C. J. (1980). *A clinical and educational manual for use with the Uzgiris and Hunt Scales of Infant Psychological Development.* Austin, TX: pro-ed.

DUNST, C. J. (1981). *Infant learning.* Allen, TX: DLM/Teaching Resources.

DUNST, C. J., COOPER, C. S., WEELDREYER, J. C., SNYDER, K. D., & CHASE, J. H. (1988). Family

Needs Scale. In C. J. Dunst, C. M. Trivette, and A. G. Deal (Eds.), *Enabling and empowering families: Principles and guidelines for practice* (pp. 149–151). Cambridge, MA: Brookline.

DUNST, C. J., CUSHING, P. J., & VANCE, S. D. (1985). Response-contingent learning in profoundly handicapped infants: A social systems perspective. *Analysis and Intervention in Developmental Disabilities, 5,* 33–47.

DUNST, C. J., JOHANSON, C., TRIVETTE, C. M., & HAMBY, D. (1991). Family-oriented early intervention policies and practices: Family-centered or not? *Exceptional Children, 58*(2), 115–126.

DUNST, C. J., LESKO, J. J., HOLBERT, K. A., WILSON, L. L., SHARPE, K. L., & LILES, R. F. (1987). A systematic approach to infant intervention. *Topics in Early Childhood Special Education, 7*(2), 19–37.

DUNST, C. J., & McWILLIAM, R. A. (1988). Cognitive assessment of multiply handicapped young children. In T. Wachs & R. Sheehan (Eds.), *Assessment of developmentally disabled children* (pp. 105–130). New York: Plenum.

DUNST, C. J., & TRIVETTE, C. M. (1985). *A guide to measures of social support and family behavior* (Monograph of Technical Assistance Development System, No. 1). Chapel Hill, NC: TADS.

DUNST, C. J., & TRIVETTE, C. M. (1987). Enabling and empowering families: Conceptual and intervention issues. *School Psychology Review, 16,* 443–456.

DUNST, C. J., & TRIVETTE, C. M. (1988). A family systems model of early intervention with handicapped and developmentally at-risk children. In D. P. Powell (Ed.), *Parent education and support programs: Consequences for children and families* (pp. 131–179). Norwood, NJ: Ablex.

DUNST, C. J., & TRIVETTE, C. M. (1989). An enablement and empowerment perspective of case management. *Topics in Early Childhood Special Education, 8*(4), 87–102.

DUNST, C. J., TRIVETTE, C. M., & DEAL, A. G. (1988). *Enabling and empowering families: Principles and guidelines for practice.* Cambridge, MA: Brookline.

DYKES, M. K., & VENN, J. (1983). Using health, physical, and medical data in the classroom. In J. Umbreit (Ed.), *Physical disabilities and health impairments* (pp. 259–280). Columbus, OH: Merrill.

ECKERMAN, C. O., & WHATLEY, J. L. (1977). Toys and social interaction between infant peers. *Child Development, 48,* 1645–1656.

EDGAR, E. (1988). Policy factors influencing research in early childhood special education. In S. L. Odom & M. B. Karnes (Eds.), *Early intervention for infants and children with handicaps* (pp. 51–62). Baltimore: Brookes.

EDGAR, E., HEGGELUND, M., & FISCHER, M. (1989). A longitudinal study of graduates of special education preschools: Educational placement after preschool. *Topics in Early Childhood Special Education, 8*(3), 61–74.

EDGAR, E., McNULTY, B., GAETZ, J., & MADDOX, M. (1984). Educational placement of graduates of preschool programs for handicapped children. *Topics in Early Childhood Special Education, 4*(3), 19–29.

ESPOSITO, B. G., & KOORLAND, M. A. (1989). Play behavior of hearing impaired children: Integrated and segregated settings. *Exceptional Children, 55,* 412–419.

ETZEL, B. C., & LEBLANC, J. M. (1979). The simplest treatment alternative: Appropriate instructional control and errorless learning procedures for the difficult-to-teach child. *Journal of Autism and Developmental Disorders, 9,* 361–382.

FALVEY, M. A. (1989). *Community-based curriculum: Instructional strategies for students with severe handicaps* (2nd ed.). Baltimore, MD: Brookes.

FALVEY, M., BROWN, L., LYON, S., BAUMGART, D., & SCHROEDER, J. (1980). Strategies for using cues and correction procedures. In W. Sailor, B. Wilcox, & L. Brown (Eds.), *Methods of instruction for severely handicapped students* (pp. 109–133). Baltimore, MD: Brookes.

FARBER, S. D. (1982). *Neurorehabilitation—A multisensory approach.* Philadelphia: Saunders.

FARRAN, D. C., CLARK, K. S., & RAY, A. R. (1990). Measures of parent-child interaction. In E. D. Gibbs & D. M. Teti (Eds.), *Interdisciplinary assessment of infants* (pp. 227–248). Baltimore, MD: Brookes.

FAW, G. D., REID, D. H., SCHEPIS, M. M., FITZGERALD, J. R., & WELTY, P. A. (1981). Involving institutional staff in the development and maintenance of sign language skills with profoundly retarded persons. *Journal of Applied Behavior Analysis, 14,* 411–423.

FEDERAL REGISTER, Nov. 18, 1987, p. 44355.

FERSTER, C. B., CULBERTSON, S., & BOREN, M. C. P. (1975). *Behavior principles* (2nd ed.). Englewood Cliffs, NJ: Prentice-Hall.

FEWELL, R. (1986). The measurement of family functioning. In L. Bickman & D. L. Weatherford (Eds.), *Evaluating early intervention programs for severely handicapped children and their families* (pp. 263–307). Austin, TX: pro-ed.

FEY, M. (1986). *Language intervention with young children.* San Diego, CA: College-Hill Press.

FINK, W. T., & SANDALL, S. R. (1978). One-to-one versus group academic instruction with handicapped and nonhandicapped preschool children. *Mental Retardation, 16,* 236–240.

FIORENTINO, M. R. (1973). *Reflex testing methods for evaluating central nervous system development* (2nd ed.). Springfield, IL: Charles C Thomas.

FOLEY, G. M. (1990). Portrait of the arena evaluation: Assessment in the transdisciplinary approach. In E. D. Gibbs & D. M. Teti (Eds.), *Interdisciplinary assessment of infants* (pp. 271–286). Baltimore: Brookes.

FOLIO, M. R., & FEWELL, R. R. (1983). *Peabody Developmental Motor Scales and Activity Cards.* Allen, TX: Developmental Learning Materials.

FORD, F. (1975). Normal development in infancy. In E. E. Bleck & D. A. Nagel (Eds.), *Physically handicapped children: A medical atlas for teachers* (pp. 161–172). New York: Grune & Stratton.

FOSTER, G., SCHMIDT, C., & SABATINO, D. (1976). Teacher expectancies and the label "learning disabilities." *Journal of Learning Disabilities, 9,* 58–61.

FOSTER, G., YSSELDYKE, J., & REESE, J. (1974). I wouldn't have seen it if I hadn't believed. *Exceptional Children, 41,* 469–473.

FOWLER, S. A., CHANDLER, L. K., JOHNSON, T. E., & STELLA, M. E. (1988). Individualized family involvement in school transitions: Gathering information and choosing the next program. *Journal of the Division for Early Childhood, 12,* 208–216.

FOWLER, S. A., SCHWARTZ, I., AND ATWATER, J. (1991). Perspectives on the transition from preschool to kindergarten for children with disabilities and their families. *Exceptional Children, 58*(2), 136–145.

FOXX, R. M., & AZRIN, N. H. (1973). *Toilet training the retarded: A rapid program for day and nighttime independent toileting.* Champaign, IL: Research Press.

FRASER, B. A., & HENSINGER, R. N. (1983). *Managing physical handicaps—A practical guide for parents, care providers, and educators.* Baltimore: Brookes.

FULLARD, W., McDEVITT, S. C., & CAREY, W. B. (1978). *Toddler Temperament Scale.* Unpublished Manuscript.

FURMAN, W., RAHE, D., & HARTUP, W. (1979). Rehabilitation of socially withdrawn preschool children through mixed-age and same-age socialization. *Child Development, 50*(4), 915–922.

FURUNO, S., O'REILLY, K. A., HOSAKA, C. M., INATSUKA, T. T., ALLMAN, T. L., & ZEISLOFT, B. (1979). Hawaii Early Learning Profile. Palo Alto, CA: VORT.

GACKOWSKI, C. R., KOBE, K., & McCORMICK, L. (1991). *Cooperative learning: A means to enhance the social interactions of preschoolers with special needs and typically developing peers.* Unpublished manuscript, University of Hawaii, Department of Special Education, Honolulu.

GARLAND, C., WOODRUFF, G., & BUCK, D. M. (June, 1988). *Case management* (Division for Early Childhood White Paper). Reston, VA: Council for Exceptional Children.

GARWOOD, G. (1982). (Mis)use of developmental scales in program evaluation. *Topics in Early Childhood Special Education, 1*(4), 61–69.

GAUSSIN, T. (1984). Developmental milestones or conceptual milestones? Some practical and theoretical limitations in infant assessment procedures. *Child: Care, Health and Development, 10,* 99–115.

GESELL, A., & AMATRUDA, C. S. (1947). *Developmental diagnosis.* New York: Paul B. Holder.

GIBBS, E. D., & TETI, D. M. (Eds.) (1990). *Interdisciplinary assessment of infants.* Baltimore, MD: Brookes.

GILLIAM, J., & COLEMAN, M. (1981). Who influences IEP committee decisions. *Exceptional Children, 47,* 642–644.

GLENDENNING, N. J., ADAMS, G. L., & STERNBERG, L. (1983). Comparison of prompt sequences. *American Journal of Mental Deficiency, 88,* 321–325.

GLOVER, M. E., PREMINGER, J. L., & SANFORD, A. R. (1978). *The Early Learning Accomplishment Profile for Developmentally Young Children.* Winston-Salem, NC: Kaplan.

GOETZ, L., GEE, K., & SAILOR, W. (1985). Using a behavior chain interruption strategy to teach communication skills to students with severe disabilities. *Journal of the Association for Persons with Severe Handicaps, 10,* 21–30.

GOETZ, L., SCHULER, A., & SAILOR, W. (1983). Motivational considerations in teaching language to students with severe handicaps. In M. Hersen, V. Van Hasselt, & J. Matson (Eds.), *Behavior therapy for the developmentally and physically disabled* (pp. 55–77). New York: Academic Press.

GOLD, M. W. (1980). *Try another way. Training manual.* Champaign, IL: Research Press.

GOLDFARB, W. (1945). Psychological deprivation in infancy and subsequent adjustment. *American Journal of Orthopsychiatry, 15,* 247–255.

GOLDFARB, W. (1949). Rorschach test differences between family-reared, institution-reared, and schizophrenic children. *American Journal of Orthopsychiatry, 19,* 624–633.

GOLDFARB, W. (1955). Emotional and intellectual consequences of psychologic deprivation in infancy: A re-evaluation. In P. H. Hoch & J. Zubin (Eds.), *Psychopathology of childhood.* New York: Grune & Stratton.

GOODENOUGH, F., & MAURER, K. (1961). The relative potency of the nursery school and the statistical laboratory in boosting I.Q. In J. Jenkins & D. Paterson (Eds.), *Studies in individual differences.* New York: Appleton-Century-Crofts.

GRAYSON, M. F. (1962). *Let's do fingerplays.* Bridgeport, CT: Luce.

GUESS, D. (1988). Problems and issues pertaining to the transmission of behavior management technologies from researchers to practitioners. In R. H. Horner & G. Dunlap (Eds.), *Behavior management and community integration for individuals with developmental disabilities and severe behavior problems* (pp. 19–46). Eugene: Specialized Training Program, University of Oregon.

Guess, D., Horner, D., Utley, B., Holvoet, J., Maxon, D., Tucker, D., & Warren, S. (1978). A functional curriculum sequencing model for teaching the severely handicapped. *AAESPH Review, 3,* 202–215.

Guess, D., & Noonan, M. J. (1982). Curricula and instructional procedures for severely handicapped students. *Focus on Exceptional Children, 14*(5), 1–12.

Guralnick, M. (1988). Efficacy research in early childhood intervention programs. In S. L. Odom & M. B. Karnes (Eds.), *Early intervention for infants and children with handicaps: An empirical base* (pp. 75–88). Baltimore: Brookes.

Guralnick, M. (1989). Recent developments in early intervention efficacy research: Implications for family involvement in P. L. 99-457. *Topics in Early Childhood Special Education, 9*(3), 1–17.

Guralnick, M. J. (1978). *Early intervention and the integration of handicapped and nonhandicapped children.* Baltimore: University Park Press.

Guralnick, M. J. (1981). The efficacy of integrating handicapped children in early education settings: Research implications. *Topics in Early Childhood Education, 1,* 57–71.

Guralnick, M. J. (1984). The peer interactions of young developmentally delayed children in specialized and integrated settings. In T. Field, J. Roopnarine, Y. M. Segal (Eds.), *Friendships in normal and handicapped children* (pp. 139–152). Norwood, NJ: Ablex.

Guralnick, M. J. (1990a). Major accomplishments and future directions in early childhood mainstreaming. *Topics in Early Childhood Special Education, 10*(2), 1–17.

Guralnick, M. J. (1990b). Social competence and early intervention. *Journal of Early Intervention, 14*(1), 3–14.

Guralnick, M. J., & Groom, J. M. (1985). Correlates of peer-related social competence of developmentally delayed preschool children. *American Journal of Mental Deficiency, 90,* 140–150.

Guralnick, M. J., & Groom, J. M. (1987). The peer relations of mildly delayed and nonhandicapped preschool children in mainstreamed playgroups. *Child Development, 58,* 1556–1572.

Guralnick, M. J., & Groom, J. M. (1988). Peer interactions in mainstreamed and specialized classrooms: A comparative analysis. *Exceptional Children, 5,* 415–425.

Guralnick, M. J., & Weinhouse, E. M. (1984). Peer-related social interactions of developmentally delayed children: Development and characteristics. *Developmental Psychology, 20,* 815–827.

Hafen, B. Q., & Karren, K. J. (1984). *First aid and emergency care workbook* (3rd ed. with 1986 respiratory and CPR standards). Englewood, CO: Morton.

Hains, A. H., Fowler, S. A., Schwartz, I. S., Kottwitz, E., & Rosenkoetter, S. (1989). A comparison of preschool and kindergarten expectations for school readiness. *Early Childhood Research Quarterly, 4,* 75–88.

Haley, S. M., Hallenborg, S. C., & Gans, B. M. (1989). Functional assessment in young children with neurological impairments. *Topics in Early Childhood Special Education, 9*(1), 106–126.

Halle, J. (1982). Teaching functional language to the handicapped: An integrative model of natural environment teaching techniques. *Journal of the Association for the Severely Handicapped, 7*(4), 29–37.

Halle, J. W., Alpert, C., & Anderson, S. (1984). Natural environment language assessment and intervention with severely impaired preschoolers. *Topics in Early Childhood Special Education, 4,* 1–14.

Halle, J. W., Baer, D., & Spradlin, J. E. (1981). Teachers' generalized use of delay as a stimulus control procedure to increase language use in handicapped children. *Journal of Applied Behavior Analysis, 14*, 389–411.

HANLINE, M. F., & DEPPE, J. (1990). Discharging the premature infant: Family issues and implications for intervention. *Topics in Early Childhood Special Education, 9*(4), 15–25.

HANLINE, M. F., & HANSON, M. J. (1989). Integration considerations for infants and toddlers with multiple disabilities. *Journal of the Association for Persons with Severe Handicaps, 14*, 178–183.

HANSON, M. J. (1984). Parent-infant interaction. In M. J. Hanson (Ed.), *Atypical infant development* (pp. 361–384). Baltimore, MD: University Park Press.

HANSON, M. J. (1987). *Teaching the infant with Down syndrome: A guide for parents and professionals* (2nd ed.). Austin, TX: pro-ed.

HANSON, M. J., & LYNCH, E. W. (1989). *Early intervention: Implementing child and family services for infants and toddlers who are at-risk or disabled.* Austin, TX: pro-ed.

HANSON, M. J., LYNCH, E. W., & WAYMAN, L. I. (1990). Honoring the cultural diversity of families when gathering data. *Topics in Early Childhood Special Education, 10*(1), 112–131.

HARBIN, G., DANAHER, J., BAILEY, D., & ELLER, S. (1991). *Status of states' eligibility policy for preschool children with disabilities.* Chapel Hill: University of North Carolina, Carolina Policy Studies Program.

HARBIN, G. L., GALLAGHER, J. J., & TERRY, D. V. (1991). Defining the eligible population: Policy issues and challenges. *Journal of Early Intervention, 15*(1), 13–20.

HARING, N., LIBERTY, K., & WHITE, O. (1981). *Final report: Field initiated research studies of phases of learning and facilitating instructional events for the severely/profoundly handicapped.* (U. S. Department of Education, Contract No. G007500593.) Seattle: University of Washington, College of Education.

HARING, T. G., & LOVINGER, L. (1989). Promoting social interaction through teaching generalized play initiation responses to preschool children with autism. *Journal of the Association for Persons with Severe Handicaps, 14*(1), 58–67.

HART, B., & RISLEY, T. R. (1978). Establishing the use of descriptive adjectives in the spontaneous speech of disadvantaged preschool children. *Journal of Applied Behavior Analysis, 1*, 109–120.

HART, B., & RISLEY, T. R. (1980). In vivo language intervention: Unanticipated general effects. *Journal of Applied Behavior Analysis, 13*, 407–432.

HART, B., & ROGERS-WARREN, A. K. (1978). A milieu approach to teaching language. In R. L. Schiefelbusch (Ed.), *Language intervention strategies* (pp. 193–235). Baltimore: University Park Press.

HART, B. M. (1985). Naturalistic language training techniques. In S. F. Warren & A. K. Rogers-Warren (Eds.), *Teaching functional language* (pp. 63–88). Austin, TX: pro-ed.

HART, B. M., REYNOLDS, N. J., BAER, D. M., BRALEY, E. R., & HARRIS, F. (1968). Effect of contingent and non-contingent social reinforcement on the cooperative play of a preschool child. *Journal of Applied Behavior Analysis, 1*, 73–76.

HART, B. M., & RISLEY, T. R. (1974). Using preschool materials to modify the language of disadvantaged children. *Journal of Applied Behavior Analysis, 7*, 243–256.

HARTUP, W. W. (1983). Peer relations. In P. H. Mussen (Ed.), *Handbook of child psychology. Vol. 4: Socialization, personality, and social development.* New York: Wiley.

HAWAII STATE DEPARTMENT OF HEALTH. (1986). *Latest facts about AIDS: AIDS and children.* Honolulu, HI: Author.

HAYDEN, A. H., & HARING, N. G. (1976). Early intervention for high risk infants and young children: Programs for Down syndrome children. In T. D. Tojessem (Ed.), *Intervention strategies for high risk infants and young children* (pp. 573–607). Baltimore: University Park Press.

HEBBELER, K. M., SMITH, B. J., & BLACK, T. L. (1991). Federal early childhood special education policy: A model for the improvement of services for children with disabilities. *Exceptional Children, 58*(2), 104–111.

HELMSTETTER, E., & DURAND, V. M. (1991). Nonaversive interventions for severe behavior problems. In L. H. Meyer, C. A. Peck, & L. Brown (Eds.), *Critical issues in the lives of people with severe disabilities* (pp. 559–600). Baltimore: Brookes.

HOLLAND, J. G., & SKINNER, B. F. (1961). *The analysis of behavior.* New York: McGraw-Hill.

HOLVOET, J., GUESS, D., MULLIGAN, M., & BROWN, F. (1980). The individualized curriculum sequencing model (II): A teaching strategy for severely handicapped students. *Journal of the Association for the Severely Handicapped, 5,* 337–351.

HOLVOET, J., O'NEIL, C., CHAZDON, L., CARR, D., & WARNER, J. (1983). Hey, do we really have to take data? *Journal of the Association for the Severely Handicapped, 8*(3), 56–70.

HORNER, R. H., DUNLAP, G., KOEGEL, R. L., CARR, E. G., SAILOR, W., ANDERSON, J., ALBIN, R. W., & O'NEILL, R. E. (1990). Toward a technology of "nonaversive" behavioral support. *Journal of the Association for Persons with Severe Handicaps, 15,* 125–132.

HORNER, R. H., & MCDONALD, R. S. (1982). Comparison of single instance and general case instruction in teaching a generalized vocational skill. *Journal of the Association for the Severely Handicapped, 7*(3), 7–20.

HORNER, R. H., SPRAGUE, J., & WILCOX, B. (1982). General case programming for community activities. In B. Wilcox & G. T. Bellamy (Eds.), *Design of high school programs for severely handicapped students* (pp. 61–98). Baltimore: Brookes.

HORSTMEIER, D. S., & MACDONALD, J. D. (1978). *Environmental Prelanguage Battery.* Columbus: Merrill.

HUNT, J. M. (1961). *Intelligence and experience.* New York: Ronald Press.

HUNT, P., GOETZ, L., ALWELL, M., & SAILOR, W. (1986). Using an interrupted chain strategy to teach generalized communication responses. *Journal of the Association for Persons with Severe Handicaps, 11,* 196–204.

HUTCHINSON, D. (1974). *A model for transdisciplinary staff development. (A nationally organized collaborative project to provide comprehensive services for atypical infants and their families.* (Technical Report #8). New York: United Cerebral Palsy.

ILLINGWORTH, R. S. (1980). *The development of the infant and young child: Abnormal and normal* (7th ed.). New York: Churchill Livingstone.

IMMUNIZATION PRACTICES ADVISORY COMMITTEE. (1985). Recommendations for protection against viral hepatitis. *Morbidity and Mortality Weekly Report, 34,* 313–334.

INDIVIDUALS WITH DISABILITIES EDUCATION AMENDMENTS OF 1991. Final Report. 102 Congress. September 11, 1991.

INNOCENTI, M. S., RULE, S., KILLORAN, J., & STOWITSCHEK, J. J. (1983). *The let's be social home program.* Logan: Outreach, Development, and Dissemination Division, Utah State University Affiliated Developmental Center for Handicapped Persons.

IRETON, H., & THWING, E. (1980). *Minnesota Infant Development Inventory.* Minneapolis, MN: Behavior Science Systems, Inc.

JOHNSON, T. E., CHANDLER, L. K., KERNS, G. M., & FOWLER, S. A. (1986). What are parents saying about family involvement in school transitions: A retrospective transition interview. *Journal of the Division for Early Childhood, 11*(1), 10–17.

JOHNSON, D., & JOHNSON, R. (1975). *Learning together and alone: Cooperation, competition, and individualization.* Englewood Cliffs, NJ: Prentice-Hall.

JOHNSON, D., & JOHNSON, R. (1983). The socialization and achievement crisis: Are cooperative learning experiences the solution? In L. Bickman (Ed.), *Applied Psychology Annual 4* (pp. 159–164). Beverly Hills, CA: Sage.

JOHNSON, D., & JOHNSON, R. (1986). Mainstreaming and cooperative learning strategies. *Exceptional Children, 52*(6), 553–561.

JOHNSON, N. M., JENS, K. G., & ATTERMEIER, S. A. (1979). *Carolina curriculum for handicapped infants.* Chapel Hill: University of North Carolina, Frank Porter Graham Child Development Center.

JOHNSON, R., & JOHNSON, D. (1981). Building friendships between handicapped and nonhandicapped students: Effects of cooperative individualistic instruction. *American Education Research Journal, 18,* 415–423.

JOHNSON, R., & JOHNSON, D. (1982). Cooperation in learning: Ignored but powerful. *Lyceum, 5,* 22–26.

JOHNSON-MARTIN, N. M., ATTERMEIER, S. M., & HACKER, B. (1990). *The Carolina Curriculum for Preschoolers with Special Needs.* Baltimore: Brookes.

JOHNSON-MARTIN, N., JENS, K. G., & ATTERMEIER, S. M. (1986). *Carolina Curriculum for Handicapped Infants and Infants at Risk.* Baltimore: Brookes.

KAISER, A. P., & WARREN, S. F. (1988). Pragmatics and generalization. In R. L. Schiefelbusch (Ed.), *Language intervention strategies.* Baltimore: University Park Press.

KARNES, M. B. (1977). Exemplary early education programs for handicapped children: Characteristics in common. *Educational Horizons, 56*(1), 47–54.

KAUFMAN, A. F., & KAUFMAN, N. L. (1983). *Kaufman Assessment Battery for Children, Interpretive Manual.* Circle Pines, MN: American Guidance Service.

KAYSER, J. E., BILLINGSLEY, F. F., & NEEL, R. S. (1986). A comparison of in-context and traditional instructional approaches: Total task, single trial versus backward chaining, multiple trials. *Journal of the Association for Persons with Severe Handicaps, 11,* 28–38.

KEOGH, B. K., & SHEEHAN, R. (1981). The use of developmental test data for documenting handicapped children's progress: Problems and recommendations. *Journal of the Division for Early Childhood, 3,* 42–47.

KILGO, J. L., RICHARD, N., & NOONAN, M. J. (1989). Teaming for the future: Integrating transition planning with early intervention services for young children with special needs and their families. *Infants and Young Children, 2*(2), 37–48.

KINGORE, B. W., & HIGBEE, G. M. (1988). *We care: A preschool curriculum for children ages 2–5.* Glenville, IL: Scott, Foresman.

KIRK, S. (1958). *Early education of the mentally retarded.* Urbana: University of Illinois Press.

KLIEWER, D., BRUCE, W., & TREMBATH, J. (1977). *The Milani-Comparetti motor development screening test.* Omaha, NE: Meyer Children's Rehabilitation Institute.

KNOBLOCH, H., STEVENS, F., & MALONE, A.F. (1980). *Manual of developmental diagnosis: The administration and interpretation of the revised Gessell and Amatruda Developmental and Neurologic Examination.* Hagerstown, MA: Harper & Row.

KOEGEL, R. L., & RINCOVER, A. (1974). Treatment of psychotic children in a classroom environment: I. Learning in a large group. *Journal of Applied Behavior Analysis, 7,* 45–49.

KOHLER, F. W., STRAIN, P. S., MARETSKY, S., & DeCESARE, L. (1990). Promoting positive and supportive interactions between preschoolers: An analysis of group-oriented contingencies. *Journal of Early Intervention, 14,* 327–341.

KOSTELNIK, M. J. (1992). Myths associated with developmentally appropriate programs. *Young Children, 47*(4), 17–23.

KRANTZ, P., & RISLEY, T. R. (1977). Behavioral ecology in the classroom. In K. D. O'Leary & S. G. O'Leary (Eds.), *Classroom management: The successful use of behavior modification* (2nd ed.) (pp. 349–367). New York: Pergamon Press.

LANGLEY, M. B. (1989). Assessing infant cognitive development. In D. B. Bailey & M. Wolery (Eds.). *Assessing infants and preschoolers with handicaps* (pp. 249–274). Columbus, OH: Merrill.

LANGLEY, M. B. (1991). Assessment: A multidimensional process. In M. B. Langley & L. J. Lombardino (Eds.), *Neurodevelopmental strategies for managing communication disorders in children with severe motor dysfunction* (pp. 199–250). Austin, TX: pro-ed.

LAZAR, I., & DARLINGTON, R. (1978). *Lasting effects after preschool* (DHEW Publication No. 79-30178). Washington, DC: U.S. Department of Health, Education, and Welfare, Office of Human Development Services, Administration for Children, Youth, and Families.

LeBLANC, J. M., & RUGGLES, R. R. (1982). Instructional strategies for individual and group teaching. *Analysis and Intervention in Developmental Disabilities, 2,* 129–137.

LEHR, D. H., & NOONAN, M. J. (1989). Issues in the education of students with complex health care needs. In F. Brown & D. H. Lehr (Eds.), *Persons with profound disabilities: Issues and practices* (pp. 139–160). Baltimore: Brookes.

LeLAURIN, K., & RISLEY, T. R. (1972). The organization of day care environments: "Zone" versus "man-to-man" staff assignments. *Journal of Applied Behavior Analysis, 5,* 225–232.

LeMAY, D. W., GRIFFIN, P. M., & SANFORD, A. R. (1977). *Learning accomplishment profile: Diagnostic edition (Rev.).* Chapel Hill, NC: Chapel Hill Training and Outreach Project.

LEONARD, L. (1990). Language disorders in preschool children. In G. H. Shames & E. H. Wiig (Eds.), *Human communication disorders* (pp. 159–192). Columbus, OH: Merrill.

LEVINE, S., ELZEY, F. F., & LEWIS, M. (1969). *California Preschool Social Competency Scale.* Palo Alto, CA: Consulting Psychologist Press.

LINDER, T. (1990). *Transdisciplinary Play-Based Assessment.* Baltimore, MD: Brookes.

LOO, C. M. (1972). The effects of spatial density on the social behavior of children. *Journal of Applied Social Psychology, 2,* 372–381.

LOWENTHAL, B. (1991). A new role for the early interventionist: Case Manager. *Infant Toddler Intervention, 1*(3), 191–198.

LYNCH, E. W., & HARRISON, P. J. (1986). *Interagency collaboration: Making magic happen.* San Diego, CA: San Diego State University.

LYON, S., & LYON, G. (1980). Team functioning and staff development: A role release approach to providing integrated educational services for severely handicapped students. *Journal of the Association for the Severely Handicapped, 5*(3), 250–263.

MAGER, R. F. (1962). *Preparing instructional objectives.* Belmont, CA: Fearon.

MacDONALD, J. (1978). *Environmental Language Intervention Program Manual.* Columbus: Merrill.

MacDONALD, J. D. (1985). Language through conversation: A model for intervention with language delayed persons. In S. F. Warren & A. K. Rogers-Warren (Eds.), *Teaching functional language* (pp. 89–122). Austin, TX: pro-ed.

McCARTHY, D. (1972). *Manual for the McCarthy Scales of Children's Abilities.* New York: The Psychological Corp.

McCARTHY, D., BOS, C., LUND, K., GLATKE, J., & VAUGHN, S. (1984). *Arizona Basic Assessment and Curriculum Utilization System (ABACUS) for young children.* Denver: LOVE.

McCOLLUM, J. A., & STAYTON, V. D. (1985). Infant/parent interaction: Studies and intervention guidelines based on the SIAI Model. *Journal of the Division for Early Childhood, 9*(2), 125–135.

McCORMICK, L. (1987). Comparison of the effects of a microcomputer activity and toy play on social and communication behaviors of young children. *Journal of the Division of Early Childhood, 11*(3), 195–205.

McCORMICK, L. (1990a). Bases for language and communication development. In L. McCormick & R. L. Schiefelbusch (Eds.), *Early language intervention: An introduction* (2nd ed.) (pp. 37–70). Columbus, OH: Merrill.

McCORMICK, L. (1990b). Extracurricular roles and relationships. In L. McCormick & R. L. Schiefelbusch (Eds.), *Early language intervention: An introduction* (2nd ed.) (pp. 261–302). Columbus, OH: Merrill.

McCORMICK, L. (1990c). Intervention processes and procedures. In L. McCormick & R. L. Schiefelbusch (Eds.), *Early language intervention: An introduction* (2nd ed.) (pp. 216–260). Columbus, OH: Merrill.

McCORMICK, L. (1990d). Terms, concepts, and perspectives. In L. McCormick & R. L. Schiefelbusch (Eds.), *Early language intervention: An introduction* (2nd ed.) (pp. 1–36). Columbus, OH: Merrill.

McCORMICK, L., & GOLDMAN, R. (1979). The transdisciplinary model: Implications for service delivery and personnel preparation for the severely and profoundly handicapped. *AAESPH Review, 4*(2), 152–161.

McCORMICK, L., & KAWATE, J. (1982). Kindergarten survival skills: New directions for preschool special education. *Education and Training of the Mentally Retarded, 17,* 247–252.

McCORMICK, L., & SCHIEFELBUSCH, R. L. (Eds.). (1990). *Early language intervention: An introduction* (2nd ed.). Columbus, OH: Merrill.

McCORMICK, L., & SHANE, H. (1990). Communication system options for students who are nonspeaking. In L. McCormick & R. L. Schiefelbusch (Eds.), *Early language intervention: An introduction* (2nd ed.) (pp. 427–471). Columbus, OH: Merrill.

McDONNELL, A., & HARDMAN, M. (1988). A synthesis of "best practice" guidelines for early childhood services. *Journal of the Division for Early Childhood, 12,* 328–341.

McGEE, G. G., DALY, T., IZEMAN, S. G., MANN, L. H., & RISLEY, T. R. (1991). Use of classroom materials to promote preschool engagement. *Teaching Exceptional Children, 23*(4), 44–47.

McGREW, P. L. (1970). Social and spatial density effects on spacing behavior in preschool children. *Journal of Child Psychology and Psychiatry, 2,* 197–205.

McGONIGEL, M. J., & GARLAND, C. (1988). The individualized family service plan and the early intervention team: Team and family issues and recommended practices. *Infants and Young Children, 1*(1), 10–12.

McGONIGEL, M. J., KAUFMANN, R. K., & JOHNSON, B. H. (Eds.) (1991). *Guidelines and recommended practices for the Individualized Family Service Plan* (2nd ed.). Bethesda, MD: Association for the Care of Children's Health.

McGONIGEL, M. J., KAUFMANN, R. K., & HURTH, J. L. (1991). The IFSP sequence. In M. J. McGonigel, R. K. Kaufmann, & B. H. Johnson (Eds.), *Guidelines and recommended practices for the Individualized Family Service Plan* (2nd ed.) (pp. 15–24). Bethesda, MD: Association for the Care of Children's Health.

McLOUGHLIN, J., NOLL, M., ISAACS, B., PETROSKO, J., KARIBO, J., & LINDSEY, B. (1983). The relationship of allergies and allergy treatment to school performance and student behavior. *Annals of Allergy, 51,* 506–510.

McLEAN, M., & HANLINE, M. F. (1990). Providing early intervention services in integrated environments: Challenges and opportunities for the future. *Topics in Early Childhood Special Education, 10*(2), 62–77.

McLean, M., & Odom, S. (1988). *Least restrictive environment and social integration*. Reston, VA: Division for Early Childhood White Paper.

McReynolds, L. V. (1986). Functional articulation disorders. In G. H. Shames & E. H. Wiig (Eds.), *Human communication disorders* (2nd ed.) (pp. 139–182). Columbus, OH: Merrill.

McWilliam, R. A. (1991). Targeting teaching at children's use of time. *Teaching Exceptional Children, 23*(4), 42–43.

Meisels, S. J., & Provence, S. (1989). *Screening and assessment: Guidelines for identifying young disabled and developmentally vulnerable children and their families*. National Center for Clinical Infant Programs. Washington, DC.

Meyer, L. H., & Evans, I. M. (1989). *Nonaversive intervention for behavior problems: A manual for home and community*. Baltimore: Brookes.

Miller, J. (1981). *Assessing language production in children: Experimental procedures*. Baltimore, MD: University Park Press.

Molnar, G. E. (Ed.) (1985). *Pediatric rehabilitation*. Baltimore: Williams & Wilkins.

Montes, F., & Risley, T. R. (1975). Evaluating traditional day care practice: An empirical approach. *Child Care Quarterly, 4,* 208–215.

Moore, G. T. (1986). Effects of the spatial definition of behavior settings on children's behavior: A quasi-experimental field study. *Journal of Environmental Psychology, 6,* 205–231.

Morris, S. E. (1982). *Pre-speech assessment scale: A rating scale for the assessment of pre-speech behaviors from birth through two years*. Clifton, NJ: Preston.

Morris, S. E. (1984). *Pre-speech Assessment Scale*. Clifton, NJ: Preston.

Mudd, J. M., & Wolery, M. (1987). Training Head Start teachers to use incidental teaching. *Journal of the Division of Early Childhood, 11,* 124–134.

Mueller, E., & Lucas, T. (1975). A developmental analysis of peer interaction among toddlers. In M. Lewis & L. A. Rosenblum (Eds.), *Friendship and peer relations* (pp. 220–239). New York: Wiley.

Muma, J. (1978). *Language handbook: Concepts, assessment, intervention*. Englewood Cliffs, NJ: Prentice-Hall.

Murphy, M., & Vincent, L. J. (1989). Identification of critical skills for success in day care. *Journal of Early Intervention, 13,* 221–229.

Nash, J. K. (1990). Public Law 99-457: Facilitating family participation on the multidisciplinary team. *Journal of Early Intervention, 14*(4), 318–326.

National Academy of Early Childhood Programs. (1984). *Accreditation criteria and procedures*. Washington, DC: National Association for the Education of Young Children.

National Association for the Education of Young Children. (1991). *Guidelines for appropriate curriculum content and assessment in programs serving children 3 through 8 years of age*. Washington, DC: Author.

Neisworth, J. T., & Fewell, R. R. (1990). Forward. *Topics in Early Childhood Special Education, 10*(3), ix–x.

Newborg, J., Stock, J., Wnek, L., Guidubaldi, J., & Svinicki, J. (1984). *Battelle Developmental Inventory*. Allen, TX: DLM Teaching Resources.

Newell, A., & Simon, H. (1972). *Human problem solving*. Englewood Cliffs, NJ: Prentice-Hall.

Nirje, B. (1985). The basis and logic of the normalization principle. *Australia and New Zealand Journal of Developmental Disabilities, 11*(2), 65–68.

Noonan, M. J., Ratokalau, N. B., Lauth-Torres, L., McCormick, L., Esaki, C. A., & Claybaugh,

K. W. (1992). Validating critical skills for preschool success. *Infant-Toddler Intervention, 2*(3), 187–202.

NOONAN, M. J., & SIEGEL-CAUSEY, E. (1990). Special needs of students with severe handicaps. In L. McCormick & R. L. Schiefelbusch (Eds.), *Early language intervention: An introduction* (pp. 383–425). Columbus, OH: Merrill.

NORTHCOTT, W. H. (1978). Integrating the pre-primary hearing-impaired child: An examination of the process, product, and rationale. In M. J. Guralnick (Ed.), *Early intervention and the integration of handicapped and nonhandicapped children* (pp. 207–238). Baltimore, MD: University Park Press.

ODOM, S. L. (1988). *The integrated curriculum.* Seattle, WA: University of Washington Press.

ODOM, S. L. & DUBOSE, R. F. (April, 1981). *Peer rating assessments of integrated preschool classes: Stability and concurrent validity of the measure and efficacy of the peer model.* Paper presented at the National Conference for the Council for Exceptional Children, New York.

ODOM, S. L., & McCONNELL, S. R. (1989). Assessing social interaction skills. In D. B. Bailey & M. Wolery (Eds.), *Assessing infants and preschoolers with handicaps* (pp. 390–427). Columbus, OH: Merrill.

ODOM, S. L., McCONNELL, S. R., KOHLER, F., & STRAIN, P. S. (1987). *Social interaction skill curriculum: Unpublished curriculum manuscript.* Pittsburgh: Early Childhood Research Institute, University of Pittsburgh.

ODOM, S. L., & STRAIN, P. S. (1984). Peer-mediated approaches to increasing children's social interactions: A review. *American Journal of Orthopsychiatry, 54,* 544–557.

OFFICE OF SPECIAL EDUCATION TENTH ANNUAL REPORT TO CONGRESS ON THE IMPLEMENTATION OF THE EDUCATION OF THE HANDICAPPED ACT. (1988). Washington, DC: U. S. Government Printing Office.

OLDS, A. F. (1987). Designing settings for infants and toddlers. In C. S. Weinstein & T. G. David (Eds.), *Spaces for children: The building environment and child development* (pp. 117–138). New York: Plenum.

OLIVER, C. B., & HALLE, J. W. (1982). Language training in the everyday environment: Teaching functional sign use to a retarded child. *Journal of the Association for the Severely Handicapped, 7*(3), 50–62.

O'NEILL, R. E., HORNER, R. H., ALBIN, R. W., STOREY, K., & SPRAGUE, J. R. (1990). *Functional analysis of problem behavior: A practical assessment guide.* Sycamore, IL: Sycamore.

PAGET, K. D. (1989). Assessment of cognitive skills in the preschool-aged child. In D. B. Bailey & M. Wolery (Eds.), *Assessing infants and preschoolers with handicaps* (pp. 273–300). Columbus, OH: Merrill.

PARKER, J. G., & ASHER, S. R. (1987). Peer relations and later personal adjustment: Are low-accepted children at risk? *Psychological Bulletin, 102,* 357–389.

PARTEN, M. B. (1932). Social participation among preschool children. *Journal of Abnormal and Social Psychology, 27,* 243–269.

PASS, R. F., & KINNEY, J. S. (1985). Child care workers and children with congenital cytomegalovirus infection. *Pediatrics, 75,* 971–973.

PATHFINDER & SCHOOL NURSE ORGANIZATION OF MINNESOTA. (1986). *Managing the student with a chronic health condition: A practical guide for school personnel.* St. Paul, MN: Medical Education and Research Association of Gillette Children's Hospital.

PATTON, J. R., BEIRNE-SMITH, M., & PAYNE, J. S. (1990). *Mental retardation* (3rd ed.). Columbus, OH: Merrill.

PECK, C. A. (1985). Increasing opportunities for social control by children with autism and severe handicaps: Effects on student behavior and perceived classroom climate. *Journal of the Association for the Severely Handicapped, 10,* 183–193.

PECK, C. A., APOLLONI, T., COOKE, T. P., & RAVER, S. (1978). Teaching retarded preschool children to imitate nonhandicapped children: Training and generalized effects. *Journal of Special Education, 12,* 195–207.

PETERSON, A. L., & HARING, K. (1989). Self-care skills. In C. Tingey (Ed.). *Implementing early intervention* (pp. 243–263). Baltimore, MD: Brookes.

PETERSON, N. L. (1987). *Early intervention for handicapped and at-risk children.* Denver: Love.

PETERSON, N. L. (1991). Interagency collaboration under Part H: The key to comprehensive, multidisciplinary, coordinated infant/toddler intervention. *Journal of Early Education, 15,* 89–105.

PETERSON, N. L., & HARALICK, J. G. (1977). Integration of handicapped and non-handicapped preschoolers: An analysis of play and social interaction. *Education and Training of the Mentally Retarded, 12,* 235–245.

PIAGET, J. (1950). *The psychology of intelligence.* San Diego, CA: Harcourt Brace Jovanovich.

PIAGET, J. (1952). *The origins of intelligence in children.* New York: International Universities Press.

PIAGET, J. (1954). *The construction of reality in the child.* New York: Basic Books.

PUBLIC LAW 102-119. (1991). P. 51, Sec. 677.1.

PUTNAM, J. W., RYNDERS, J. E., JOHNSON, R., & JOHNSON, D. (1989). Collaborative skill instruction for promoting positive interactions between mentally handicapped and nonhandicapped children. *Exceptional Children, 55*(6), 550–557.

QUILITCH, H. R., & RISLEY, T. R. (1973). The effects of play materials on social play. *Journal of Applied Behavior Analysis, 6,* 573–578.

RATNER, N., & BRUNER, J. (1978). Games, social exchange and the acquisition of language. *Journal of Child Language, 5,* 391–401.

ROGERS-WARREN, A. K. (1982). Behavioral ecology in classrooms for young, handicapped children. *Topics in Early Childhood Special Education, 2*(1), 21–32.

ROGERS-WARREN, A., & WARREN, S. F. (1980a). Mands for verbalization: facilitating the display of newly trained language in children. *Behavior Modification, 4,* 361–382.

ROGERS-WARREN, A. K., & WARREN, S. F. (1980b). Pragmatics and generalization. In R. L. Schiefelbusch & J. Pickar (Eds.). *Communicative competence* (pp. 189–219). Baltimore: University Park Press.

ROSSETTI, L. M. (1990). *Infant-toddler assessment.* Boston: Little, Brown.

RULE, S., FIECHTL, B. J., & INNOCENTI, M. S. (1990). Preparation for transition to mainstreamed post-preschool environment: Development of a survival skills curriculum. *Topics in Early Childhood Special Education, 9*(4), 78–90.

RULE, S., STOWITSCHEK, J. J., INNOCENTI, M., STRIEFEL, S., KILLORAN, J., SWEZEY, K., & BOSWELL, C. (1987). The social integration program: An analysis of the effects of mainstreaming handicapped children into day care centers. *Education and Treatment of Children, 10*(2), 175–192.

RUSCH, F. R. (1979). Toward the validation of social/vocational survival skills. *Mental Retardation, 17,* 143–145.

SAILOR, D., & GUESS, W. (1983). *Severely handicapped students: An instructional design.* Boston: Houghton Mifflin.

SAINATO, D. M., & LYON, S. R. (1983, December). A descriptive analysis of the requirement for independent performance in handicapped and nonhandicapped preschool class-rooms. In P. L. Strain (Chair), *Assisting behaviorally handicapped preschoolers in mainstreaming settings: A report of research from the Early Childhood Research Institute.* Paper presented at the HCEEP/DEC Conference, Washington, DC.

SAINATO, D. M., & LYON, S. R. (1989). Promoting successful mainstreaming transitions for handicapped preschool children. *Journal of Early Intervention, 13*(4), 305–314.

SALISBURY, C. L., & VINCENT, L. J. (1990). Criterion of the next environment and best practices: Mainstreaming and integration 10 years later. *Topics in Early Childhood Special Education, 10,* 78–89.

SALZBERG, C. L., & VILLANI, T. V. (1983). Speech training by parents of Down syndrome toddlers: Generalization across settings and instructional contexts. *American Journal of Mental Deficiency, 87,* 403–413.

SAVAGE, S. (1983). *Individualized critical skills model (ICSM).* Alameda, CA: Training and Resources Group, California Department of Education, Personnel Development Section.

SCHAFER, D. S., & MOERSCH, M. S. (Eds.). (1981). *Developmental programming for infants and young children.* Ann Arbor: University of Michigan Press.

SCHALOCK, R. L., HARPER, R. S., & GENUNG, T. (1981). Community integration of mentally retarded adults: Community placement and program success. *American Journal of Mental Deficiency, 85,* 478–488.

SEIBERT, J. M., & HOGAN, A. E. (1982). A model for assessing social and object skills and planning intervention. In D. McClowry, A. Guilford, & A. Richardson (Eds.), *Infant communication: Development, assessment, and intervention* (pp. 21–53). New York: Grune and Stratton.

SEIBERT, J. M., HOGAN, A. E., & MUNDY, P. C. (1982). Assessing interactional competencies: The Early Social-Communication Scales. *Infant Mental Health Journal, 3,* 244–258.

SEIBERT, J. M., HOGAN, A. E., & MUNDY, P. C. (1987). Assessing social and communication skills in infancy. *Topics in Early Childhood Special Education, 7*(2), 38–48.

SELIGMAN, M. (1975). *Helplessness: On depression, development and death.* San Francisco: W. H. Freeman.

SEMON, D. A., & BRASHEARS, F. L. (1989). *Case management for families with children with special health care needs: A family centered perspective.* (Project Report, Grant #MCJ000944). Lawrence, KS: The University of Kansas School of Social Welfare.

SHEA, G. P., & GUSSO, R. A. (1987). Group effectiveness: What really matters: *Sloan Management, 3,* 25–31.

SHEARER, M., & SHEARER, D. (1972). The Portage Project: A model for early childhood. *Exceptional Children, 39,* 210–217.

SHEEHAN, R. (1989). Implications of P.L. 99-457 for assessment. *Topics in Early Childhood Special Education, 8*(4), 103–115.

SHERMAN, K. (1989). (Personal communication).

SHORES, R. E., HESTER, P., & STRAIN, P. S. (1976). The effects of amount and type of teacher-child interaction on child-child interaction. *Psychology in the Schools, 13,* 171–175.

SHULMAN, B. B. (1986). *Test of Pragmatic Skills* (Rev.). Tucson, AZ: Communication Skill Builders.

SIEGEL-CAUSEY, E., & GUESS, D. (1989). *Enhancing nonsymbolic communication interactions among learners with severe disabilities.* Baltimore: Brookes.

SILVERMAN, F. (1980). *Communication for the speechless.* Englewood Cliffs, NJ: Prentice-Hall.

SIMEONSSON, R. J. (1988). Assessing family environments. In D. B. Bailey & R. J. Simeonsson (Eds.), *Family assessment in early intervention.* Columbus, OH: Merrill.

SIMEONSSON, R. J., & BAILEY, D. B. (1989). Essential elements of the assessment process. In

D. Bailey & M. Wolery (Eds.), *Assessment of preschool children* (pp. 25–41). Columbus, OH: Merrill.

Simeonsson, R. J., Huntington, G. S., Short, R. J., & Ware, W. B. (1982). The Carolina Record of Individual Behavior: Characteristics of handicapped infants and children. *Topics in Early Childhood Special Education, 2*(2), 43–55.

Sirignano, S. W., & Lachman, M. E. (1985). Personality change during the transition to parenthood: The role of perceived infant temperament. *Developmental Psychology, 21*(3), 558–567.

Skeels, H. M. (1966). Adult status of children with contrasting early life experiences. *Monographs of the Society for Research in Child Development, 31* (Serial No. 105).

Skeels, H. M., & Dye, H. (1939). A study of the effects of differential stimulation on mentally retarded children. *Proceedings and Addresses of the American Association on Mental Deficiency 44,* 114–136.

Skinner, B. F. (1938). *The behavior of the organism.* Englewood Cliffs, NJ: Prentice-Hall.

Skinner, B. F. (1957). *Verbal behavior.* New York: Appleton-Century-Crofts.

Slentz, K. L., & Bricker, D. (1992). Family-guided assessment for IFSP development: Jumping off the family assessment band wagon. *Journal of Early Intervention, 16*(1), 11–19.

Slobin, D. T. (1968). Imitation and grammatical development in children. In N. S. Endler, L. Boulton, & H. Osser (Eds.), *Contemporary issues in developmental psychology.* New York: Holt, Rinehart and Winston.

Smith, P. D. (1989). Assessing motor skills. In D. B. Bailey & M. Wolery, *Assessing infants and preschoolers with handicaps* (pp. 301–338). Columbus, OH: Merrill.

Snell, M. E. (1987). *Systematic instruction of persons with severe handicaps.* Columbus, OH: Merrill.

Snell, M. E., & Browder, D. (1987). Domestic and community skills. In M. E. Snell (Ed.) *Systematic instruction of persons with severe handicaps* (3rd ed.) (pp. 390–434). Columbus, OH: Merrill.

Snell, M. E., & Gast, D. L. (1981). Applying time delay procedure to the instruction of the severely handicapped. *Journal of the Association for Persons with Severe Handicaps, 6*(3), 3–14.

Snell, M. E., & Zirpoli, T. J. (1987). Intervention strategies. In M. E. Snell (Ed.) *Systematic instruction of persons with severe handicaps* (3rd ed.) (pp. 110–149). Columbus, OH: Merrill.

Sparrow, S. S., Balla, D. A., & Cicchetti, D. V. (1984). *Vineland Adaptive Behavior Scales.* Circle Pines, MN: American Guidance.

Spellman, C., DeBriere, T., Jarboe, D., Campbell, S., & Harris, S. (1978). Pictorial instruction: Training daily living skills. In M. E. Snell (Ed.), *Systematic instruction of the severely and profoundly handicapped* (pp. 391–411). Columbus, OH: Merrill.

Spencer, Z. A. (1976). *150 plus: Games and activities for early childhood.* Carthage, IL: Fearon.

Spiegel-McGill, P., Zippiroli, S. M., & Mistrett, S. G. (1989). Microcomputers as social facilitators in integrated preschools. *Journal of Early Intervention, 13*(3), 249–260.

Spitz, R. A. (1945). Hospitalism: An inquiry into the genesis of psychiatric conditions in early childhood. *Psychoanalytic studies of the child* (Vol. 1). New York: International Universities Press.

Spitz, R. A. (1946). Anaclitic depression. *Psychoanalytic Study of the Child, 2,* 313–342.

Spitz, R. A. (1947). Hospitalism: A follow-up report. *Psychoanalytic Studies of the Child* (Vol. 2). New York: International Universities Press.

SPODEK, B., SARACHO, O. N., & DAVIS, M. D. (1991). *Foundations of early childhood education.* Englewood Cliffs, NJ: Prentice-Hall.

STAATS, A. W., & STAATS, C. K. (1963). *Complex human behavior.* New York: Holt, Rinehart & Winston.

STERNAT, J., MESSINA, R., NIETUPSKI, J., LYON, S., & BROWN, L. (1977). Occupational and physical therapy services for severely handicapped students: Toward a naturalized public school service delivery model. In E. Sontag (Ed.), *Educational programming for the severely and profoundly handicapped* (pp. 263–278). Reston, VA: Division on Mental Retardation, Council for Exceptional Children.

STILLMAN, R., & BATTLE, C. (1985). *Callier-Azusa Scale-H: Scales for the Assessment of Communicative Abilities.* Dallas: University of Texas.

STOKES, T. F., & BAER, D. M. (1977). An implicit technology of generalization. *Journal of Applied Behavior Analysis, 10,* 349–367.

STONEMAN, Z., CANTRELL, M. L., & HOOVER-DEMPSEY, K. (1983). The association between play materials and social behavior in a mainstreamed preschool: A naturalistic investigation. *Journal of Applied Developmental Psychology, 4,* 163–174.

STOWITSCHEK, J. J., CZAJKOWSKI, L., RULE, S., STRIEFEL, S., INNOCENTI, M. S., & BOSWELL, C. (1985). *Systematic programming of social interaction through coincidental teaching.* Logan: Outreach, Development, and Dissemination Division, Utah State University Affiliated Developmental Center for Handicapped Persons.

STRAIN, P. S. (1983). Identification of social skill curriculum targets for severely handicapped children in mainstream preschools. *Applied Research in Mental Retardation, 4,* 369–382.

STRAIN, P. S., & KOHLER, F. W. (1988). Social skill intervention with young children with handicaps. In S. L. Odom & M. B. Karnes (Eds.), *Early intervention for infants and children with handicaps* (pp. 129–144). Baltimore, MD: Brookes.

STRAIN, P. S., & ODOM, S. L. (1986). Peer social initiations: Effective intervention for social skills development of exceptional children. *Exceptional Children, 52,* 543–551.

SULZER-AZAROFF, B., & MAYER, G. R. (1977). *Applying behavior analysis procedures with children and youth.* New York: Holt, Rinehart & Winston.

SUMMERS, J. A., DELL'OLIVER, C., TURNBULL, A. P., BENSON, H. A., SANTELLI, E., CAMPBELL, M., & SIEGEL-CAUSEY, E. (1990). Examining the Individualized Family Service Plan process: What are family and practitioner preferences? *Topics in Early Childhood Special Education, 10*(1), 78–99.

SUTTER, P., MAYEDA, T., CALL, T., YANAGI, G., & LEE, S. (1980). Comparison of successful and unsuccessful community placed mentally retarded persons. *American Journal of Mental Deficiency, 85,* 262–267.

TAYLOR, O. L. (1990). Language and communication differences. In G. H. Shames & E. H. Wiig (Eds.) *Human communication disorders* (3rd ed.) (pp. 127–158). Columbus, OH: Merrill.

TAYLOR, S. (1988). Caught in the continuum: A critical analysis of the principle of the least restrictive environment. *Journal of the Association for Persons with Severe Handicaps, 13,* 25–36.

THOMAN, E. B., DENENBERG, V. H., SIEVEL, J., ZEIDNER, L., & BECKER, P. (1981). State organization in neonates: Developmental inconsistency indicates risk for developmental dysfunction. *Neuropaediatrie, 12,* 45–54.

THOMPSON, T., & HANSON, R. (1983). Overhydration: Precautions when treating urinary incontinence. *Mental Retardation, 21,* 139–143.

THORNDIKE, R. L., HAGEN, E. P., & SATTLER, J. M. (1986). *Manual for the third revision (Form L-M) of the Stanford-Binet Intelligence Scale.* Boston: Houghton-Mifflin.

TOUCHETTE, P. E. (1971). Transfer of stimulus control: Measuring the moment of transfer. *Journal of the Experimental Analysis of Behavior, 15,* 347–354.

TREMBLAY, A., STRAIN, P. S., HENDRICKSON, J. M., & SHORES, R. E. (1981). Social interactions of normal preschool children. *Behavior Modification, 5,* 237–253.

TURNBULL, A. P. (1991). Identifying children's strengths and needs. In M. J. McGonigel, R. K. Kaufmann, & B. H. Johnson (Eds.), *Guidelines and recommended practices for the Individualized Family Service Plan* (2nd ed.) (pp. 39–46). Bethesda, MD: Association for the Care of Children's Health.

TURNBULL, H. R., & TURNBULL, A. P. (1990). The unfulfilled promise of integration: Does Part H ensure different rights and results than Part B of the Education of the Handicapped Act? *Journal of Early Intervention, 10*(2), 18–32.

TWARDOSZ, S., NORDQUIST, V. M., SIMON, R., & BOTKIN, D. (1983). The effect of group affection activities on the interaction of socially isolate children. *Analysis and Intervention in Developmental Disabilities, 13,* 311–338.

U. S. DEPARTMENT OF HEALTH AND HUMAN SERVICES, PUBLIC HEALTH SERVICES, CENTER FOR DISEASE CONTROL. (1992, April). *HIV and AIDS surveillance report.* Atlanta, GA: Author.

UZGIRIS, I. C., & HUNT, J. McV. (1975). *Assessment in infancy: Ordinal scales of psychological development.* Chicago: University of Illinois Press.

VANDELL, D. L., WILSON, K. S., & BUCHANAN, N. P. (1980). Peer interaction in the first year of life: An examination of its structure, content, and sensitivity to toys. *Child Development, 51,* 481–488.

VANDERCOOK, T., & YORK, J. (1990). A team approach to program development and support. In W. Stainback & S. Stainback (Eds.), *Support networks for inclusive schooling* (pp. 95–122). Baltimore: Brookes.

VINCENT, L., BROWN, L., & GETZ-SCHEFTEL, M. (1981). Integrating handicapped and typical children during the preschool years: The definition of best educational practice. *Topics in Early Childhood Special Education, 1*(1), 17–24.

VINCENT, L. J., LATEN, S., SALISBURY, C., BROWN, P., & BAUMGART, D. (1981). Family involvement in the educational processes of severely handicapped students: State of the art and directions for the future. In B. Wilcox & R. York (Eds.), *Quality education for the severely handicapped: The federal investment* (pp. 130–182). Washington, DC: U.S. Dept. of Education.

VINCENT, L. J., SALISBURY, C., WALTER, G., BROWN, P., GRUENEWALD, L. J., & POWERS, M. (1980). Program evaluation and curriculum development in early childhood special education: Criteria of the next environment. In W. Sailor, B. Wilcox, & L. Brown (Eds.), *Methods of instruction for severely handicapped students* (pp. 303–328). Baltimore, MD: Brookes.

VOELTZ, L. M., & EVANS, I. M. (1983). Educational validity. *Journal of the Association for Persons with Severe Handicaps, 8*(1), 3–15.

WACHS, T. D. (1979). Proximal experience and early cognitive-intellectual development: The physical environment. *Merrill-Palmer Quarterly, 25*(1), 3–41.

WALKER, H., & HOPS, H. (1976). Increasing academic achievement by reinforcing direct academic performance and/or facilitative nonacademic responses. *Journal of Educational Psychology, 68,* 218–225.

WALTER, G., & VINCENT, L. J. (1982). The handicapped child in the regular kindergarten classroom. *Journal of the Division for Early Childhood, 6,* 84–95.

WARREN, S. F., & KAISER, A. P. (1986). Incidental language teaching: A critical review. *Journal of Speech and Hearing Disorders, 51,* 291–299.

WARREN, S. G., McQUARTER, R. J., & ROGERS-WARREN, A. K. (1984). The effects of teacher mands and models on the speech of unresponsive language-delayed children. *Journal of Speech and Hearing Research, 49,* 43–52.

WECHSLER, D. (1967). *Manual for the Wechsler Preschool and Primary Scale of Intelligence.* New York: The Psychological Corp.

WEIKART, D. P., ROGERS, L., ADCOCK, C., & McCLELLAND, D. (1971). *The cognitively oriented curriculum.* Washington, DC: National Association for the Education of Young Children.

WESTLING, D. L., FERRELL, K., & SWENSON, K. (1982). Intraclassroom comparison of two arrangements for teaching profoundly mentally retarded children. *American Journal of Mental Deficiency, 86,* 601–608.

WHITE, O. R. (1980). Adaptive performance objectives: Form versus function. In W. Sailor, B. Wilcox, & L. Brown (Eds.), *Methods of instruction for severely handicapped students* (pp. 47–69). Baltimore: Brookes.

WHITE, O. R., & HARING, N. G. (1976). *Exceptional teaching.* Columbus, OH: Merrill.

WILCOX, B., & BELLAMY, G. T. (1982). *Design of high school programs for severely handicapped students.* Baltimore: Brookes.

WILCOX, J., SBARDELLATI, E., & NEVIN, A. (1987). Cooperative learning groups aid integration. *Teaching Exceptional Children, 20*(1), 61–63.

WINTON, P., TURNBULL, A., & BLACHER, J. (1985). Expectations for and satisfaction with public school kindergarten: Perspectives of parents of handicapped and nonhandicapped children. *Journal of the Division of Early Childhood, 9,* 116–124.

WOLERY, M., BAILEY, D. B., & SUGAI, G. M. (1988). *Effective teaching: Applied behavior analysis with exceptional students.* Boston: Allyn and Bacon.

WOLERY, M., & BROOKFIELD-NORMAN, J. (1988). (Pre) Academic instruction for handicapped preschool children. In S. L. Odom & M. B. Karnes (Eds.), *Early intervention for infants and children with handicaps* (pp. 109–128). Baltimore: Brookes.

WOLERY, M., & DYK, L. (1984). Arena assessment: Description and preliminary social validity data. *Journal of the Association for the Severely Handicapped, 3,* 231–235.

WOLERY, M., & SMITH, P. D. (1989). Assessing self-care skills. In B. Bailey & M. Wolery (Eds.), *Assessing infants and preschoolers with handicaps* (pp. 447–477). Columbus, OH: Merrill.

WOLF, M. M. (1978). Social validity: The case for subjective measurement, or how applied behavior analysis is finding its heart. *Journal of Applied Behavior Analysis, 11,* 203–214.

WOLFE, B. L., GRIFFIN, M. L., ZEGER, J. D., & HERWIG, J. (1982). *Portage Project TEACH: Training for educators and administrators of children with handicaps: Development and implementation of the individual service plan in Head Start.* Portage, WI: Cooperative Education Service #12.

WOLFENSBERGER, W. (1972). The principle of normalization and its implications to psychiatric services. *American Journal of Psychiatry, 127,* 291–297.

WOLFENSBERGER, W. (1972). *The principle of normalization in human services.* Toronto: National Institute on Mental Retardation.

WRAY, L. D., & WIECK, C. A. (1985). Moving persons with developmental disabilities toward less restrictive environments through case management. In K. C. Lakin & R. H. Bruininks (Eds.), *Strategies for achieving community integration of developmentally disabled citizens* (pp. 219–235). Baltimore, MD: Brookes.

WUTZ, S. V., MEYERS, S. P., KLEIN, M. D., HILL, M. K., & WALDO, L. J. (1982). Unobtrusive training: A home-centered model for communication training. *Journal of the Association for the Severely Handicapped, 7,* 36–48.

Name Index

Subject Index

Kaufman Assessment Battery for Children (K-ABC), 108
Kindergarten
  integrated, 19
  program differences in, 370–371
  resource room for, 19
  segregated, 18–19
  survival skills for, 114, 149, 273, 361, 366–367, 369
  transition from preschool to, 355–356

Language
  assessment of, 62–66, 103–107
  defined, 104
  specific language impairment, 105
Language delay, 105
Language disorder, 105
Language sampling, 107
LAP (Learning Accomplishments Profile), 112, 151
LEA (local education agency), 14, 21
Lead agency, 10
Learning
  cooperative, 297–301
  guided, 141
  observational, 109, 282
  social, 109
Learning Accomplishments Profile (LAP), 112, 151
Learning centers, 313
Least intrusive procedures, and independence, 307, 327
Least restrictive environment (LRE), 8, 14, 21, 332
Legislation (see Federal policies; names of specific laws)
Local education agency (LEA), 14, 21
LRE (least restrictive environment), 8, 14, 21, 332

Mainstreaming, 288, 355–356 (see also Normalization)
Management (see Program management)
Mand-model procedure, 239, 241–242
Materials, 334–338
  adaptation for natural environments, 250
  engagement with, 247–248
  independence and, 309–310
  promoting interaction with, 294–295
McCarthy Scales of Children's Ability, 108
Mealtime intervention, 225–233
Mediational techniques, 185, 311

Milieu teaching, 239 (see also Naturalistic teaching approaches and techniques)
Minnesota Infant Development Inventory, 46
Modality sampling, 206
Modeling, peer, 282
Model-lead-test procedure, 242
Model Preschool Program (University of Washington), 8
Monitoring of children, 342
Montessori preschool program, 3, 252
Morphology, 104
Motivation, 173–178
Motor skills
  assessment of, 59–62, 110–111
  fine, 316–318, 319–320
  functional, 110
  gross, 314–316
  independence and, 314–318, 319–320
Multidisciplinary team, 27–28
Muscle tone, abnormal, 213

NAEYC (National Association for the Education of Young Children), 288
Nasogastric tube, 233
National Academy of Early Childhood Programs, 249
National Association for the Education of Young Children (NAEYC), 288
Natural environment, 238
Natural environment adaptations, 248–263
  data collection, 260, 262
  instructional methods, 253–262
  physical environment, 249–251
  planning goals and objectives, 251–253
Naturalistic curriculum, 20–21, 133–159
  content of instruction in, 134–138
  context for instruction in, 139–140
  ecological assessment and, 143–149
  evaluation methods in, 142–143, 158–159
  goal of, 133, 149–153
  implementing, 143–159
  instructional goals and, 149–153
  instructional methods in, 140–142
  instructional plans and, 153–155, 158
  instructional schedule and, 155–158
  model for, 133–143

Naturalistic teaching approaches and techniques, 22, 238–248
  adaptations for natural environments (see Natural environment adaptations)
  behavior trapping, 248
  helping others use, 262–263
  incidental teaching, 239, 240–241
  independence and, 307–308, 327–328
  interesting materials, 247–248
  interrupted behavior chains, 177, 201–202, 245–247
  interrupted routines, 243–245
  time-delay prompts, 242–243
  verbal prompts, 241–242
Naturalistic trends, 131–133
Natural maintaining contingencies, 183, 310
NDT (Neurodevelopmental Training), 217
Negative reinforcement, 212
Neonatal Behavioral Assessment Scale, 67
Neurodevelopmental Training (NDT), 217
Newborns
  home environment and, 139, 351–353
  instructional procedures for, 140–141
Nonrestrictiveness (see Restrictiveness)
Normalization, 33–34
  of experiences, 333–334
  in family support and participation, 346–347
  scheduling and, 343–344
Norm-referenced tests, 45–46, 102, 103
North Carolina, Individual Family Service Plan in, 69, 74–82
Notes, anecdotal, 97
Novelty, use of, 141–142

Objective(s)
  adaptation for natural environments, 251–253
  general case, 180–182
  guidelines for, 126
  independence and, 323, 327
  short-term, 323
  writing, 124, 126–127
Objective-referenced tests, 46, 102–103
Observation(s), 46–47, 48, 97–101
Observational learning, 109, 281–282